GUYNECOLOGY

THE MISSING SCIENCE OF
MEN'S REPRODUCTIVE HEALTH

RENE ALMELING

UNIVERSITY OF CALIFORNIA PRESS

University of California Press
Oakland, California

Library of Congress Cataloging-in-Publication Data

Names: Almeling, Rene, author.
Title: GUYnecology : the missing science of men's reproductive health /
    Rene Almeling.
Description: Oakland, California : University of California Press, [2020] |
    Includes bibliographical references and index.
Identifiers: LCCN 2020000751 (print) | LCCN 2020000752 (ebook) |
    ISBN 9780520289246 (cloth) | ISBN 9780520289253 (paperback) |
    ISBN 9780520963986 (ebook)
Subjects: LCSH: Male reproductive health—Research—United States—
    History. | Male reproductive health services—United States—History.
Classification: LCC QP253.A46 2020 (print) | LCC QP253 (ebook) |
    DDC 612.6/1—dc23
LC record available at https://lccn.loc.gov/2020000751
LC ebook record available at https://lccn.loc.gov/2020000752

Manufactured in the United States of America

29 28 27 26 25 24 23 22 21 20
10 9 8 7 6 5 4 3 2 1

Contents

List of Figures and Tables   vii

Acknowledgments   ix

List of Abbreviations   xiii

Introduction   1

PART I   **MEDICAL SPECIALIZATION AND THE MAKING OF BIOMEDICAL KNOWLEDGE**

1. Whither GUYnecology?   27

2. Andrology Again   54

PART II   **CIRCULATING KNOWLEDGE ABOUT MEN'S REPRODUCTIVE HEALTH**

3. Making Knowledge about Paternal Effects   73
   with Jenna Healey

4. Reproductive Health for Half the Public   91

PART III   MEN'S VIEWS OF REPRODUCTION

5. Sex, Sperm, and Fatherhood   119

6. Healthy Sperm?   142

   Conclusion: The Politics of Men's Reproductive Health   165

   Appendix A: Methods   183

   Appendix B: Interviewees   195

   Notes   201

   Bibliography   231

   Index   269

Figures and Tables

FIGURES

1. Photographer focusing on figure in foreground   19
2. Photographer adjusting aperture to bring background figure slightly more into focus   19
3. *JAMA* article "Andrology as a Specialty," 1891   34
4. Advertisement for the Heidelberg Medical Institute   49
5. Sign-up sheet for the inaugural meeting of the American Society of Andrology, 1975   64
6. Evolution of the American Society of Andrology logo, 1980–2013   66
7. Google Ngram for "andrology or andrologist," 1800–2008   74
8. Google Ngram for "women's reproductive health" and "men's reproductive health," 1800–2008   74
9. Google Ngram for "obstetrics," "gynecology," "urology," and "andrology," 1800–2008   75
10. Reproductive Equation   88

11. Number of *New York Times* articles discussing paternal effects on sperm versus on children, 1968–2018   94

12. Screenshot of CDC website on men's preconception health, 2015   106

13. March of Dimes brochure for Men Have Babies Too campaign, 1993   110

14. Men with more gender-egalitarian views are more likely to tell second sperm story   139

15. "Healthy Sperm" leaflet   143

TABLES

A. Demographic characteristics of interviewees   121

B. Proportion of men mentioning actions they could take to increase the chances of having a healthy child   147

C. Interviewees   196

Acknowledgments

Thank you to the people and institutions who made this research possible. Of all those who provided guidance, assistance, and support, I appreciate this opportunity to specifically acknowledge . . .

. . . *The teachers who taught me how to think and write:* Cindy Burgett, debate coach at Washburn Rural High School in Topeka, Kansas; Elizabeth Long, sociology professor and my senior essay adviser at Rice University; Gail Kligman, Ruth Milkman, Abigail Saguy, Carole Browner, and Stefan Timmermans, my graduate advisers at UCLA.

. . . *The amazing people who cared for our children during the six years it took to research and write this book:* At Tender Care in Hamden, Connecticut: Lori Osber, Stephanie Scala, Karen D., Elaina Cerilli, Kaleena Kafka, Marisa Montalto, Karen Cortezano, Kara Ventriglio, Jessica Marcolini, Jennifer Mingo, Shannon D., Kaitlin DeFelice, Stephanie P., and Holly Rosa. At United Community Nursery School in New Haven: Betty Baisden, Laurine "Reenie" Wilson, Vonceil Floyd, Barbara Gagliardi, Lori Esposito, Lindsay Brelsford, Lance E. Ligon, Linda Sisson, Naomi Wilson, and Becky Baisden. At Sequoia Children's Center in Redwood City, California: Carol McLalan, Rebecca Mayfield, and Maria Adriano.

. . . The interviewees who took time from their own lives to discuss their experiences and views with me. Without their generosity and engagement, this research would not have been possible.

. . . The graduate student research assistants who helped to gather data and generously shared their insights as we talked through the project: Celene Reynolds, Jenna Healey, Megann Licskai, Todd Madigan (who also supplied the title for the book when brainstorming a password we could both remember), Dana Hayward, Vanessa Bittner, Elisabeth Becker, and Ufuk Topkara.

. . . The librarians and archivists who shared their immense knowledge and pointed me to materials: David Rose at the March of Dimes, Arlene Shaner at the New York Academy of Medicine, and especially Melissa Grafe at Yale.

. . . The staff at Yale, who provided excellent administrative support: Pam Colesworthy, Lauren Gonzalez, Ellen Stevens, Cathy Volpe, and Bess Connolly.

. . . The members of my sociology writing group, every month for seven years and counting: Laura Carpenter, Joanna Kempner, and Jennifer Reich.

. . . The colleagues and friends who commented on drafts and talked through various aspects of this project with me: Chitra Ramalingam, Isaac Nakhimovsky, Lani Keller, Topher Carroll, Laura Barraclough, Dan HoSang, Julia Adams, Vida Maralani, Mark Schlesinger, Scott Boorman, Phil Gorski, Jeff Alexander, Jonathan Wyrtzen, Emily Erikson, Fred Wherry, Andy Papachristos, Alka Menon, Eli Anderson, Julia DiBenigno, Jaimie Morse, John Evans, Andrew Deener, Marcia Inhorn, Joanna Radin, Naomi Rogers, Henry Cowles, Anna Bonnell Freidin, Vanessa Agard-Jones, Gretchen Berland, Sean Brotherton, Danya Keene, Philipp Ziesche, Adele Clarke, Krista Luker, Ali Miller, Rayna Rapp, Emily Martin, Helena Hansen, Hannah Landecker, Angela Creager, Keith Wailoo, Christine Williams, Charles Bosk, Wanda Ronner, Margaret Marsh, Elizabeth Roberts, Stan Honig, Pierre Jouannet, Bill Petok, Rob Jansen, Nick Wilson, Owen Whooley, Charles Rosenberg, Kara Swanson, Jennifer Croissant, Jennifer Merchant, Janelle Lamoreaux, Anita Hardon, Ruth Levine, and especially Sarah Richardson. Special thanks to Steve Epstein, Miranda Waggoner, John Warner, Linda Sebastian, and Jeff Ostergren for

reading the complete manuscript and offering such wonderfully constructive comments.

... *My very patient and phenomenally supportive editor:* Naomi Schneider at the University of California Press.

... *The institutions that provided financial support and time to do the research and writing:* Yale University, the National Science Foundation, and the Center for Advanced Study in the Behavioral Sciences at Stanford University.

... *My parents:* Guy Almeling and Linda Sebastian.

... *My family:* Jeff, Clare, and Cecil.

Abbreviations

AAGUS	American Association of Genito-Urinary Surgeons
ACOG	American College of Obstetricians and Gynecologists
AMA	American Medical Association
ASA	American Society of Andrology
ASRM	American Society for Reproductive Medicine
AUA	American Urological Association
BMI	body mass index
CDC	Centers for Disease Control and Prevention
CIDA	Comité Internacional de Andrología
DBCP	dibromochloropropane
DDT	dichlorodiphenyltrichloroethane
DNA	deoxyribonucleic acid
DoD	Department of Defense
DOHaD	developmental origins of health and disease
EPA	Environmental Protection Agency
FDA	Food and Drug Administration

ICSI	intracytoplasmic sperm injection
IQ	intelligence quotient
IRB	institutional review board
ISA	International Society of Andrology
IVF	in vitro fertilization
JAMA	*Journal of the American Medical Association*
MSM	men who have sex with men
NICHD	National Institute of Child Health and Human Development
NIH	National Institutes of Health
NIOSH	National Institute for Occupational Safety and Health
NYT	*New York Times*
OSHA	Occupational Safety and Health Administration
SES	socioeconomic status
STD; STI	sexually transmitted disease; sexually transmitted infection
WHO	World Health Organization

Introduction

Imagine the following scenario . . .

The alarm clock is beeping, and John's eyes creak open, landing on the book he was reading the night before: *A Man's Guide to Producing Healthy Sperm*. He and his wife, Jen, have been trying for months to have a baby, and they are both doing all they can to improve their chances. Rolling out of bed, he hops in the shower, keeping the water lukewarm to avoid cooking his sperm. He brushes his teeth with a natural toothpaste he is using to avoid excess exposure to chemicals. Throwing on a shirt and pair of pants he washed with a new detergent stripped of all dyes and scents, he and Jen say their goodbyes and head off for the day.

As John makes his way through the morning commute, he notices a billboard warning passersby about the pernicious effects of aging sperm. Next to an hourglass trickling sand, boldface type cautions men about the male biological clock. Feeling a twinge of anxiety because he waited until his late thirties to have children, he rushes on to work. Soon it is lunch: time to take his pill. Fumbling with the childproof top, John notes the ubiquitous red warning label: "Men: Do not take this medication if you might conceive a child in the next three months." Worried how it might affect the baby he and Jen hope to have, John had called his doctor, who advised him to continue with the medication because it was so crucial for John's own health.

After eating a superfood sandwich of avocado and organic cheese, John munches on blueberries and flips through a men's health magazine someone left behind. Skimming the feature article on how guys can grow strong sperm, he reads that sperm take about three months to mature in the male body. Not only that, nearly everything a man does during that time can damage these cells: eating unhealthy food, drinking alcohol, taking drugs, coming into contact with chemicals at work or home, and so on. And from his own reading, John already knows that damaged sperm can lead to miscarriage, birth defects, and even childhood illnesses. Back at his desk, the afternoon passes quickly, and one of his friends stops in to see about a drink after work. He joins the happy hour crew but opts for juice, thinking about all the times he has seen the standard-issue government label on beer bottles, warning that excessive alcohol consumption can damage sperm. John does not want to take any chances.

.   .   .   .   .

Not only is John not real, the world I have just described does not exist. Men going about their daily lives are not subject to endless advice about their sperm. They do not encounter books and billboards and warning labels about how their health might affect their children's health. And even when they do contemplate becoming a father, men do not experience anxiety about every last morsel they eat or product they consume.

But they could. In recent years, biomedical researchers have been amassing evidence that the health of men's bodies—including factors such as their age, behaviors, and toxic exposures—can affect sperm and in turn their children's health.[1] The headline of one front-page story in the *New York Times* announced "Father's Age Is Linked to Risk of Autism and Schizophrenia," and some physicians now argue that men too have a biological clock.[2] Health websites have begun posting basic information about how to produce "healthy sperm," encouraging men to eat right, quit smoking, avoid alcohol and drugs, and maintain a healthy weight.[3] The "news" here is that it is not just women's bodies that affect reproductive outcomes. Indeed, many of the warnings women receive about pregnancy—regarding their age, watching what they eat and drink, and avoiding chemicals—also appear to apply to men, particularly during the ten weeks it takes sperm to grow inside their bodies.

Now that scientists are learning just how important men's health is for reproductive outcomes, the question is, What took so long? After all, researchers spent more than a century scrutinizing every tiny aspect of women's lives for potential effects on children's health.[4] Gynecology was one of the first specialties to emerge during the first major wave of medical specialization at the end of the nineteenth century, and professional associations, medical journals, and clinics all devoted to the "diseases of women" soon followed.[5] Today, women are encouraged to schedule regular visits to have their reproductive organs examined, and public health campaigns remind them of their constantly ticking biological clocks.[6] Women who are pregnant or planning to become so are bombarded with information about what to ingest and how to behave. They hear advice from friends and relatives, receive long lists of dos and don'ts from clinicians, and see warning labels pasted on medicines and alcoholic beverages.[7] In contrast, there is still no cohesive medical specialty devoted solely to men's reproductive health, no recommendations that men have their reproductive organs examined regularly, no public health campaigns about the male biological clock, and no government labels warning men about the toxic effects of alcohol and drugs on sperm.

The lack of medical attention to men's reproductive health is particularly surprising given the claim that, for twentieth-century medical researchers, male bodies served as the "standard" body. Beginning in the 1960s, activists in the women's health movement pointed to the lack of women in clinical trials and argued that medical research on middle-aged White men could not simply be generalized to other demographic groups, such as women and racial minorities. Federal agencies, such as the National Institutes of Health and the Food and Drug Administration, responded to this critique in the 1990s by issuing requirements that women and people of color be systematically included in biomedical research and clinical trials.[8] Taken together, then, there is a disjuncture between the historical centrality of men's bodies to medical research and *inattention* to how the health of those bodies matters for reproduction. There is a puzzle here: If the male body is standard, how is so little known about its contributions to reproductive outcomes?

This book examines how cultural ideas about gender led to a missing science, that of men's reproductive health. I build on social scientific theories of medical specialization, gendered bodies, and knowledge-making to analyze how this gap in biomedical knowledge came to be, and I examine its social, clinical, and policy consequences. In the first part of the book, I use a wide range of historical materials dating to the mid-1800s to excavate the making of non-knowledge about men's reproductive bodies. Following a *longue-durée* look at the relationship between medical specialization and knowledge-making, part 2 of the book zooms in on the topic of paternal effects, the emerging science of how men's age, behaviors, and exposures can affect reproductive outcomes. Using paternal effects as a case to examine what happens when knowledge about men's reproductive health goes from unmade to made, I scrutinize reporting in the news media and pronouncements from health officials to assess whether this new knowledge is being circulated among the broader public. Then, turning to the general public, the last part of the book is based on interviews with individual men and women, which reveal how the historical lack of attention to men's reproductive health profoundly shapes contemporary beliefs about reproduction. In short, this book offers an explanation for why John's world does not exist. In the Conclusion, I reflect on what it would mean to try to bring it to life.

THE POLITICS OF REPRODUCTION

Dictionary definitions of *reproduction* routinely refer to the biological process of generating offspring. Scholars in the social sciences take a different approach, arguing that reproduction is not only fundamentally biological but also fundamentally social. In their classic article on the politics of reproduction, the anthropologists Faye Ginsburg and Rayna Rapp argue that no aspect of reproduction "is a universal or unified experience, nor can such phenomena be understood apart from the larger social context that frames them."[9] By *social context*, they mean the power of nations, markets, sciences, religions, social movements, cultural norms, and social inequalities to influence reproduction at every level, from individual experiences to state policies.

Following Ginsburg and Rapp's crystallization of the field, there was an outpouring of research on topics such as pregnancy and birth, contraception and abortion, and infertility and assisted reproductive technologies, such as surrogacy, in vitro fertilization (IVF), and egg and sperm donation. Yet, while many of these processes involve men at some point and to some degree, most social scientific analyses of reproduction limit their focus to women. In a comprehensive review of the literature, I argue that this has resulted in an implicit conceptualization of reproduction as something that occurs in women's bodies.[10] Even Ginsburg and Rapp specify women, writing that "no aspect of *women's* reproduction is a universal or unified experience."[11] I excerpted their definition in such a way as to make it more broad, to emphasize the importance of encompassing men in research on reproduction.

One of the core goals of this book is to begin sketching answers to some of the unasked questions about the politics of men's reproduction: How do scientists and clinicians and states and markets approach the topic of men's reproduction? What is the relationship between cultural norms of masculinity and understandings of the male reproductive body? How do social inequalities—such as those around gender, race, class, and sexuality—affect men's experiences of reproduction?

GENDERED BODIES AND MEDICAL KNOWLEDGE

Within the broad rubric of men and reproduction, my focus in this book is on men's reproductive health. To construct an analytic framework, I bring together social scientific theories of gendered bodies with recent developments in historical inquiry about the making of *non*-knowledge. A second core goal of this book is to use the case of men's reproductive health to retheorize the relationship between gender and medical knowledge-making.

Sex/Gender

Since the mid-twentieth century, gender scholars have grappled with how best to conceptualize the relationship between bodies and societies. Indeed, they are part of a broader academic debate about just what is encapsulated in that tiny slash between phrases like *sex/gender, nature/*

nurture, and *genes/environment.* In 1975, the anthropologist Gayle Rubin published an influential conceptualization of sex/gender, delineating the biological attributes of males and females (*sex*) from the cultural processes associated with masculinity and femininity (*gender*). Using this distinction, gender scholars offered numerous demonstrations of how the cultural construction of femininity and masculinity produced inequalities in various realms of social life, such as families and schools, workplaces, and the law.[12] At the same time, scholars of race developed the crucial insight that gender cannot be studied in isolation; it "intersects" with cultural processes around other social categories, including race, class, and sexuality.[13]

In effect, though, social scientists treated the slash between sex/gender as a distinct line separating the realm of biology, with its chromosomes and gonads, from the realm of culture, with its ideas and meanings about the significance of biological sex differences. Starting in the 1990s, gender scholars began to raise concerns about focusing solely on the cultural side of the slash, noting that assumptions about biology were returning to "haunt" theories of gender inequality.[14] Responding to these epistemological concerns, one empirical approach taken by gender scholars is to examine directly some of the biological processes previously understood as off limits. Exemplary is Emily Martin's groundbreaking study of eggs and sperm, in which she analyzed how cultural norms of femininity and masculinity led to beliefs about passive eggs and aggressive sperm.[15] She demonstrated how these beliefs influenced not only the questions that biomedical scientists asked in the laboratory but also portrayals of their research in medical textbooks. Likewise, historians documented the influence of cultural gender norms on the twentieth-century discoveries of "male" and "female" hormones and the X and Y chromosomes.[16] In my first book, I too compared eggs and sperm, but in terms of how gendered norms influence the cultural and economic value of egg and sperm donors in a twenty-first-century medical market.[17]

To underscore the irreducibility of sex and gender, of biology and society, Anne Fausto-Sterling suggested the metaphor of nesting dolls, which I adapted to illustrate reproduction as a biological and social process.[18] The innermost doll represents bodily processes, such as those associated with genes, cells, and organs. The next larger dolls represent processes at the level of the individual (identities, experiences, etc.) and then the inter-actional (family, friends, educators, employers, clinicians, etc.). Finally, the outermost doll represents historical, structural, and cultural processes, such as those associated with nations, economies, social movements, sciences, and the media. Importantly, a change in the shape of any one doll necessarily affects the shapes of all the other dolls. For example, cellular alterations can reverberate up to the level of institutional configurations and vice versa. As a result, the nesting-dolls metaphor allows for a visualization of how biological and social processes may be analytically distinguishable but are actually indissoluble.

Studies like the ones described above—about hormones, chromosomes, and gametes—document the interweaving of biological and social processes in particular areas of scientific research or in particular medical markets. For the most part, though, scholars writing in this tradition have focused on science that exists, on knowledge that has been produced, on markets that have been created. In this book, I take a different approach. By looking to a *gap* in biomedical knowledge, I analyze how and why knowledge about men's contributions to reproductive outcomes mostly did *not* exist and was *not* produced (until recently). To do so, I turn to the interdisciplinary science studies literature, where scholars have begun asking questions about the relationship between knowledge and non-knowledge.

The Making of Non-knowledge

Just as gender scholars have worked to elucidate the relationship between bodies and societies, science studies scholars have been engaged in an analogous project on sciences and societies. Many of the historians and social scientists working on these issues cite Sheila Jasanoff's conceptualization of "co-production," finding it useful for thinking about how scientific processes and social processes each simultaneously produce one another.[19] In short, neither science nor society is separable from nor reducible to the other.

But in recent decades, as science studies scholars offered more and more fine-grained analyses of scientific knowledge-making, it became clear that a new item needed to be added to the intellectual agenda: non-knowledge. As the historian Nancy Tuana puts it, "If we are to fully understand the complex practices of knowledge production and the variety of features that account for why something is known, we must also understand the practices that account for *not* knowing, that is, for our *lack* of knowledge."[20] This epistemological endeavor has been assigned various labels, such as agnotology, undone science, and even ignorance studies.[21]

While cracking the inevitable jokes about being experts in ignorance, researchers have quickly assembled a wide variety of case studies. To mention just a few: Charles Mills examines how "white ignorance" allows people to avoid knowledge about oppression; Naomi Oreskes and Erik Conway reveal how just a few scientists have sown doubt about the hazards of climate change or smoking tobacco; and Joanna Kempner and colleagues analyze how scientists avoid producing "forbidden knowledge" deemed too sensitive or dangerous.[22]

As the number and kinds of non-knowledge identified by scholars have proliferated, so too have typologies designed to catalogue them. Particularly helpful is Jennifer Croissant's framework, which enables rigorous comparisons across disparate cases of non-knowledge. With a close eye to the importance of social power in shaping processes around knowledge-making, she identifies five properties of ignorance:

1. *Presence or absence* of knowledge, particularly in relation to uncertainty. Is it a known unknown that can be made more certain, perhaps with more data, or is it fundamentally uncertain?

2. *Chronicity and time*, including the prospective and retrospective elements of identifying knowledge and non-knowledge. Is it not yet known, forgotten, obliterated?

3. *Granularity*. Are specific facts or a broad domain of knowledge missing?

4. *Scale* at which one can identify origins, causal processes, and consequences—from individual cognitive processes to cultural formations.

5. *Intentionality*. Does the non-knowledge result from direct intent, such as fraud or censorship, or is it inadvertently or unconsciously produced?[23]

I draw on this framework in posing specific empirical questions about the gap in biomedical knowledge regarding men's reproductive health. What kind of non-knowledge is it? Is it truly an absence, or has knowledge been produced and forgotten (or erased) over time? Are there just specific facts missing, or does it constitute a broad domain of knowledge that has been overlooked? What are the causes and consequences of non-knowledge about men's reproductive health?

CRAFTING A NEW THEORETICAL APPROACH TO GENDER AND MEDICAL KNOWLEDGE-MAKING

Bringing together social scientific theories of gendered bodies and non-knowledge to study men's reproductive health offers an opportunity to rethink existing approaches to gender and medicine. In this section, I describe how assumptions about the male as standard and the female as reproductive influenced the kinds of research questions asked by biomedical scientists and social scientists alike. As scholars began to point out asymmetries in the resulting knowledge, they focused primarily on medical knowledge about *women*, even as they made claims about *gender*. I argue that attending to this slippage and developing truly comparative analyses of women and men will make possible a new approach to the relationship between dualistic conceptions of gender and medical knowledge-making.

Standard Body : Male :: Reproductive Body : Female

Pick up any book by a historian or social scientist who studies gender and medicine, and you are likely to encounter one or both of the following claims: (1) biomedical scientists and clinicians positioned male bodies as standard while (2) they considered female bodies primarily in terms of reproduction. These divergent approaches to the human body are made possible in part by a cultural belief in sex as a dualism, as consisting of two non-overlapping categories: male and female. It is not just that they do not overlap; they are perceived to be opposites, as in the phrase "the opposite sex." (See "Note on Terminology.")

As Fausto-Sterling has noted, dualisms rarely remain separate but equal.[24] Instead, they are typically imbued with a sense of hierarchy and are often associated with inequalities. Moreover, bodily hierarchies and inequalities are never just gendered; they are simultaneously raced,

NOTE ON TERMINOLOGY

Dualistic (or binary) conceptions of sex and gender have been challenged in recent years by intersex and trans scholars and activists, who offer a range of alternatives for thinking about gender and bodies, from spectrums to fluidity. However, during the period I discuss in this book, from the late nineteenth century to the early twenty-first century, medical researchers and individuals typically conceived of sex as dualistic, so I refer to "male bodies" and "men's experiences." A more precise rendering would be "bodies that society has historically defined as a particular kind of body—namely, male." However, that is unwieldly to write every time, so I would kindly ask readers to keep this preamble in mind whenever I use the words *male* or *men* (or *female* or *women*). In the Conclusion, I return to these issues and consider how changing approaches to sex and gender might shift the conceptual ground on which reproductive knowledge is produced.

classed, and sexualized. Indeed, there is a large body of research demonstrating how bodies that diverge from the White, male, heterosexual "standard" are marked as inherently pathologized.[25] In the realm of reproduction, this pathologization has manifested in numerous state and clinical abuses of poor people and people of color, including forced and coercive sterilization.[26]

Women's health activists have also made the argument that White male bodies served as the "standard" for biomedical researchers. While Steven Epstein has suggested this claim is not universally true of twentieth-century biomedicine, it does accurately describe some domains of research at particular times.[27] One infamous example is the lack of biomedical knowledge about cardiovascular disease in women. Heart attacks were associated with stress, which was associated with masculinity and the workplace, and research on the symptoms and effects of heart disease was conducted primarily on male bodies. It was not until the past few decades that clinicians realized the symptoms of heart attacks manifest differently in women's bodies.[28] In my view, this is another example of a gap in knowledge created through systematic inattention, in this case to women's bodies.

When biomedical researchers do study women's bodies, they tend to focus on their reproductive capacity. Since the inception of modern-day medicine in the late nineteenth century, scientists and physicians sought to exert control over women's reproduction, building large medical specialties around gynecology and obstetrics, inventing countless interventions during pregnancy and birth, developing new forms of female contraception, and using their political clout to influence abortion politics, sometimes to ban the procedure and other times to legalize it.[29]

In contrast, men's reproductive bodies are largely ignored, hovering around the edges of established areas of medicine—urology, fertility, sexual health—without serving as the primary focus of any one of them.[30] When definitions of men's reproductive health do appear, the topics are generally limited to "contraception, avoiding sexually transmitted diseases, and preserving fertility," as on the National Institutes of Health website.[31] Yet, there are still only two forms of male contraception: condoms and vasectomy. The male contraceptive pill remains a "technology-in-the-making" after more than a half century of efforts to develop it.[32] Most fertility treatments are still directed at women's bodies; one of the few exceptions is intracytoplasmic sperm injection (ICSI), which involves locating and injecting a single sperm into a single egg. However, the use of ICSI necessitates IVF, so women still have to undergo hormonal stimulation, an egg retrieval operation, and embryo transfer. Moreover, this abbreviated list of topics makes no mention of new knowledge about how men's age and health prior to conception can affect reproductive outcomes. In short, men's reproductive health is not really a topic either in medicine or politics.

Biomedical researchers are not the only ones who position men as standard and women as reproductive. Social scientists do the same. The voluminous literature on the politics of reproduction I mentioned above is devoted almost entirely to women's experiences, whether in the realm of contraception and abortion, pregnancy, prenatal testing, or birth.[33] It was not until recently that scholars even noticed the gap in social scientific knowledge about men and reproduction.[34] Now there are a few studies on male contraception, male infertility, men's experiences of birth, and sperm donation.[35]

A large social scientific literature on masculinity does exist, but it is mostly concerned with issues of sexuality, identity, violence, and sport.

Indeed, men's *sexuality,* including their sexual health, receives far more attention than their involvement in reproduction.[36] In introductory texts on masculinity, there are numerous discussions of various aspects of men's sexual practices and sexual identities but almost no mention of reproduction or even fatherhood. *None* of the twenty-two contributions in *The Masculinity Studies Reader* or thirty-two contributions in *Exploring Masculinities* explore these latter topics, reinforcing the notion that there is little connection between men and reproduction.[37]

At this point, some readers may be thinking it makes sense that biomedical researchers and social scientists have focused on women's bodies when studying reproduction, given that it is women who become pregnant and give birth. However, these kinds of biological explanations only go so far. It may make sense that there has been *more* attention to women, but it does not follow that there should be almost *no* attention to men. To illustrate, think back to the example of biomedical research on heart disease: it is not as though women did not have a heart that could become diseased. It was that the production of knowledge about heart disease was entangled in notions of male bodies and masculinity. Likewise, the production of knowledge about reproduction has been so enmeshed in beliefs about female bodies and femininity that questions about how male bodies might matter go unasked.

Considering the Relationality of Claims about Gendered Bodies

Suffice it to say that both claims—about the male as standard and the female as reproductive—are long-standing and deeply rooted. However, they appear to have developed as somewhat separate claims, which precludes seeing the subtle tensions that appear when they are placed alongside one another. For example, activists in the women's health movement mobilize the trope of the standard body to argue that women are ignored by medical researchers.[38] But they also contend that women's reproductive bodies have been subjected to unending medical interventions.[39] Women's bodies cannot be both completely ignored and completely medicalized. Another tension, indeed, the central puzzle motivating this book, arises from the disjuncture between the idea of the male as standard and yet largely unknown when it comes to reproduction. Men's bodies cannot both be the standard object of medical research and virtually ignored.

Rather than continuing to repeat a distinct claim about male bodies and a distinct claim about female bodies, I suggest that both claims be considered simultaneously and perceived relationally. Both approaches are fundamentally about which kinds of bodies are understood as necessary for producing which kinds of knowledge. And placing side by side beliefs about the male as standard and the female as reproductive makes it possible to see how these approaches to the human body *combine* to produce consequential gaps in biomedical knowledge, such as about women's heart attacks or men's reproductive contributions.

To return to the notion of sex as a dualism, this is how and why the combining occurs. The content of one side of the binary has been defined by the content of the other side of the binary. Historically, in both biomedicine and the broader culture, people are categorized as *either* male *or* female. Their bodies are *either* standard *or* reproductive. The conceptual result can be summarized as the following:

If male bodies are standard, then female bodies are not.
If female bodies are reproductive, then male bodies are not.

This, I argue, is the basic conceptual process through which dualistic beliefs about "opposite" sexes have combined to shape knowledge-making, both in medicine and social science. This is why there are fully developed medical specialties devoted solely to women's reproduction, while knowledge about men's reproductive health is thin and scattered among disparate specialties. This is why historians and social scientists have thoroughly studied women's experiences of reproduction and know almost nothing about men in this realm.

Shifting the Focus from Women (or Men) to Gender

So how is it that the "male as standard" and the "female as reproductive" evolved as two separate claims when one is clearly related to, and even predicated, on the other? Here, I suggest this is a specific instance of a broader pattern: social scientific researchers claiming to be studying "gender" when they are actually studying only women or, less often, only men. The slippage between studying women and calling it gender has conceptual consequences and often results in empirical claims that cannot be substantiated and may even be flat-out wrong.[40] Rather than just looking at one side of the binary or the other, I argue that shifting the analytical lens to gender, examining how this dualism has shaped medical knowledge-making and individual lives, enables a more thorough and precise theorization of the relationship between knowledge and bodies.

The first thing to notice about much of the literature on gender and medicine is that it is primarily composed of research on *women* and medicine. This pattern of studying women but calling it gender is not unique to the social scientific study of medicine. It is part of a broader historical legacy of the 1960s-era feminist movement and, in particular, the creation of "women's studies" programs in academia. As leading universities opened their doors to women undergraduates in the mid-twentieth century and women began joining the faculty, professors began calling for specialized departments focused on women.[41]

In newly developed courses, degree programs, speaker series, and conferences, women's studies faculty sought to spotlight women's voices and examine women's experiences. Historians unearthed forgotten women scientists, English professors wrote about ignored women writers, and musicologists identified little-known women musicians. But as time passed, the focus on women raised new questions about the "unmarked category" of men and how the social organization of masculinity contributed to gender inequality.[42] In response, women's studies programs began inserting the term *gender* into their names, becoming Departments of Women's and Gender Studies or simply Gender Studies.

Yet, even as academic programs and social scientific theorists shifted their attention from the category of woman to a more relational concept of gender, most of the empirical research on "gender" remained primarily about women. This is not to malign the profound contributions of classic studies on women's bodily experiences and medical specialties such as gynecology. However, the focus on women in these studies means they are actually limited to offering conceptualizations of *women* and medical knowledge, not *gender* and medical knowledge.

The same is true of research focused solely on men, such as Cynthia Daniels's *Exposing Men,* which brought early attention to the lack of biomedical research about men's reproductive health. To explain this lack, she offers the concept of "reproductive masculinity," which is defined as a set of cultural beliefs positioning men as invincible, secondary to reproduction, and far removed from the health problems of their children.[43] However, inconsistencies emerge when one looks more closely at particular elements of this definition. For example, men are not always perceived as secondary to reproduction; sometimes they are seen as primary, such as when they are considered to be the active agents who "cause" pregnancy. At other times, men are understood as neither primary nor secondary, but equal to women, such as when people think in terms of genetic contributions to offspring as being fifty-fifty.[44] And if men are perceived as far removed from the health problems of their children, how did biomedical researchers even begin to ask the questions that led to recent revelations about the effects of men's age and bodily health on reproductive outcomes? Ultimately, Daniels's portrayal of reproductive masculinity is too static, unable to account for variation in time and place. It is also, by definition, limited to a conceptualization of *men* and medical knowledge, not *gender* and medical knowledge.[45]

It bears repeating that this research about women/medicine and men/medicine has led to important insights about the relationship between bodies and biomedical knowledge, and it is the foundation on which I am standing to write this book. But my approach diverges in that I want to shift the focus from women *or* men to *gender,* a shift that emphasizes the relational, the comparative, the processual. As R. W. Connell succinctly puts it, gender "is a process rather than a thing."[46] Studying women *or* men (or female *or* male, femininity *or* masculinity) means studying one thing, one category, one half of the binary without explicitly taking into account the other half. Studying *gender* means studying the dynamic processes through which women *and* men, male *and* female, masculinity *and* femininity, have been constructed in relation to one another over time. It allows for more than just pointing to the gap in knowledge about men's reproductive health; it enables a broader question about how and why such gaps come to be. How is medical knowledge-making about men (as standard) *related* to medical knowledge-making about women (as reproductive)? How do these social and scientific processes *combine* to create consequential gaps in knowledge?

From Conceptual Insight to Empirical Approach

Rather than focusing exclusively on women or men, researchers can incorporate theoretical insights about gender as relational by including both women and men (or female and male bodies) in the same study, examining how the conceptualization of gender as a dualism shapes the process of making medical knowledge. Nelly Oudshoorn takes this approach in her classic study of the discovery of estrogen and testosterone in the 1920s. Through a careful excavation of historical records, she shows how scientists came to understand these bodily substances as "sex hormones." Even though both estrogen and testosterone appear in male and female bodies, they became associated primarily with one sex and were assigned responsibility for stereotypically masculine and feminine traits.[47] Steven Epstein's historical analysis of what he calls the "inclusion and difference paradigm" demonstrates how the push to incorporate women and racial minorities into biomedical research ended up reinforcing the idea that their bodies are biologically different from those of White men.[48] Sarah Richardson's *Sex Itself* examines the history of how the X and Y became "sex chromosomes" and were portrayed as the biological bedrock for a binary conception of male and female.[49]

Each of these studies underscores the point that biomedical knowledge about men and women is not separable and should not be treated as such. These scholars take a gendered approach in that they compare women and men (or body parts and substances associated with female and male bodies), but the first two position gender more as content, while Richardson also uses gender to theorize the *process* of medical knowledge-making. By *content*, I mean that Oudshoorn and Epstein analyze how particular cultural understandings of gender are mobilized in making knowledge and influence which knowledge is made. In these studies, gendered norms and beliefs are more an *object* of analysis and less a *mechanism* for how knowledge-making happens. In contrast, one of Richardson's explicit goals is to "model gender in science," by which she means taking into account the *"constructive* role of gender conceptions" in shaping which questions are asked, which theories and models are proposed, which research practices are used, and how the results are rendered in descriptive language.[50] As a result, both her theoretical apparatus and empirical analysis are driven by attention to how sex as a relational dualism shapes knowledge-making about the X and Y chromosomes.

Together, these studies underscore the theoretical and empirical significance of studying *gender* and medical knowledge, and not just women or men and medical knowledge. Including both women and men in the same study makes possible a relational analysis of how gender shapes the process of medical knowledge-making. I extend this line of research by flipping the question: how does the relationality of gender shape the making of *non*-knowledge?

A THEORETICAL PROPOSITION: THE RELATIONALITY OF KNOWLEDGE-MAKING ABOUT MEN'S AND WOMEN'S BODIES

Because gender is relational, medical knowledge-making about men's and women's bodies is relational. Since gender has historically been constructed as consisting of dualistic, opposite categories, I argue that focusing attention on one kind of body results in *not* focusing attention on "the other" kind of body. And in determining which kind of body should be used for answering which kinds of questions, scientists and clinicians are deeply influenced by the cultural norms and institutional structures of their time.

As I discuss in more detail in chapter 1, since at least the nineteenth century, scientists and clinicians interested in reproduction have foregrounded women's bodies: designing interventions into their bodily processes, organizing research projects about how their age and health affect reproductive outcomes, and creating extensive professional infrastructures to foster future knowledge-making and more clinical interventions. Within the conceptual architecture of gender as dualism, all of this attention to women and reproduction necessarily shifts attention *away* from men and reproduction. Put another way, the relationality of gender results in extensive knowledge-making about women and reproduction and non-knowledge-making about men and reproduction.

To illustrate this dynamic, consider the following metaphor. Imagine a photographer standing in front of two figures, one in the foreground and one in the background. Both figures are in the frame, but the photographer has been trained to focus on the figure in the foreground, leaving the second figure blurry, as in figure 1. Now imagine something shifts in the milieu, making the photographer curious about what that second figure looks like. Adjusting the aperture, the figure in the background becomes a little more distinct, as in figure 2. However, there is not enough detail to capture the photographer's gaze, so the photographer returns the camera's focus to the figure in front (not shown).[51]

This metaphor represents ways of seeing and knowing about the human body. The figure in the foreground is a female body, and the figure in the background is a male body. The "photographer" could be a scientist, clinician, reporter, policy maker, or person from the general public. An important part of the metaphor is that any of these individuals will have been "trained" to view the body, to focus their gaze, in a particular way. That training is the result of a complex interaction over time between biological processes, cultural processes, and institutional processes (think back to the nested dolls). And when it comes to gendered bodies, part of this training will be rooted in beliefs about male and female bodies as dichotomous, such that focusing on one means not focusing on the other.

To complete the metaphor, it is important to consider the photographer's output, the "picture" that is produced, which could be medical knowledge, clinical guidelines, a news report, a policy brief, or individual beliefs. Those outputs can then shape and reshape biological, cultural, and institutional processes, which may affect the photographer's approach in the future. What I am describing here is a feedback loop, which incorporates the crucial element of temporality and demonstrates how change might be possible.[52]

When applying this metaphor to particular times and places, it is also important to consider how the photographer's own characteristics—gender, race, and so on—might affect the images produced. For example, the historical narrative in the first part of the book makes clear that the kinds of knowledge (aka "pictures") that are made is affected not only by the social context but also the demographic characteristics of the people producing them. And as for the human figures about which the knowledge is being made, they are always more than just gendered; they are also raced, classed, aged, and imbued with sexuality.

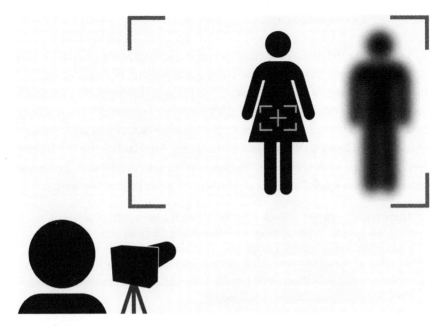

Figure 1. Photographer focusing on figure in foreground.

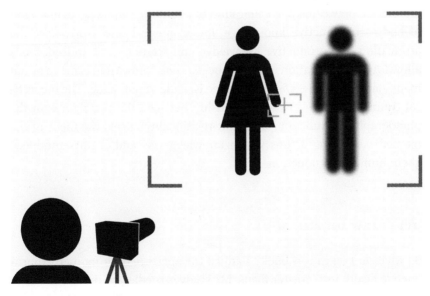

Figure 2. Photographer adjusting aperture to bring background figure slightly more into focus.

The "seeing" part of this metaphor will be familiar across disciplines, as it has affinities with sociological conceptualizations of framing and art historical analyses of the "male gaze."[53] Similarly, the concept of feedback loops has been widely used by scholars in biology, economics, psychology, and history to describe processes as disparate as heart rates and episodes of conflict.[54] Closer to the subject of this book, Ian Hacking has mobilized feedback loops to describe the "making up" of people, the social creation of new "human kinds," such as alcoholics or child abusers. He writes:

> There is a looping or feedback effect involving the introduction of classifica-
> tions of people. New sorting and theorizing induces changes in self-
> conception and in behavior of the people classified. Those changes demand
> revisions of the classification and theories, the causal connections, and the
> expectations. Kinds are modified, revised classifications are formed, and the
> classified change again, loop upon loop.[55]

One could certainly apply this description to the way women have been classified as a "reproductive" kind, but it cannot easily accommodate an analysis of classifications that are *not* made, of knowledge that is not produced.

Hence, my argument centers on how a feedback loop producing an association between a particular kind of knowledge and a particular kind of body—reproductive knowledge and women's bodies—*precludes* the association of reproductive knowledge and men's bodies. Indeed, loops allow for an examination of both process—*how* knowledge is made or not made—and content—*what* knowledge is made or not made. The theoretical contribution lies in the relationship between the two figures in the photographer's frame and how that relationality affects the focus of the biomedical gaze and thus which knowledge is—and is not—produced about human reproduction.

OVERVIEW OF THE BOOK

So what do I do in this book? I adjust the aperture to bring men's reproductive health into greater focus. My study is predicated on the existence of an enormous literature about women and reproduction, which I use as a comparative case, an analytic backdrop. Indeed, it is difficult to identify what is unknown about men's reproductive contributions without assessing what *is* known about women's reproductive contributions. In that way, the book offers a truly relational analysis of knowledge-making about men's and women's bodies.

I organize the chapters around three intertwining processes: the production (or lack thereof) of biomedical knowledge about men's reproductive health, the circulation of such knowledge among the broader public, and the reception of such knowledge by individual men and women. Sociologists of culture have developed this tripartite framework for analyzing cultural objects of all sorts, from novels or paintings to various kinds of knowledge, emphasizing the importance of attending not only to the production but also the circulation and reception of culture.[56] Including all three processes in a single study involves emphasizing breadth over depth, which is preferable in this instance for two reasons. First, as Barbara Duden has observed, it is important to analytically separate medical knowledge and individual experiences, because there is no easy equivalence between the two.[57] One must examine if, when, and how biomedical knowledge influences individual beliefs and vice versa. Second, emphasizing breadth over depth also makes sense for topics on which there has been little research, and, as discussed above, the topic of men's reproductive health certainly qualifies. When little is known, it can be advantageous for an initial study to take a broad view in mapping the contours of a subject.

Part 1 of the book examines the relationship between medical specialization around reproduction and the making of biomedical knowledge. Drawing on historical documents from the past two centuries, including archival materials from professional associations, treatises, journal articles, and memoirs, each of the first two chapters examines an attempt to create a new medical specialty called andrology that would "parallel" gynecology. The first such attempt, in the late 1880s, came from physicians in the United States who wanted to wrest the treatment of then-rampant venereal disease from disreputable providers they derided as "quacks." Although their efforts took place during a massive wave of professional specialization, the notion that men's reproductive bodies merited a specialty was ridiculed by their colleagues. I argue that this was a crucial moment in which the potential for linking male bodies and reproduction was stymied, further reinforcing the link between female bodies and reproduction for decades to come.

Without the infrastructure provided by a cohesive medical specialty, knowledge-making about men's reproduction lagged throughout the first half of the twentieth century. Chapter 2 analyzes a second attempt to launch a specialty called andrology in the late 1960s, this time an international and interdisciplinary effort that did achieve some success, albeit more limited than the organizers hoped. In contrasting this outcome to that of the late-nineteenth-century attempt, I argue that 1960s-era social movements, such as those for women's rights and patients' rights, altered the conceptual possibilities for thinking about how men matter for reproduction. As the process of medical specialization can vary widely from country to country,[58] the remaining two parts of the book—about the circulation and reception of knowledge about men's reproductive health— are primarily about the United States, where andrology remains an almost unheard-of area of medicine.

To this day, there are only a handful of topics associated with the subject of men's reproductive health, such as contraception, STIs, sexual health, and infertility. In recent decades, an important new addition to this list is paternal effects. A pair of chapters in part 2 of the book uses paternal effects as a case to analyze whether and how newly made knowledge about men's reproductive bodies circulates among the broader public. Chapter 3 offers a detailed scientific literature review tracing the making of biomedical knowledge about how a man's bodily health affects sperm. For most of the twentieth century, scientists and clinicians assumed that fertile sperm was healthy sperm. In other words, if a sperm could "cause" a pregnancy, it was considered unmarred.[59] It was not until researchers began distinguishing between sperm's fertility and its "health" that they began asking questions about how damaged sperm might affect reproductive outcomes, such as miscarriage and childhood diseases. As a result, the still small field of researchers studying paternal effects continues to work to accumulate evidence about the risks to children posed by men's age, health, and exposures prior to conception.

Now that knowledge about paternal effects is being produced, chapter 4 assesses whether it is being circulated to the broader public by organizations in a position to publicize the new findings. I compare reports in the news media, including fifty years of articles about sperm in the *New York Times* and consumer websites on health and parenting, to official statements issued by federal health agencies and professional medical associations. The news media do occasionally cover this aspect of men's reproductive health but tend to limit reporting to how a man's age, behaviors, and exposures can affect *sperm* (including its count, shape, or motility), less often mentioning that these same factors may also affect the health of *children.*

Pivoting to the general public, part 3 of the book is about reception and draws on in-depth interviews with forty men and fifteen women regarding their views of men's reproduction in general and paternal effects in particular. Given the lack of qualitative research with men about reproduction, chapter 5 is devoted to the basic empirical question of how individuals describe a man's role in reproduction. I find that both men and women define a man's involvement as having sex, providing sperm, and providing for one's family. Digging deeper into how they describe reproductive cells, I learn that individuals tell two different biological stories about sperm, the first a more traditional narrative of active sperm and passive egg and the second a more egalitarian narrative that is often couched in the language of genetics.

Returning to the topic of paternal effects, chapter 6 examines how individuals react to new biomedical research showing that a man's age, behaviors, and exposures can pose risks to his children's health. I designed a leaflet titled "Healthy Sperm" and asked people to walk me through their reactions. Their surprise at learning this information, most of them for the first time, is just one legacy of the non-production and non-circulation of biomedical knowledge about men's reproductive health. While every single man voiced a ready willingness to do everything possible to give his children the best start in life, interviewees also pointed to numerous structural and environmental barriers standing between individual men and the goal of "healthy sperm." The insights gleaned from these interviews can be applied more broadly to public health messaging around reproduction, especially efforts to avoid further stigmatizing those in already marginalized communities.

In the Conclusion, I detail the contributions of this study to social scientific debates about gender, medicine, and non-knowledge before drawing out some of the themes that run through the book: how the organizational infrastructure provided by a medical specialty can affect the production and accumulation of biomedical knowledge, how the distinction between reproductive and sexual bodies has shifted over time, the significance of humor and embarrassment in shaping everything from scientific research to doctor-patient interactions, and the eugenic undertones of contemporary calls for reproductive responsibility. Turning to the implications of this research, I make recommendations for the general public, biomedical researchers, healthcare providers, and public health policy makers. In particular, I note how the ramifications of non-knowledge about men's reproductive health extend far beyond the realm of medicine into white-hot political debates around contraception and abortion. The notion that reproduction is women's business—that it occurs primarily in women's bodies and is solely women's responsibility—is buttressed by biomedical and social processes that continually position women as reproductive and men as not-reproductive. Bringing men's reproductive health into focus would not only likely improve their lives and the lives of their children, it also has the potential to influence gender politics more broadly.

PART I Medical Specialization and the
Making of Biomedical Knowledge

1 Whither GUYnecology?

I almost think we are all of us ghosts. . . . It is not only what
we have inherited from our father and mother that "walks"
in us. It is all sorts of dead ideas, and lifeless old beliefs,
and so forth. They have no vitality, but they cling to us all
the same, and we cannot shake them off.

Mrs. Helen Alving, Henrik Ibsen's *Ghosts*

In 1891, Henrik Ibsen's play *Ghosts* had its English-language premiere at
the Royalty Theater in London. It had been published in Norwegian a
decade before and already riled audiences in Denmark, Sweden, and
Norway.[1] Like Ibsen's other well-known play, *A Doll's House*, this production too presented a clear denunciation of traditional social mores. But it
was the frank portrayal of syphilis that provoked such a vituperative
response among British critics, who labeled it "foul and filthy"; "morbid,
unhealthy, unwholesome"; "a dirty act done in public"; and "repulsive."[2]
Venereal disease, to use the parlance of the time, was epidemic at the end
of the nineteenth century,[3] so even though the play never once mentions
syphilis by name, critics and audiences alike would have been fully aware
of what was plaguing the characters on stage. And as is clear from the
media's response, the disease was enormously stigmatized because of its
association with illicit sexuality.[4]

At the same time, without a clear diagnostic test on hand, it was often
difficult for physicians of the day to distinguish the rashes and lesions of
syphilis from other common genital conditions.[5] Indeed, in a prominent
genito-urinary textbook, Doctors William H. Van Buren and Edward L.
Keyes wrote disparagingly of a commonplace medical proverb: "If you do

not know what to do, treat the patient for syphilis."[6] If even doctors had trouble specifying the cause of men's ills, then how did the average man decide when and where to seek treatment?

The answer to this question in the United States varied enormously by a man's geographic location, race, class, and nationality. Compare the situation of a White, Northern man of means who lived in a city and had access to various highly trained medical specialists with that of a poor Polish immigrant living in the rural Midwest far from any physician, who had to wait in line at the county fair for five minutes with a traveling "doctor."[7] Or with a Black sharecropper living in the South during the years after the Civil War, who had little access to formal health care and was fearful of being subjected to medical experiments, similar to men who would enroll in the US Public Health Service's infamous Tuskegee Study just a few decades later.[8] Hanging over all these men, though, was the moral opprobrium associated with such diseases.

The shame and stigma associated with genital conditions were not limited to venereal disease. From swelling and pain to impotence and sterility, men facing a wide range of sexual and reproductive issues might experience embarrassment, worry about their virility, delay asking for help, and seek relief from salesmen hawking miracle cures. Indeed, Thomas Blizard Curling, consulting surgeon to the London Hospital and author of the definitive Victorian textbook on testicles,[9] writes about just these concerns when describing men suffering from spermatorrhea, a condition marked by seminal loss that was believed to be brought on by masturbation:[10]

> The condition of these persons is melancholy enough. Aware of the abhorrence with which their practices are regarded, they hesitate to consult the regular practitioner, and fly for relief to ignorant but artful quacks, by whom their pecuniary resources are drained, for which they only meet in return with bitter disappointment. Such is the heavy penalty often paid by man for gross indulgence in sensuality—a degraded nature and a ruined constitution embittering the best days of his existence, and sometimes leading to insanity or suicide.[11]

As Ibsen's play spotlighting syphilis was making the rounds, the genitourinary specialist Dr. Keyes led an effort to address these ongoing issues by launching a new medical specialty called "andrology." He and his colleagues hoped to bring the treatment of male reproductive organs out of the shadows and into the realm of respectability. This chapter describes those efforts and explains why they failed.

MEDICAL SPECIALIZATION AND REPRODUCTION

Modern-day medicine is characterized by a truly dizzying array of specialties, populated by scientists and clinicians whose sole focus is trained on a particular body part or demographic. For example, cardiologists specialize in the heart, pediatricians specialize in children, and pediatric cardiologists specialize in the hearts of children. It was not always so. While there have always been healers, it was not until the middle of the nineteenth century that physicians began to organize themselves into an autonomous profession, differentiating their learned services from those of midwives and others they labeled as "quacks."[12]

The American Medical Association was founded in 1847. Over the next several decades, it became a common rite of passage for elite physicians-in-training to travel to Europe, where specialization had already begun to take hold. Pointing to the rapid proliferation of medical knowledge and declaring it impossible to keep abreast, physicians inspired by their educational forays returned to America and began forming new professional subgroups around particular body parts and processes: eyes, ears, brains, and birth, among others.[13] Scholars chronicling the history of medical specialization likewise point to the increase in medical knowledge as an *explanation* for why the profession began to subdivide.[14] But as the body was carved into turf for different specialties, not all of its parts were claimed.

In this chapter, I argue that the late nineteenth century—and in particular the late 1880s—was a "critical juncture" in the history of medical specialization around reproduction.[15] During this period, it is certainly possible to imagine a scenario in which reproduction, which involves both women and men, could have become the basis for a unified medical specialty encompassing both female and male bodies. That is not what happened. Instead, gynecology and obstetrics, both specialties oriented solely to the female reproductive body, emerged early and were thoroughly and quickly institutionalized in the last decades of the nineteenth century.[16] In effect, women's reproductive parts and processes were hived off from general practice and designated a distinct realm of medical knowledge and treatment. So what happened with men's reproductive bodies? Were they truly ignored, as some scholars have claimed? If not, then when and how did scientists and clinicians attend to men's reproductive parts and processes?

To answer these questions, I pull together disparate historical threads from the period in which the medical profession began assuming the basic shape it holds to this day. The threads include indictments of epidemic venereal disease, the rise of "men's specialty clinics," the burgeoning professional interest in sexology and eugenics, and scientific research on now-unfamiliar conditions like spermatorrhea. Compared to the enormous and sustained efforts to initiate and develop medical specialties oriented to women's reproduction, I find that attempts to launch a parallel specialty for men are halting and ridiculed. Drawing on the metaphor of the photographer I sketched in the Introduction, I argue that the relative ease and success of specialization around women's reproductive bodies is profoundly related to the difficulty of establishing such a specialty for men. Indeed, despite periodic efforts over the past century, there is still no vibrant, thriving specialty oriented solely to men's reproductive health.

Medical Specialization around Women's Reproductive Bodies

Here I offer a brief overview of the development of gynecology and obstetrics to demonstrate how the organizational infrastructure provided by these early medical specialties contributed to later research on hormones and the contraceptive pill, which, in turn, further reinforced the idea of women's bodies as reproductive. While not an exhaustive history of medical approaches to the reproductive aspects of women's bodies, my goal is to provide a "proof of concept" for the idea that there is a pattern—the reinforcement of a feedback loop—in the continual linking of women's bodies and reproduction from the nineteenth century to the present. Then, turning to men, I describe how the failed attempt to establish a medical specialty oriented to men's bodies resulted in a lack of organizational infrastructure, which, in turn, impeded the making of medical knowledge about men and reproduction. This part of the feedback loop reinforces the notion of men's bodies as *not* reproductive.

In the last decades of the nineteenth century, gynecology emerged as one of the earliest medical specialties, complete with hospitals and clinics, professional associations, and journals all focused on the "diseases of women." Ornella Moscucci argues that, before 1800, women's diseases were not seen as the province of any one group of medical practitioners.[17] That started to change in midcentury, when clinicians began to argue that women's reproductive functions dominated their physiology and psychology. One prominent physician contended that the "physical attributes which indelibly stamp her as a woman, which direct, control, and limit the exercise of her faculties [are] of infinitely more importance in the pathological history of woman than it is in that of man."[18]

While the uterus was initially the organ of interest, the ovaries soon took center stage.[19] By 1870, it had become accepted clinical practice to surgically remove women's ovaries to treat all manner of physical and emotional problems, from menstrual pain to insanity.[20] The twin assumptions that women and men were profoundly different and that women's pathologies derived from her unique biology both defined and legitimized the specialty of gynecology. And the concentration of a large number of "similar cases under the same roof" of newly established women's hospitals contributed to biomedical research on women's reproductive bodies.[21] From the very inception of medical specialization, then, a powerful feedback loop was instantiated that located womanhood in the reproductive tract and reproduction within women.

This feedback loop was continually reinforced throughout the twentieth century. Adele Clarke chronicles the emergence of a field called the reproductive sciences in the 1910s, spanning medicine, biology, and agriculture. Within medicine, the focus was squarely on women's bodies, with the population of obstetricians and gynecologists growing exponentially and formally merging into a single specialty in the 1930s.[22] These and other specialists conducted study after study of women's reproduction, on topics ranging from menstruation, birth, and menopause to contraception and abortion. Research on infertility, a condition that is now believed to strike men and women in equal proportions,[23] also tended to emphasize the diagnosis and treatment of female bodies, sometimes to the exclusion of even a simple sperm count.[24]

While researchers were busy producing new knowledge about women's reproductive bodies, they were also producing dense networks of scientists, clinicians, and clinics focused on this issue. Nelly Oudshoorn underscores the infrastructural significance of these networks in analyzing the rise of the hormone model in the 1920s and '30s. Drawing on old ideas about the roots of femininity in the ovaries and masculinity in the testicles, biomedical researchers posited that these organs emitted female and male substances.[25] To identify and isolate what they termed "sex hormones," scientists could turn to the large number of preexisting gynecological clinics, which made women's bodies, and in particular their urine and ovaries, readily available to researchers. In contrast, Oudshoorn points to the *lack* of men's clinics and male-focused clinicians as rendering men's biological material much less accessible, which, she argues, delayed the identification of testosterone by several years.[26] Then, despite the surprise of finding "female hormones" in men and "male hormones" in women, the early endocrinologists continued to associate estrogen with women and testosterone with men, a link that continues to this day.[27]

Fast forwarding a few decades, one result of the hormone model and the extensive research on women's bodies (and not on men's) was the development of a female contraceptive pill for women and none for men.[28] As Oudshoorn puts it, men "gradually disappeared" as an object of research in endocrinology. Underscoring the significance of organizational infrastructure, she argues that "knowledge claims linking men with reproduction could not be stabilized because there did not exist an *institutional context* for the study of the process of reproduction in men."[29] Consequently, there is still no male pill, and the ubiquity of the female pill has further inscribed women's bodies as reproductive entities.

These links between women's bodies and reproduction were further reinforced by women themselves, as activists placed the issue of reproduction on the agenda of feminist movements throughout the twentieth century. Margaret Sanger's early-twentieth-century efforts were centered on enabling women to "plan parenthood."[30] Feminists in the 1960s and '70s sought to make new knowledge about women's reproductive bodies and argued for abortion rights.[31] And contemporary activists advocating "reproductive justice" use an intersectional approach to expand the focus beyond abortion, pointing to state and clinical abuses of marginalized populations to argue that women need not only the right *not* to have a child but also the right to *have* a child and parent in a safe and healthy environment.[32] In each of these cases, scholars and activists have underscored the social and political significance of pregnancy occurring within women's bodies.

Pulling together these historical moments, it becomes possible to see a pattern repeating itself: the instantiation and reinforcement of a feedback loop linking women's bodies and reproduction. The initial emergence of a medical specialty for women's reproductive bodies in the late nineteenth century forged biological, cultural, and organizational ties on which numerous twentieth-century research agendas were built. In turn, those research agendas—on hormones, fertility, and contraception, to name just a few— each reinforced the links between women's bodies, cultural norms of femininity, and biomedical infrastructure for producing yet more knowledge about women and reproduction. In contrast, as I describe in the remainder of this chapter, the opposite was true of men. The cultural terrain of the late nineteenth century made it difficult to launch andrology as a specialty, which resulted in a lack of biomedical infrastructure, which inhibited medical knowledge-making about men's reproductive bodies. Indeed, this gap, this lack of attention, this production of non-knowledge proves nearly impossible to interrupt, even when there are explicit calls to do so.

Andrology as a Specialty?

In the 1880s, as physicians watched new specialties spring up all around them, a small group of doctors came together in New York City to launch a new association oriented to men's bodies. Within a few years, their efforts landed them in the pages of the *Journal of the American Medical Association,* where an unsigned editorial published in 1891 lauded the inception of andrology as a new medical specialty (see figure 3). Just about 500 words, it is sandwiched between an editorial on caesarean sections and another titled "Physiology of Vomiting."

A detailed exegesis of this brief statement makes it possible to begin mapping the contours—and fault lines—of clinical approaches to the male in the other case of death there was a complication in the fact that the surgeon at the same time removed a fibroid tumor.

ANDROLOGY AS A SPECIALTY.

The first step in the right direction as far as the differentiation of the department of genito-urinary diseases into a separate and distinct specialty, was the formation of the Section of Andrology in the Congress of American Physicians and Surgeons. Much adverse criticism and some ridicule were excited by the nomenclature which the American Association of Genito-Urinary Surgeons constituting this Section finally adopted. But the American Andrological Association—now an important integral part of the Congress—is a complete success, and has demonstrated its ability to place the specialty of andrology upon as high a plane as that occupied by gynecology, ophthalmology, or dermatology. The parallelism between andrology and gynecology is especially well marked. The exigencies of general practice, which finally demanded the establishment of a department of surgery devoted exclusively to the study and treatment of diseases peculiar to women, are well recognized. The crude and imperfect work—and, we were going to say, surgical barbarity—characterizing this highly respectable special branch of surgical art prior to its differentiation into a specialty, are difficult to realize in the light of the magnificent work that is being done in this department at the present day. There is no question but that those affections peculiar to the male have been more neglected, less fully understood, and more frequently treated "for what there is in it," rather than a desire to benefit the patient, than was ever true of the diseases of women. We believe that to-day fully as barbarous, slipshod, and dishonest work is being done in this class of affections as was ever to be observed in gynic disease. Diseases of men have ever been the fruitful field of the quack and charlatan, and it must be confessed, that of certain physicians who in other directions, perhaps, may exhibit comparative honesty of purpose and practical skill. They have been the fruitful soil wherein the noxious principles of professional prejudice and popular ignorance have thrived and waxed luxuriant in the development of a crop of error, quackish pre-

tense, and incompetent surgery. Fostered by the indifference and neglect of the respectable physician, the practices of the quack have flourished like a poisonous fungus at the roots of the mighty oak of medical science. It is high time that a special association for the study of andrology should be encouraged by the sentiment of the profession at large. The time will come when the new departure in specialistic practice and nomenclature will be looked upon with quite as much favor as is gynecology to-day.

But andrology will never occupy the position it deserves until the average doctor ceases to think himself competent to treat the most complicated case of genito-urinary disease—as long as the patient's money lasts. There is no part of the body that so quickly and painfully resents incompetency and tinkering as does the genito-urinary apparatus of the male.

PHYSIOLOGY OF VOMITING.

There is no more common symptom of disease, with the possible exception of pain, than vomiting. It occurs in such a variety of conditions both general and local, and is, withal of such importance in the differential diagnosis of many morbid conditions, that clear ideas of the mechanism of its production are a desideratum. Our standard works on physiology present some rather wide discrepancies. Foster says that the varying impulses presented in the act of vomiting may best be considered as starting from a centre located in the medulla, near the respiratory centre. Landois and Sterling state that the centre for the movements concerned in vomiting lie in the medulla oblongata. Mills says that the vomiting centre is usually located in the medulla; he believes, however, that the doctrine of centres in its present form, especially with such precise limitations physiologically and anatomically, cannot be maintained. In this matter, he thinks we have been overlooking the connection of parts while occupied with defining their limits, and it is more than likely that our explanations of the entire process are quite inadequate to unravel its real complexity. Hlasko (Inaug. Dis. Dorpat., 1887) after a large number of experiments, came to the conclusion that there was no centre in the bulb, but that contractions of the cardia were determined by impulses pro-

Figure 3. JAMA article "Andrology as a Specialty," 1891.

reproductive body during this period. The first sentence of the editorial identifies the subject of andrology as "genito-urinary diseases" and calls it a "step in the right direction" that it should become a "separate and distinct specialty." Listing a few other specialties that had emerged in previous years—"gynecology, ophthalmology, or dermatology"—the author notes that the "parallelism between andrology and gynecology is especially well marked." Just as improvements in the "surgical art" of treating "diseases peculiar to women" followed when gynecology became a specialty separate from general practice, the author hopes the same will occur for "affections peculiar to the male," for which the available treatments are "barbarous, slipshod, and dishonest." Indeed, the editorial states bluntly that "there is no question" the diseases of men have been "more neglected, less fully understood, and more frequently treated 'for what there is in it,' rather than a desire to benefit the patient, than was ever true of the diseases of women."

As to how this situation came to be, the editorialist blames the "indifference and neglect of the respectable physician," who consigns men to the "quack and charlatan," a "noxious" confluence of "professional prejudice and popular ignorance." Underscoring how lucrative these treatments can be, the author also indicts "the average doctor" who "think[s] himself competent to treat the most complicated case of genito-urinary disease— as long as the patient's money lasts." The editorial concludes ominously: "There is no part of the body that so quickly and painfully resents incompetency and tinkering as does the genito-urinary apparatus of the male."

As an entry point into a particular moment in history, the *JAMA* editorial raises a number of fascinating questions. First, the term *andrology*— the roots of which mean "science of man"—and the repeated phrases "diseases of men" or "peculiar to men" suggest the founders of the specialty intended their focus to be on male bodies. At the same time, they also defined their subject as "genito-urinary diseases." Since both men and women have what was then often called "a genito-urinary apparatus," this leads to a question about how these first andrologists drew the line between their domain and that of gynecology? Was it simply the sex of the diseased body that determined which specialist should treat it?

Beyond the phrase "genito-urinary diseases," it is also intriguing the editorial never explicitly states *which* diseases are "peculiar to men." The discussion of respectability and references to "quacks" suggest the list probably includes sexually transmitted diseases such as syphilis and gonorrhea, as well as conditions such as impotence and spermatorrhea. While these diseases have received some scholarly attention, it typically comes from historians of sexuality, who focus more on sexual practices than on issues of reproduction and fatherhood.[33] I place these conditions and the clinicians who sought to specialize in them within a historical frame of gendered and reproductive politics, an analytical shift that reveals new aspects of the relationship between male bodies and medical specialization.

WHO, WHAT, WHERE, WHEN, WHY

I begin with basic queries about who was involved in the nascent specialty of andrology, how they defined the scope of their subject, and what their goals were. While a few scholars have briefly noted the existence of the *JAMA* editorial,[34] I could not find any in-depth historical studies of the organization it mentions—the American Andrological Association—nor the people who started it. As a result, I combed through medical journals and meeting transactions, as well as personal letters, memoirs, and obituaries, to answer two questions: What was andrology at the end of the nineteenth century? And why did it disappear?

It turns out the andrological organization mentioned in the editorial was initiated by a newly constituted group of elite physicians who had originally named themselves the Association of Genito-Urinary Surgeons. This group came together under the leadership of Edward Lawrence Keyes (1843–1924), one in a long line of physicians and a star student of William H. Van Buren, a professor specializing in the genito-urinary system at Bellevue Hospital Medical College in New York.[35] That is where Keyes encountered him as a medical student in New York following his graduation from Yale and a brief stint in the Civil War.[36] Upon completing his medical degree at the age of twenty-three, Keyes followed Van Buren's advice and sailed for Paris in 1866, where he studied with prominent venereologists such as Philippe Ricord.[37] Upon his return, Keyes joined Van Buren's practice, and in 1874, the two published what would become one of the leading genito-urinary textbooks of the late nineteenth century. In addition to the textbook, Keyes was well-known for his method of treating syphilis (introduced in 1876) and for establishing the first ward for genito-urinary surgery in the United States at Bellevue.[38] He continued to teach there until 1890, and his dramatic lecturing style left quite an impression on his students. Keyes's opening lecture would begin with a patient coming in on a stretcher. Turning to the patient, Keyes "whips a sheet off the ulcerated nakedness" and proclaims, "Gentlemen, this is syphilis!"[39]

Given Keyes's prominence as a genito-urinary specialist, he received a letter in 1886 asking if he would be interested in starting a new professional association. Dr. Claudius Mastin of Mobile, Alabama, was in the process of initiating the Congress of American Physicians and Surgeons,[40] a short-lived competitor to the American Medical Association.[41] One of Mastin's goals was to simplify travel by grouping together the many and multiplying professional meetings resulting from the increasing number of medical specialties.[42] The first triennial meeting of the Congress was to take place in Washington, DC, in 1888, and there was not yet an association for genito-urinary surgeons. Mastin wrote Keyes asking if he would be willing to found one.[43]

On letterhead from No. 1 Park Avenue, where he lived and worked,[44] Keyes initially demurred, responding in May 1886, "I personally, am no organizer. . . . I fear I am not the best man to take the initiative."[45] Keyes did offer to suggest names and write letters in support of such an organization. Mastin must have seized on the opening, because just a few months later, Keyes wrote him back to finalize who ought to be invited to the first organizational meeting of an "American Society which shall have for its object the advancement of our knowledge of matters genito-urinary and syphilitic." To form the "nucleus" of this society, Keyes invited twenty-four men: fifteen he categorized as "surgeons known especially for genito-urinary work," and nine as "gentlemen especially known in relation to syphilitic practice, teaching or research." Most hailed from the Northeast, but there were also physicians from Chicago, St. Louis, San Francisco, and even Hot Springs, Arkansas, the "mecca of the American syphilitic."[46] Just one physician declined involvement, stating as his reason that "syphilis belongs to dermatology."[47] Indeed, the scope of the new specialty, including which diseases and body parts would be included in its domain, as well as the basic matter of its name were discussed repeatedly during the organization's first years.

Debating the Scope and Name of the New Specialty

As Keyes and his colleagues worked to arrange their first meeting, they did so within a context of rapid medical specialization. The boundaries between newly formed specialties could be a little blurry, but it was no accident that Keyes sought to bring together physicians with expertise in genito-urinary conditions and venereal disease, the latter of which could produce skin lesions, hence the overlap with dermatology. However, Keyes intended the new specialty to be broader than just venereal disease.

On October 16th, 1886, ten men gathered at Keyes's home to discuss the formation of the new professional society.[48] On the agenda: a name, a governing structure, and a method for electing new members.[49] After some discussion, those present voted to call themselves the Association of Genito-Urinary Surgeons. With its grouping of genital and urinary, this locution—which drew commentary from more than one medical journal reporting the appearance of the new organization—was an explicit attempt at breadth. Indeed, the prominent syphilologist Prince Albert Morrow, who attended that first meeting, penned an editorial just two months later announcing that the four-year-old journal he edited, the *Journal of Cutaneous and Venereal Diseases*, would henceforth be known as the *Journal of Cutaneous and Genito-Urinary Diseases* to reflect the "*broadening* of the scope of the journal, so as to embrace the consideration of a large class of genito-urinary diseases."[50] While many of the articles Morrow would go on to publish continued to focus on dermatology and venereal disease, the distinctive phrasing of "genito-urinary diseases" was viewed as being more "broad."

As to which specific organs and conditions the Association for Genito-Urinary Surgeons sought to include within its purview, Keyes, who had been elected temporary chairman and served as the organization's first president, rattled off the following at its first annual meeting in Lakewood, New Jersey: the kidney, urethra, bladder, cord, testis, and syphilology, the latter of which he described as "a flowery kingdom full of surprises."[51] Many of these same body parts appeared in the table of contents in his textbook with Van Buren, and while some are specific to men, such as the [spermatic] cord and testis, women too have kidneys, a urethra, and a bladder. From the earliest days, then, there was a lack of clarity about the precise bodily basis of this new specialty. Did genito-urinary surgeons intend to treat both male bodies and female bodies? If so, how did they distinguish themselves from the already existing and thoroughly institutionalized specialty of gynecology?

A Parallel to Gynecology?

Papers presented at the earliest genito-urinary conferences and articles published in their journals indicate that Keyes and his colleagues did discuss the diagnosis and treatment of both male and female bodies, as well as the bodies of children. In the *Journal of Cutaneous and Genito-Urinary Diseases,* images of rash-covered women's genitals appeared alongside those of men's (I am sparing the reader a reprint). At the same time, however, it is clear that these early specialists were struggling to carve out a professional space distinct from gynecology. Gynecology and obstetrics had so fully claimed dominion over women's "genito-urinary apparatus" that the newly formed association of genito-urinary surgeons was left, by default, the terrain of the male body.

This dynamic is especially clear in the repeated rhetoric of parallelism, in which andrology is described as a "parallel" to gynecology. For example, the *JAMA* editorial mirrors the language of "diseases of women" by referring to "diseases of men" and points out that the "parallelism" of specialties oriented to each is "especially well-marked." An expectation of parallelism is also revealed in the occasional comments of nineteenth-century authors who point to the discrepancy in attention to female and male bodies.[52] For example, prefacing a textbook on "urinary and reproductive organs," Glasgow physician Donald Campbell Black notes that "male sexual derangements" have not been treated with "sufficiently scientific spirit" in previous works, but that "strangely enough, corresponding diseases in the female have suffered rather from a *nimia diligentia*" (excessive diligence).[53] Making a similar point, a review of three books on the "diseases of women" in the *Ohio Medical Journal* includes an early use of the term *andrology*:

> The vastness of gynecological literature is becoming disproportionate to its importance as compared with general medicine.... [There are many treatises and] innumerable monographs, not to mention the journals devoted to

this specialty. Gynecology is having its "boom." Pedology is fairly represented. It is only andrology that is a little in the background; possibly
because man's special diseases do not present so attractive a field for medical
eloquence.[54]

One of the most colorful examples appears at the beginning of
Moscucci's history of gynecology, where she quotes the British surgeon
Thomas Spencer Wells describing the different levels of attention to wom-
en's genitals versus men's. Railing against the common practice of remov-
ing women's ovaries, he raises the improbable image of female clinicians
"promulgating the doctrine that most of the unmanageable maladies of
men were to be traced to some morbid change in their genitals, founding
societies for the discussion of them and hospitals for the cure of them, one
of them sitting in her consultation chair, with her little stove by her side
and her irons all hot, searing every man as he passed before her."[55]

Keyes himself engaged in parallelism during the third annual meeting
of the American Association of Genito-Urinary Surgeons in 1889, when he
made a motion to change the group's name to the American Andrological
Association.[56] The term *syphilology* was added, and his motion was formally approved the following year at the annual meeting for what was
now called the American Association of Andrology and Syphilology.[57] I
searched in vain for any mention of Keyes's rationale for the change, but
by constructing a name in which the root *andro-* means "man," he evoked
a comparison to gynecology, in which the root *gyneco-* means "woman."[58]
The term *andrology* had been used by German physicians since at least
1837 to describe those who addressed diseases of the male reproductive
system, and they too would often refer to gynecology as a foil for andrology.[59] It is possible that the busy traffic of physicians-in-training between
the United States, Paris (where Keyes studied), and Germany carried this
term back to American shores.[60] Although nineteenth-century physicians
would never have put it this way, the rhetorical move of positioning
andrology as a parallel to gynecology is possible only because gender was
constructed as a dualism. But the new terminology of andrology did not
settle the question of what exactly was meant by the language of parallelism. Were male and female bodies similar enough to be treated by the
same specialty, or were they so different as to require distinct specialties?

Similarity and Difference in Male and Female Bodies

Whether they called themselves "genito-urinary surgeons" or "andrologists," there was a continuing lack of clarity about which body parts they wanted to claim as professional turf. One example of this uncertainty appears in *The American Lancet*'s report that "the genito-urinary surgeons have formed a National Association. We *presume* this means the genito-urinary organs of males. These gentlemen are to men what gynaecologists are to the women."[61] Indeed, Keyes and others had identified andrology as a "parallel" to gynecology, suggesting their focus would be on male bodies instead of female bodies. But at the same time, their day-to-day practices included seeing female patients and sometimes publishing articles about women's bodies. This kind of question—Which body parts go together and make sense in a single specialty?—is core to any process of medical specialization. However, the genito-urinary surgeons were—perhaps unknowingly—also grappling with a related query: When those parts are sexed, do they require distinct specialties?

The answer to this question was not clear then, nor, as I will discuss in the Conclusion, is it always clear now. And the reason for the uncertainty is not that scientists have yet to figure out the "real" truth about sex and gender. Instead, the lack of clarity derives from the fact that the body cannot ever be seen or known outside of particular historical contexts; there is no "acultural" or ahistorical body.[62] As beliefs about the body change, so do definitions about what constitutes male bodies and female bodies. And in this particular time and place, among late-nineteenth-century Euro-American scientists and clinicians, there were raging debates over what was similar and what was different about male and female bodies (as well as Black and White bodies or heterosexual and homosexual bodies).[63] Working within the dominant paradigm, which took a somewhat mechanistic parts- or organs-based approach to the body (the hormonal model was still decades away), experts paid particular attention to what they referred to as "reproductive organs" or "sexual organs" or "organs of generation." The varying descriptors are due to a rhetorical shift that began in the eighteenth century, when the biologically tinted term *reproduction* began to appear in lieu of the religiously tinted term *generation*.[64] However, nineteenth-century authors continued to use these terms almost interchangeably.[65]

To address the question of whether such organs were essentially similar for women and men or whether they were better understood as "parallel" but different, one place to look is contemporaneous medical treatises. There are numerous ponderous tomes with titles such as *A Practical Treatise on the Surgical Diseases of the Genito-Urinary Organs including Syphilis, Functions and Disorders of the Reproductive Organs*, and *System of Genito-Urinary Diseases, Syphilology, and Dermatology*.[66] Often, the texts concentrated on either the "male organs of generation" or the "female organs of generation," sometimes to the complete exclusion of the other sex or considering men's and women's body parts in separate chapters.[67] Such texts typically detailed the male anatomy by describing the penis, urethra, testicles, scrotum, cord, prostate, and so on before devoting entire chapters to specific diseases, including syphilis, gonorrhea, impotence, spermatorrhea, varicocele, sterility, and chimney sweep's cancer (the latter is cancer healthy young men developed on their scrotum after repeated exposure to soot).[68] Thus, while both women and men were understood to have reproductive organs, those organs were not gender-neutral; the necessity of stating whether they were male or female implies it was difficult to consider these parts separately from the sexed body in which they were located.

When textbook writers did explicitly compare women's and men's bodies, they sometimes emphasized similarity and other times difference.[69] For example, in his textbook on testicles, Curling analogizes the structure and function of male and female organs:

> In the normal course of human development, the proper genital organs are in either sex developed in two distinct pieces: namely, the part for the formation of the generative substance, the testicle or ovary, and the part for the conveyance of that substance out of the body, the seminal or oviduct.[70]

Others pointed to these exact same parts while underscoring difference. James George Beaney, echoing the old Aristotelian metaphor of (male) seed and (female) soil,[71] contends that "the leading difference between the organs of the two sexes is that, whilst those of the male are constituted to secrete and give, those of the female are adapted entirely to receptivity."[72]

Debates about difference and similarity were also playing out at the level of the cell, as biologists used microscopy to examine sperm and eggs.[73] Scientists, including those who took positions as "spermists" or "ovists," differed as to men's and women's contributions to generation.[74] Florence Vienne argues that by the end of the nineteenth century, though, embryologists had begun to adopt a view of eggs and sperm "as cells containing *equal* shares of hereditary material."[75] Beliefs about what was then called sterility followed suit. Whereas, historically, most of the responsibility for childless unions had been placed on women, late-nineteenth-century physicians began assessing male partners alongside their female patients, counting sperm and examining external genitalia.[76]

However, even as some experts noted similarities between women's and men's bodies, one profound difference persisted: men's genitals were never seen as core to their health and psychology like women's genitals were. Indeed, even as Moscucci calls it "striking" that the development of gynecology was not paired with a "complementary 'science of masculinity' or 'andrology,'" she notes that "the physiology and pathology of the male sexual system simply *were not seen* to define men's nature."[77] While gender politics had rendered it linguistically and conceptually possible for Keyes to call his new specialty andrology, they also proved its undoing. By proposing to focus on men's genitals and the conditions plaguing them, the andrologists were ridiculed mercilessly by their colleagues, forcing them to beat a hasty retreat.

Ridiculed Far and Wide

As the members of the nascent association worked to define their domain and settle on a moniker, they faced criticism on both fronts. The editorial pages of medical journals wondered about the need for such a specialty and raised pointed questions about its name. One of the most prominent—and scathing—critiques appeared in *The Lancet* in 1888. The brief commentary notes the arrival of a preliminary program for the upcoming annual meeting of the American Association of Genito-Urinary Surgeons, and reflecting, in part, greater British reluctance to medical specialization,[78] it objects to both the name of the association and its intentions: "The expression 'genito-urinary' surgeons, which does not seem to us a happy one, indicates the disposition to erect a new specialty, which we trust will be reconsidered." It goes on to mock the "diversity of the complaints" represented in the program, wondering how they could possibly form the basis of a coherent specialty. Specifically, it asks, "Is syphiloma of the vulva to be regarded as something apart and special?"[79] Returning to these themes several times in the next few months, *The Lancet* called the name of the association "unsavoury"[80] and asked why, in reporting on the first Congress of American Physicians and Surgeons, the "palpation of the ureters in the female" was being discussed at the American Gynecological Society and not in the Association of Genito-Urinary Surgeons.[81]

Keyes and his colleagues did not let *The Lancet's* attacks go unanswered. They took to the pages of the *Journal of Cutaneous and Genito-Urinary Diseases* to defend themselves in an editorial published in January 1889. With the epigraph "He laughs best who laughs last," the editorial derides the "sneers that have been heaped upon [the association] since its inception by the London '*Lancet*'" and accuses "that venerable sheet" of "decay." It points to the recently published transactions of the American Association of Genito-Urinary Surgeons to note that the quality of members and research speaks for itself:

> If the profession in England is not up to the age and cannot recognize that a grouping of the maladies of a special set of organs form a legitimate field of special research, it is to be regretted. . . . In this country the advantage of grouping genito-urinary surgical matters with a study of the general subject of syphilis has long been recognized.[82]

Perhaps it was insults such as *The Lancet's* labeling the phrase "genito-urinary" as "unsavoury" that inspired Keyes to rename the specialty andrology; just months after the editorial appeared, he was making his motion at the association's annual meeting. Yet, the new terminology only provoked more criticism. Invoking Shakespeare, the *British Medical Journal* issued a brief comment titled "What's in a Name?" to report that the association "is henceforth to be known by the surprising and ponderous title of 'The American Andrological and Syphilographical Association.'"[83] While the *BMJ* accidentally added a few extra syllables, the mockery was not limited to the British. Indeed, *JAMA's* editorial "Andrology as a Specialty" noted that "much adverse criticism and ridicule were excited by the nomenclature" of the "American Andrological Association" at the Congress of American Physicians and Surgeons in 1891.[84]

Indeed, the andrological association had organized its fifth annual meeting in Washington, DC, to coincide with the physicians' and surgeons' congress in 1891, thereby allowing its members to attend both. They must have felt the sting of ridicule in person. At their next meeting the following June, Dr. Robert W. Taylor, who had served as the association's first secretary, proposed changing the name back to its original "on the ground that the present name made the Association a laughing-stock, 'andrology' meaning the 'science of men.'"

Unfortunately, the brief references to the association's name change in medical journals and meeting transactions do not reveal precisely what made *andrology* a laughingstock. It does not appear to be a matter of overspecialization; the leaders of the congress had concerns about that very issue and still continued to include the genito-urinary surgeons on their program.[85] So it may have been something specific to the language of andrology in referring to the bodily domain genito-urinary surgeons wanted to claim. At the time, *andrology* was also a term used in philosophical and anthropological circles, which may have led physicians to mock its extension to the male reproductive organs.

In any case, Keyes objected to Taylor's proposal because "members of the association were not genito-urinary *surgeons*, but rather, investigators of the genito-urinary *organs*, or *system*."[86] In the end, Keyes was overruled. Taylor's motion to drop the language of andrology and reinstate the original name of "American Association of Genito-Urinary Surgeons" passed nine to three.[87] As I detail below, along with this more limited name came a more limited focus, and the first real possibility of creating a specialty devoted to the "diseases of men" in all its breadth and possibility vanished into history.

FIGHTING FOR RESPECTABILITY, AND LOSING

It was not only the name—*genito-urinary* or *andrology*—or questions about which kinds of bodies the specialty intended to treat that resulted in ridicule. The New York–based organization was also trying to bring respectability to body parts long associated with venereal disease, immorality, and quackery. These associations are clear in the *JAMA* editorial, which notes that "diseases of men have ever been the fruitful field of the quack and charlatan." It emphasizes the necessity of the "profession at large" to encourage a "special association for the study of andrology" and concludes optimistically that "the time will come when the new departure in specialistic practice and nomenclature will be looked upon with quite as much favor as is gynecology today."[88] But it was not meant to be; the cultural headwinds facing the new group were too strong.

Virility and Race at the End of the Nineteenth Century

Beyond the realm of medicine, there was widespread concern about the waning virility of modern (White) men at the end of the nineteenth century.[89] Those who had once labored mightily on the family farm now sat doughily all day at desks *if* they could get a job: the process of industrialization had left many without employment prospects at all.[90] Some middle-class men were even being diagnosed with neurasthenia, a nervous disorder characterized by profound physical and mental exhaustion from contemporary life.[91] To combat the ills of being sedentary, health advocate Bernarr MacFadden evangelized about the importance of "physical culture" in popular magazines and books, writing:

> There are thousands, and perhaps millions, of boys, young men, and even old men, whose powers, mental, physical, and sexual, are fast declining. . . . The first duty of every male human adult is to be a man. All other requirements should be subordinate to this. You cannot build a house without a foundation to rest upon, and virile manhood is the foundation upon which must rest all the results that accrue from education and the refining influences of civilized life. . . . For if you are not a man, you are nothing but a nonentity!"[92]

Protestant leaders conveyed similar sentiments in their calls for "muscular Christianity," emphasizing the importance of competitive sports and physical education for men, particularly in light of the waves of Catholic immigrants arriving in America.[93]

The normativity of Whiteness meant that the specific kind of male body being discussed in these works was not always named, but masculinities are never just gendered.[94] During this same period, the emerging field of sexology, which shared many of the same methods and researchers with the "racial science" of the day, drew on scientific tropes to elucidate two categories of men that stood in contrast to that of enervated White hetero-sexuals: (1) the effeminate White homosexual male and (2) the hypersex-ual Black male "beast" believed to be prone to raping White women and controlled only by castration or lynching or both.[95] As Melissa Stein notes, concerns about weak White men were profoundly related to concerns about racial dominance.[96] The burgeoning feminist movement, populated mostly by White women and calling for women's access to higher educa-tion and the vote, only further aggravated societal concerns about the diminishment of White men.[97]

It is within this broader context that physicians such as Prince Morrow raised alarms about the spread of venereal disease. Although few health departments collected statistics, Morrow and others estimated in 1901 that 80 percent of men in New York City had been infected with gonorrhea at some point and perhaps as many as many as 18 percent were syphilitic.[98] While gonorrhea was considered no more consequential than the common cold, syphilis was seen as far more serious, and venereal disease in general was perceived as a further threat to the male constitution.[99] But it was not only men who were in danger from such diseases. Public health reports blamed men's moral fallibility for extramarital sex, which resulted in them passing contagion on to their "innocent" wives and children,[100] the very issue at the center of Ibsen's *Ghosts*. And although the genito-urinary sur-geons rarely mentioned race or immigration in their meeting transactions or in the pages of their journals, the intertwining narratives of disease and sanitation, eugenics and nativism, would likely have meant that such asso-ciations were part and parcel of their thinking about the male body.[101]

Ceding the Diseases of Men to "Quacks"

The link between venereal disease and immorality lent suspicion not only to the men who contracted such diseases but also those who deigned to treat them.[102] Indeed, diseases "peculiar to men" had long been the prov-ince of healers derided as profit-seeking amateurs by those professional doctors who considered themselves "regular" physicians.[103] As the medi-cal profession worked to consolidate its professional power in the nine-teenth century, it sought to eliminate various forms of competition by deploying the label *quack*, applying it to midwives, homeopaths, and in this case, those specializing in the diseases of men.[104] Because this derogatory epithet was not necessarily rooted in scientific evidence about the quality or efficacy of care, readers should envision each mention of *quacks* that follows as being ensconced in quotation marks.

One important distinction between the two groups is that regular physicians were less likely to promise sure cures than quacks were, and some would even grudgingly admit they did not actually have access to more efficacious treatments.[105] Quacks were also more likely to advertise widely, something regular physicians refused to do. In fact, in what was likely an attempt to differentiate themselves from quacks, the American Association of Genito-Urinary Surgeons refused to allow its members to list the specialty on their business cards, even though it would have been allowed by the American Medical Association. They did so because the "association was organized for mutual scientific advancement" and it was "an *honest* combination of workers."[106]

Given that so many men suffered from venereal disease and other stigmatized conditions affecting their reproductive organs, they understandably sought treatment. While it would be difficult to specify what proportion of nineteenth-century men visited quacks operating what were called "men's specialist clinics," Suzanne Fischer defines them as a "once-ubiquitous medical institution."[107] Some were stationary storefronts that restricted entry to "men only," and others were traveling clinics that stayed in each location for as long as patients lined up. They promised treatment for the same conditions genito-urinary specialists claimed as their purview: syphilis, gonorrhea, impotence, spermatorrhea, and sterility.[108] Tracing the fortunes of one such enterprise, Fischer finds that the Heidelberg Medical Institute, which was started by the Reinhardt brothers from St. Paul (two of whom held medical degrees from reputable institutions) grew to more than thirty clinics around the Midwest between the 1890s and the 1910s.[109] One of their ads can be seen in figure 4.[110]

Such enterprises faced harsh critiques from the medical profession. For example, those authoring textbooks about genito-urinary matters would often begin with apologies for writing about such disreputable topics, but then would go on to underscore the need for regular physicians to attend to such diseases lest men find themselves duped by quacks. James George Beaney's preface to *The Generative System* states that he is "embarrassed"

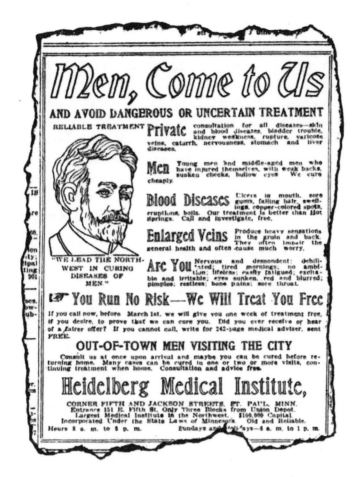

Figure 4. Advertisement for the Heidelberg Medical Institute.

by "the nature of the subject," but "imperfect knowledge" of the "organs of reproduction" induced him to write. The "sexual systems of women and men" have been neglected through "false delicacy" so the topic has been seized by "charlatans."[111] In his famous treatise on spermatorrhea, the French professor of medicine Claude-François Lallemand puts it even more starkly, pointing to the profession's ignorance of such diseases and the "common consent" to neglect such subjects that are "certainly repugnant to delicacy." The result, though, is that "sufferers finding themselves neglected by their ordinary medical attendants, rush to find relief wherever there seems to them the slightest chance of its being obtained; and the ignorant and rapacious advertising quacks have a rapid and profitable sale for their injurious nostrums."[112] It was not only individual physicians who complained about quacks. In the early decades of the twentieth century, both the American Medical Association and muckraking newspapers launched campaigns to expose the fraudulent claims of men's specialty clinics.[113]

Why did so many men pursue treatment from practitioners derided as quacks? Those who could afford a regular physician, much less a genito-urinary specialist, may not have wanted to reveal they had contracted such a condition. Given the moral blemish associated with diseases of the male organs, there is little doubt that men felt a great deal of shame, which perhaps led them to prefer the anonymity and confidentiality of practices like those run by the Reinhardt brothers. And for those with fewer economic resources, including working-class men in urban areas, men's specialist clinics offered affordable and accessible treatments and sometimes even offered care in the languages of newly arrived immigrants. For those living in rural areas where doctors were few and far between, city-based clinics would accept mailed inquiries and promised to reply from a nondescript address in discreet packaging.[114]

But even when men's genital conditions had nothing to do with illicit sexuality, physicians noted that they would hesitate to seek care. For example, two mid-century authors of textbooks about testicles included several stories of men suffering agony for months before visiting a doctor, even though they had only bumped into a drawer in the middle of the night or, that "most frequent cause of violence," mashed their testicles on the pommel of a saddle while riding a horse.[115] As Curling put it, "the mind is very readily disturbed by any appearance of imperfection in the organs of generation."[116] Both he and Cooper noted cases in which deformities or the loss of testicles constituted such a severe assault on a man's virility that it resulted in suicide or homicide.[117]

It was both this shame and the easy prey it made of men for quacks that inspired Keyes, Morrow, and the others to hope that andrology would soon obtain "as high a plane as that occupied by gynecology."[118] But despite their efforts to distinguish themselves from quacks and bring respectability to the treatment of diseases of men, they did not succeed.[119]

Excising the Genito- *to Become Urology*

Indeed, similar dynamics played out just a few years later, when the "new-fashioned" urologists waged a successful campaign to excise the *genito-* from genito-urinary surgery and focus instead on the less-stigmatized urinary tract. A full consideration of these developments is beyond the scope of this book and awaits further scholarly attention as there appear to be no comprehensive histories of urology, save for a few tracts written by urologists in the early twentieth century. Briefly, the American Urological Association (AUA) was founded in 1902, when the New York Genito-Urinary Society voted to disband and give itself a new name. In particular, they were concerned about the "black eye" that came from being considered "clap doctors."[120]

Along with the new name came an intentionally nonvenereal and nongenital focus. As the founder and first president, Harvard-trained physician Ramon Guiteras, explained in the first volume of the *American Journal of Urology,* the new association "cut out most of the genital part of genito-urinary diseases. . . . Venereal diseases, with the exception of urethral infections and lesions, were debarred and genital diseases, excepting such as have an influence over the urinary organs, were not considered." He goes on to note that some wondered whether the new urological association might be a "rival" of the American genito-urinary association, but "this was not so" because its "scope" was "quite different."[121] Indeed, physicians whose practices consisted of venereology alone would not be allowed membership in the AUA, and papers focused on venereal disease were not accepted for their scientific meeting.[122] Although both the genito-urinary association and the urological association were based in New York, they did not have a single founding member in common.[123]

Keyes's genito-urinary textbook also reflected the shift toward urology. The 1906 edition was co-authored with his son, a urologist, and their preface calls attention to the reduced focus on venereal disease as compared to previous editions.[124] The American Association of Genito-Urinary Surgeons does remain in existence to this day, and in fact, it awards the Keyes Medal in recognition of "outstanding contributions to the advancement of *urology*."[125]

MASCULINITY, MORALITY, AND THE FAILURE OF MARKET INCENTIVES

The medical profession in the late nineteenth century was in active-expansion mode, seeking to enlarge its scientific domain by claiming ever more bodily turf. In the end, though, both the push from regular physicians and the pull of men's specialist clinics—what the 1891 *JAMA* article calls the "noxious" mix of "professional prejudice and individual ignorance"— resulted in men's reproductive organs remaining mostly in the hands of quacks till well into the twentieth century. Indeed, regular physicians easily conceded the market for what was then both quite a diseased and lucrative aspect of the human body. Put another way: at a critical juncture in the incipient structuring of the medical profession, physicians ignored clear demand from half the population—namely, men. Repugnance and respectability won out over professionalization and the profit motive.

My argument in this chapter is made possible only by bringing together subjects that are typically treated separately. Venereal disease has mostly been studied by historians of sexuality, while quackery has been the province of historians of medical specialization. And historians of reproduction have mostly focused on women's bodies, women's experiences, and women's specialties, such as gynecology and obstetrics. Bringing all three topics—men's reproduction, venereal disease, and quacks—together into the same analytical frame allows for a new answer to the question of why there is no medical specialty for men's reproductive bodies.

Indeed, the version of events I offer provides a crucial corrective to conventional wisdom about the relationship between medical specialization and gendered bodies. Scholars of gender and medicine have long argued that men's bodies have not been subject to the same level of attention and intervention as women's bodies.[126] In particular, many researchers point to the early institutionalization of specialties such as obstetrics and gynecology as the cause of endless meddling in women's reproductive parts and processes. The corresponding assumption has been that male bodies were virtually ignored, their reproductive parts unattended, their bodies free from intervention. In recent years, though, historians have begun to raise questions about that long-held assumption. Digging into the history of venereology, sexology, psychology, and embryology, gender scholars are learning that, in fact, late-nineteenth-century male bodies *were* being scrutinized, poked, injected, and even electrocuted. To provide just one example, Christina Benninghaus writes that doctors treating male sterility "touched and squeezed [male genitals]; they punctured testicles and used bougies to widen the urethra. They used catheters to deal with strictures, and they applied electricity and hot and cold baths to the testicles in order to encourage sperm production."[127]

In this chapter, I join these scholars in upending the truism that the male reproductive body was largely absent as an object of scientific and medical interest in the late nineteenth century. I go one step further, though, in offering an *explanation* for how scholars developed an assumption that men's reproductive organs were ignored: men were being treated mostly by quacks. The failure to launch andrology as a medical specialty combined with the market dominance of quacks meant that there was a great deal of attention being paid to the male reproductive body, just not in the pages of professional medical journals or on the panels of professional medical societies. To return to the notion of the feedback loop, some of the key elements—such as specialty clinics, practitioners, and patients—*did* exist for men's reproductive organs, but *outside* the purview of the regular medical profession. As the saying goes, "History is written by the victors." In this case, the result is that there was no recognizable, sustainable, and later *remembered* biomedical infrastructure in which to unite the various inquiries into the male organs of generation and the diseases of men.

The failed launch of andrology in the late nineteenth century—a market failure occasioned by the combustible mix of masculinity and morality— constitutes a critical juncture in the history of professional specialization that continues to haunt medicine to this day. In the next chapter, I bring the story up to the present, arguing that the lack of a formal specialty meant there was no organizational infrastructure to unite the scanty networks of physicians and scientists interested in producing knowledge about various aspects of men's reproduction. As a result, over the course of the twentieth century, the figure of the male reproductive body remained blurry and in the shadows, even as there were attempts to bring it into focus.

2 Andrology Again

It had been nearly eighty years since Dr. Keyes lost his bid to retain the language of andrology when another editorial appeared in another medical journal titled "Andrology as a New Specialty of Medicine."[1] Authored by Carl Schirren, a German dermatologist specializing in venereal disease and male infertility, it appeared in the first volume of his newly launched journal, *Andrologie,* in October 1969. The first line of the article defines the new specialty: "Andrology is the study of man's capacity for procreation and all related disorders. It is to be regarded as the counterpart to gynecology." As the incoming president of the German Society for the Study of Fertility and Sterility, Schirren was undoubtedly familiar with that organization's new section on andrology, which was founded in 1967.[2] And with his inaugural definition of the field, Schirren drew parallels to gynecology just as Keyes had in the 1890s.[3] However, the German physician had no idea he was not the first to propose a medical specialty oriented to men's reproductive bodies called andrology.

Much had happened in the world since the first attempt to launch andrology, not least two world wars and the Great Depression. Eugenicists had risen and then fallen out of favor, as their notions of reproductive fitness were mobilized to justify mass sterilization in the United States and mass murder in Hitler's Germany.[4] Biomedicine underwent another paradigm shift as the hormonal model of the body was layered on top of the preceding organs-based model.[5] And public health rose to new prominence as basic sanitary measures yielded improvements in disease prevention and life expectancy.[6] Despite the significance of these political and medical trends, I spend relatively little time on these intervening years because one thing did not change: there was still no comprehensive, unified effort on the part of the medical profession to study and treat the male reproductive body.

That is, not until the 1960s. Not only did Schirren found the journal *Andrologie*, but physicians from Spain and Argentina teamed up to form an international association for andrologists, which was followed by regular professional meetings and even more journals devoted to the topic. How does such a specialty become thinkable, tractable, visible in the 1960s in a way it was not before? And did the (unknowing) choice of the same label for these efforts—andrology—augur similar intentions for their scope?

MEN'S REPRODUCTIVE HEALTH IN THE EARLY TWENTIETH CENTURY: A CONTINUING LACK OF TRACTION

To be clear, it is not as though there was no attention to men's reproductive health during the first half of the twentieth century.[7] Venereal disease continued to rage through the population, posing particular challenges to military leaders during World War I, who struggled to recruit men healthy enough to fight.[8] In laboratories devoted to hormonal research, scientists worked to characterize testosterone, although they did continue to focus more fully on women's bodies than men's.[9] Fertility doctors were increasingly likely to include a sperm test when evaluating couples who were having trouble getting pregnant, and they had quietly started offering what they called "artificial insemination by donor."[10] Eugenicists, too, were primarily concerned with the reproductive fitness of potential mothers but occasionally discussed the effects of fathers' constitutions.[11] And some of the "quacks" running men's specialty clinics stayed in business until well into the 1950s.[12]

As more materials from this period are digitized, it has even become possible to find a few references to andrology, including in medical dictionaries and textbooks. For example, the *American Illustrated Medical Dictionary*, first published in 1900 and followed by many subsequent editions, defined *andrology* as the "scientific study of the masculine constitution and of the diseases of the male sex."[13] However, neither the 1895 edition of *Webster's Academic Dictionary* nor the 1896 edition of *Index Medicus* had an entry for *andrology*, suggesting the term was not in wide use.

It pops up again in the subtitle of a 1910 textbook, *Male Diseases in General Practice: An Introduction to Andrology*, written by a British general surgeon named Edred Moss Corner. In the preface, he laments that "men, not being subject to a physiological process comparable to childbirth, have not been the recipients of so much attention as has been given to women" and argues the need for "a science of the diseases of men . . . termed andrology; a name comparable to gynaecology, the science of the diseases of women."[14] Obliquely referring to the feminists of his time, Corner poses a hypothesis about the lack of attention:

> In these days, when the "injustices" of woman are proclaimed so loudly, it is a relief to find a department in which she has received more attention than has been given to man. Perhaps the disparity of consideration arose from the doctors being men; their diseases being in consequence a part of every one's work, and those of women a specialty. But the profession is no longer recruited solely from men, and a special science and art of andrology must arise.[15]

The book was reviewed favorably in *JAMA* and elsewhere, but the *British Medical Journal* notes sarcastically that "Mr. Corner discloses an ardour and enthusiasm" for the topic of male diseases that led him to describe "no less than ten operations for imperfect descent of the testicles" and criticizes the "elevation of his subject into the entity 'andrology.'"[16] Likewise, the *New York Medical Journal* argued that the term *andrology* "merely adds to the already existing confusion between the old fashioned specialty 'genitourinary and venereal diseases' and the new fashioned 'urology.'"[17]

A few decades later, just after the end of World War II, another physician, this time from Bonn, Germany, called again for a medical specialty named andrology. Harald Siebke was a gynecologist who directed the women's clinic at the University of Bonn, where the historian Ralf Forsbach has determined that he performed forced sterilizations during the Nazi era.[18] Although it is unclear whether Siebke also performed sterilizations on men (given that he worked at a hospital for women), Florence Vienne has argued more generally that the male reproductive body became a particular "object of knowledge" in Germany during this period, not only in the sterilization surgeries performed by Nazis but also in the medical experiments they conducted on Holocaust victims.[19]

In a birthday tribute to a fellow German gynecologist published in 1951, Siebke editorialized about the need for physicians treating female sterility to work more closely with those treating male sterility, all with the goal of helping couples conceive children. Especially concerned that men's bodies were going completely unexamined, Siebke emphasized the need to evaluate both men's genitals and their sperm. As to how this situation came to be, he suggested that part of the blame lay with those specializing in male sterility calling themselves "dermatologists," following an earlier nomenclature when dermatology and venereology were closely linked. Instead, he proposed that such physicians adopt the title "andrologist, or a men's doctor [Männerarzt], just like a women's doctor [Frauenarzt]." He acknowledged that it is only "word play" but that it might facilitate men's visits to the doctor.[20] Just as Keyes and Corner had before him, Siebke articulated a parallel between andrology and gynecology, drawing on dualistic notions of sexed bodies to make the case for sex-specific specialties.

However, in the end, none of these periodic calls for andrology in the first half of the twentieth century gained traction. As in the photographer metaphor in the Introduction, physicians were encouraging a shift in focus to encompass the male figure, hoping to make it less blurry, but there was scant biomedical infrastructure to support such an effort for men's reproductive health. There was no cohesive community of researchers and clinicians to hear these calls, much less translate them into action in the form of knowledge production or medical care. But this dynamic started to shift in the 1960s, as male reproductive bodies slowly started to come into focus.[21] What changed?

ANDROLOGY IN THE 1960S

As even the most casual student of history knows, the 1960s and '70s were a period of extraordinary social upheaval, when people who had experienced oppression due to racism, sexism, and heteronormativity came together in powerful movements for legislative and cultural change. Civil rights activists sought the full rights of citizenship for people of color, from the voting booth to schools and on the job.[22] Feminists argued that women should be considered equal to men in every realm of society, and in particular, launched campaigns for reproductive autonomy centered on access to contraception and abortion.[23] Gays and lesbians emerged from the shadows and sought "liberation" for a plurality of sexual identities and practices, buttressed by scientific sexology studies such as the Kinsey Report.[24]

In the realm of medicine, where physicians' cultural authority had peaked in the 1950s, activists agitating for women's health and patients' rights worked to shift the uneven power dynamic between doctor and patient.[25] There was also a midcentury boom in expert discourses about the "role of men and fathers," which contributed to changing notions of masculinity and enabled various kinds of reforms, such as dads moving from the waiting room into the birthing room.[26] And just as in the 1890s, there were those who raised their voices in strong opposition to all this change, concerned about the emasculation of (White) men.[27]

These social movements did not just shift policy and practice; they also altered the conceptual ground for cultural beliefs about the human body. The "naturalness" of sex differences was under fire, as was the idea of biological race and the inevitability of heterosexuality, making it possible to ask new questions about the relationship between bodies and societies. I argue that changing cultural norms around gender and parenthood came together with emerging biomedical knowledge about reproduction and genetics, making it feasible to link men's bodies and reproductive health in a way they had not been before. Indeed, when scientists and clinicians around the globe made yet another call for andrology at the end of the 1960s, they actually had a bit of success in launching this "new" specialty.

Who, What, Where, When, Why

Even as there were new and more insistent calls for an expansion in human rights for women, people of color, and sexual minorities, there were also ongoing efforts to monitor and control their reproductive behavior. In the United States, women who were poor or a racial minority or both continued to be sterilized throughout the twentieth century, often without their consent.[28] Male prisoners, particularly men of color, were sometimes castrated as part of their "punishment," continuing and medicalizing the practice of White lynch mobs.[29]

When it came to poor and marginalized people elsewhere, American scientists took up the rhetoric of "population control" after the Second World War in lieu of straightforward eugenic language.[30] For countries deemed to have too large a population, organizations such as the Rockefeller-funded Population Council encouraged medical and social scientists to create "educational" initiatives and birth control programs.[31] In some cases, they trained their policy sights on male sterilization, arguing that "traditional values" in "developing" countries rendered men the primary decision makers within families.[32]

One of the voices calling attention to male reproductive bodies during this time was Warren O. Nelson, professor of anatomy at the University of Iowa, a perhaps unlikely hotbed of sperm research in Middle America. Among his articles is a piece in *JAMA* co-authored with Raymond Bunge, a urologist who at the same time was working with Jerome K. Sherman, a graduate student in zoology, to develop a technique for freezing and thawing human sperm.[33] Their work made possible the rise of commercial sperm banks beginning in the 1970s.[34]

In 1954, Nelson was tapped to serve as the first medical director of the newly established Population Council.[35] As an expert in the biology of spermatogenesis, his research included male fertility and male contraception, and he was involved with professional organizations for urology, endocrinology, and anatomy.[36] In the early 1960s, Nelson worked with Charles LeBlond, a cell biologist and fellow sperm expert, to form the Male Reproductive Biology Club. After Nelson's death in 1964, his colleagues gathered at the annual meeting for anatomists and renamed the club in his honor.[37]

By the end of that decade, a loosely organized international network of scientists and clinicians, including several members of the Male Reproductive Biology Club, were working to organize an interdisciplinary subfield they called "andrology." Just a year after the German dermatologist Carl Schirren published the first volume of *Andrologie* (soon renamed *Andrologia*), physicians from Spain and Argentina received funding from the Population Council to form a study group called the Comité Internacional de Andrología (CIDA). Led by Antonio Puigvert, a urologist from Barcelona who headed the Puigvert Foundation, and Roberto Eusebio Mancini, who in 1966 founded the Centro de Investigación de Reproducción in Buenos Aires, it inspired the formation of national associations for andrology all around the globe.[38] Most of these national associations then joined CIDA and also used *Andrologia* as their official publication.[39]

In addition to organizing professional associations in their own countries, the new andrologists corresponded, visited one another's labs, and came together in international workshops with titles such as "The Human Testis."[40] Held in Positano, Italy in 1970 with funding from the pharmaceutical firm Serono, that particular workshop was organized by two American scientists known for their research on male contraception: Eugenia Rosemberg of the Medical Research Institute of Worcester and C. Alvin Paulson of the University of Washington. Schirren attended, and the Argentinean scientist Mancini provided introductory remarks in which he pointed to the lack of scientific attention to "the male gonad." In the foreword to the volume containing the workshop's proceedings, Mancini concludes that if it has "excited our interest in further research and . . . opened new and original lines of study, then the organization of this gathering was amply justified."[41]

Indeed, although these scientists and clinicians hailed from different countries, they were similar in echoing their 1890s predecessors' laments about the relative lack of attention to men's reproductive bodies compared to women's. Yet, they were completely unaware of previous attempts to establish andrology as a specialty.[42] It was not until two decades after the initial volume of *Andrologie* that the new andrologists learned about Keyes's efforts at the end of the nineteenth century. Mikko Niemi, a Finnish anatomist and fertility specialist, stumbled upon the 1891 *JAMA* editorial and found it so "far-sighted and candid" with passages "relevant and valid even 95 years later" that he reprinted it in its entirety.[43] Speculating about why research into aspects of the "male reproductive system" had remained underdeveloped relative to its "counterpart," gynecology, Rune Eliasson, an endocrinologist at the Karolinska Institute in Stockholm and first president of CIDA, obliquely referred to "historical, sociological and other reasons" while addressing the first International Congress of Andrology organized by CIDA in 1976.[44]

In contrast to the 1890s-era andrologists, who were clinicians focused on particular conditions such as venereal disease, impotence, and infertility, andrologists in the 1960s and '70s built a larger umbrella, incorporating clinicians who worked on male infertility as well as basic scientists who studied particular biological processes or entities such as sperm, including those whose research was limited to animals. By the time CIDA became the International Society of Andrology in 1981, its published statutes defined *andrology* in broad terms: "the branches of science and medicine dealing with the male reproductive organs in animals and in men and with diseases of these organs."[45]

The American Society of Andrology

Inspired by the efforts of his colleagues around the world, Emil Steinberger, a protégé of Warren O. Nelson and member of the Male Reproductive Biology Club, began working to organize an American society for andrology in the early 1970s. According to Steinberger's three-volume, self-published memoir, which is dedicated in part to "W. O. the cornerstone of my career," he landed in graduate school in Iowa at Nelson's invitation.[46] Having escaped the Holocaust in Poland, he briefly attended medical school in Germany after the war before emigrating to the United States in 1948. He completed his MD and nearly all of the requirements for a PhD in 1955.[47] In 1971, he was recruited to the newly formed medical school at the University of Texas–Houston to establish and chair the Department of Reproductive Biology and Endocrinology.[48] From that perch, he began identifying potential members for the new andrology society by working the crowds at professional meetings.[49] Richard Sherins, a reproductive endocrinologist who would later serve as president of the American Society of Andrology (ASA) in the 1980s, recalled Steinberger approaching him at a conference in 1975: "With an arm on my shoulder, he said, 'Richard, I now dub you an Andrologist.' I had no idea what he was talking about, as 'Andrology' was not yet part of my scientific lexicon."[50]

Steinberger was not twisting arms all by himself. A small group of physicians and scientists that included several women worked to launch the ASA and put on its first meeting in Detroit in 1975, annexed to a symposium titled "The Human Semen and Fertility Regulation." In a series of letters exchanged over just two months, Steinberger and Eugenia Rosemberg, who was then research director at the Medical Research Institute of Worcester, hammered out both the meeting agenda and the organization's structure using The Endocrine Society as a template.[51]

Rosemberg was born in Buenos Aires and completed medical school there in the same program and around the same time as did CIDA co-founder Roberto Mancini, an early link between two scientists who came to specialize in andrology.[52] Later, Rosemberg and Mancini co-authored research articles on the testes.[53] At Worcester, which was partially funded by the Population Council, Rosemberg contributed to the development of oral contraceptives alongside Gregory Pincus and Min-Chueh Chang.[54] In 1970, she moved to the National Institutes of Health for a year to serve as chief of contraceptive development before returning to Worcester; in both posts, she emphasized the importance of male contraception.[55]

A few years later, as Rosemberg was working to organize the American Society of Andrology's first meeting in Detroit, she wrote Steinberger to suggest he serve as the first president.[56] He responded that she or Alvin Paulson, the professor of reproductive physiology at the University of Washington with whom she had organized the Italian workshop on the human testis, should be vice president.[57] Instead, Rosemberg opted to serve as program chairman (*sic*) of the ASA's first scientific meeting the following year.[58] Her ties to the organization ran so deep that, upon her death, Rosemberg bequeathed a large sum of money to it, which was used to fund the annual Distinguished Andrologist Award.[59]

At that first meeting of the ASA in 1975, Steinberger circulated a sign-up sheet that reveals the diversity of disciplinary affiliations and interests of potential members (see figure 5).[60] While some attendees hoped that andrology would become its own stand-alone medical specialty, Steinberger was not convinced it was necessary. During his inaugural presidential address to the ASA, he noted the "striking lag" in research on the male reproductive system—"It appears that the male, for whatever reason, has been neglected both by the laboratory scientist and the physician"—and described the ASA's goal of "stimulat[ing] research in male reproduction" and its "commitment to the integration of basic and clinical sciences."[61] At the same time, he believed the "interdisciplinary" nature of the ASA rendered the establishment of a specialty "inappropriate" and even "destructive."[62] He softened this position a few years later in an address to the Second International Congress of Andrology titled "The Past, Present, and Future of Andrology." Noting the importance of national distinctions in how medical specialties evolve, he described the situation in the United States:

> The urologists traditionally have claimed the area of surgery dealing with the male reproductive system and in recent years some urologists expressed also the desire to manage male infertility. . . . The gynecologists, a few years ago, established a subspecialty of Reproductive Endocrinology [which] allegedly also encompasses male reproductive disorders. But a large segment of male patients with reproductive system disorders, hypergonadism or infertility are still treated by the internist-endocrinologist. *Thus there is no single specialty that provides comprehensive care for the male patient with a reproductive system disorder.*[63]

Steinberger continued by noting that if none of these "existing established medical specialties" clearly declare "andrology as their responsibility," this impedes "appropriate training of the 'andrologist.'" He then argues that it also introduces "an element of confusion in the mind of the male patient with a reproductive system disorder and in the mind of a physician who searches for and is in need of an appropriate consultant." He concludes by stating that "if the specialties are not willing to apply the rapidly accumulating knowledge and to sacrifice the necessary time element, a clinical specialty of Andrology may have to be developed to provide appropriate modern care to males with reproductive system disorders."[64]

I heard echoes of these sentiments in conducting interviews with physicians who had been in medical school at the time and later became nationally recognized experts on men's reproductive health. A urologist who would open one of the first and eventually one of the largest commercial sperm banks in the United States described being a medical resident in the early 1970s:

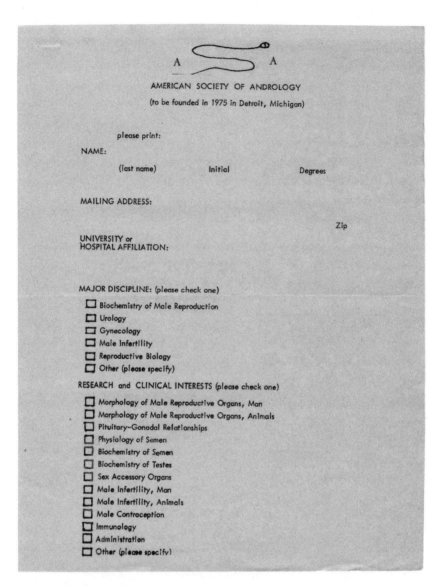

Figure 5. Sign-up sheet for the inaugural meeting of the American Society of Andrology, 1975.

There was very little known about male infertility. When I was a first-year resident, my mentor assigned each resident to study different aspects of urology. He gave me [the question of] how does sperm get from the testicle to the outside world? It was fascinating. Very little was known, absolutely nothing in humans, and everything had to be extrapolated from animal husbandry and veterinary medicine. We knew sperm developed in the testicle but weren't sure of the mechanism of the epididymis, the vas deferens, the seminal vesicle, the prostate; what actually causes sperm to go from the testicular epididymal area to the outside world to negotiate a pregnancy. The second year, he gave me the topic "mechanism of erection." We didn't know how a guy got an erection. So I spent two years of my residency studying sperm and erection. When I finished my residency, I was truly interested in the field of andrology, which did not exist. So it was the study of man like gynecology is the study of women. I was fascinated by it being a new subject, young, enthusiastic. So I decided I was going to try and specialize in male infertility. I was very fortunate because in [West Coast city], none of the urologists wanted to deal with it, and I got very busy very quickly.[65]

Ten years later, in the mid-1980s, another medical student interested in urology, who would later become president of the Society for the Study of Male Reproduction, explained to his mentors he had entered the field to focus on male infertility. "They looked at me like I was from outer space because most urologists, that's not what they do. They do BPH [i.e., enlarged prostate], prostate cancer, kidney cancer, you know, surgery like that, or stones." When he described the biomedical landscape in the 2010s, not much had changed during the preceding half century: men's reproductive health continued to fall in between specialties. "It's kind of a small part of what we do in urology. It's a small part of primary care. It's a small part of endocrinology. But most reproductive endocrinologists don't know anything about sperm; they're the 'egg doctors.'"[66]

Another thing to notice about the ASA sign-up sheet from 1975 (figure 5) is that a sperm constitutes the *S* at the top of the page, iconography the ASA returned to with its latest logo in 2013 (see figure 6).[67] There are other humorous notes buried in the organization's history. While they initially relied on *Andrologia* as their official publication, financial difficulties and communication problems with the publisher eventually led the Americans to form the *Journal of Andrology*, first published in 1980 and still in print (now as *Andrology* after merging with the *International*

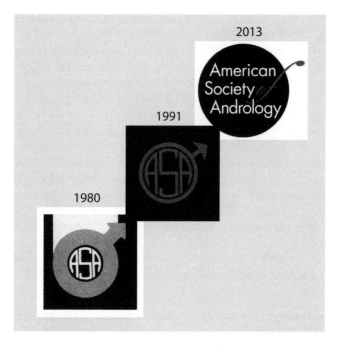

Figure 6. Evolution of the American Society of Andrology logo,
1980–2013.

Journal of Andrology in 2013).[68] The first editor recalled the administrative assistant giving delinquent reviewers a "black testis award," which was "duly noted on their index card in our address file."[69] And in celebration of its thirtieth birthday in 2005, the Archives Committee of the ASA drafted a brief history of the organization, noting that "we are the only organization that honors its young andrologist with an oversized 'condom' hat. The wearing and placing of this hat has become an important and honored tradition in the Society."[70]

Yet, despite the numerous national societies, multiple journals, and growing number of individuals identifying themselves as andrologists, the field remains small and largely unknown in the United States. At its first scientific meeting in 1976, the American Society of Andrology had 235 members.[71] Today, there are "over 600," and their specialties, as listed on the ASA website, remain quite varied: "male reproduction, endocrinology, urology, anatomy, gynecology/obstetrics, biochemistry, animal science, molecular & cell biology, and reproductive technologies."[72] Microsoft Word still places red squiggles under the word *andrology*, betraying a lack of recognition by its internal dictionary. And as the andrologists themselves admitted on the eve of the ASA's thirtieth birthday: "At every meeting, a stranger on the elevator asks, 'What is andrology?'"[73]

THE LACK OF MEDICAL SPECIALIZATION
AROUND MEN'S REPRODUCTIVE HEALTH

As reproduction received scientific and medical attention throughout the twentieth century, the cultural terrain continued to offer fertile ground for focusing primarily on women's bodies, especially in the well-established and large specialties of gynecology and obstetrics and robust biomedical research agendas around hormones and the contraceptive pill.[74] But it is not as though there was *no* attention to men's reproductive bodies during this period. Scientists were studying men, and doctors were treating them, but the lack of a singular, cohesive specialty made it difficult to sustain scientific and clinical attention to men's reproductive health.

The process of medical specialization is often accompanied by the development of organizational infrastructure: annual meetings where specialists mingle and forge collaborations, premier journals for research and discussion, and training programs to ensure the next generation of specialists. Simply put, for the first half of the century, there was none of this to unify the disparate researchers and clinicians working on various aspects of men's reproductive bodies. As a result, any attention to men's reproductive health remained diffuse and scattered amongst loosely related specialties, such as urology, infertility, and endocrinology. It is against this backdrop that one can read the periodic calls for andrology and understand why those calls fell on deaf ears. Or more precisely, the ears that might have heard the calls would have been few and far between, unlikely to be organizationally linked to others with similar interests.

It was not until the social movements of the 1960s and '70s that it became more conceptually feasible to link men's bodies to the topic of reproductive health. With sweeping changes in scientific research, clinical practice, and cultural beliefs around gender and reproduction, the topic of men's reproductive health became more thinkable, more tractable than it previously had been.[75] And it became possible to interrupt, however slightly, the strong feedback loop linking the categories of "women" and "reproduction." The emergence of another biomedical specialty called andrology in the late 1960s is emblematic of this shifting terrain during the latter half of the century. Indeed, while the 1890s-era andrologists were laughed out of the pages of medical journals, the later andrologists did successfully create and institutionalize the infrastructure of a specialty, albeit a small and narrowly defined one, with professional associations, annual meetings, and journals.

Now, as with many historical arguments, one is certainly entitled to ask about which way the causal arrow points. Did the social context enable andrology, or did andrology change the social context? In this case, I contend that it was probably the social context that enabled andrology rather than vice versa, because andrology consisted of a relatively small group of subspecialists who to this day in the United States are not widely known outside their field.

And it is also important to note that even as the andrologists of the 1890s and 1960s chose the same name, there is no clear line through history linking one to the other. They took different configurations and had different goals because each was situated in the politics of masculinity and medicine of their era. While each incarnation of andrology focused on the male body and its reproductive parts, the 1890s grouping consisted of clinicians primarily interested in venereal disease, whereas the 1960s grouping included basic scientists and clinicians primarily focused on sperm and male infertility. The earlier andrologists also faced much higher levels of stigma and shame than did the later andrologists. Yet, even as their projects were not identical, they were similar in one crucial way: andrologists at both points in time sought to define their specialty as "parallel" to gynecology, evident in their choice of Greek root as well as the content of their scientific and medical interests. And that is because both 1890s-era and 1960s-era andrologists were responding to an ongoing cultural paradigm of gender as dualism, in which female bodies are reproductive and male bodies are not reproductive.

The possibility and process of medical specialization are deeply influenced by both the biological knowledge base and cultural norms of the time. Health policy scholars point to the benefits of medical specialization, such as improvements in the diagnosis and treatment of particular conditions based on the increasing expertise that results from lengthy periods of in-depth training.[76] But researchers also raise concerns about the pathologies of specialization, including the smaller number of "generalist" clinicians who can treat the "whole person," particularly ones who are willing to live and work in rural areas, leading to reduced access to basic care.[77] To this debate, I would add a cautionary note about what happens when there is a *lack* of specialization. It can lead to a lack of focused biomedical attention, a lack of clinical care, and as I demonstrate in the next chapter, a lack of knowledge.

PART II Circulating Knowledge about Men's Reproductive Health

3 Making Knowledge about Paternal Effects

Despite ongoing struggles for professional recognition, andrology does now exist. As scientists and clinicians worked to organize the biomedical infrastructure for this new specialization, launching journals and creating professional societies, their efforts were concomitant with a general uptick in attention to men's reproductive bodies that began in the 1970s. To illustrate, figures 7–9 show a series of Ngrams, which track the number of times a word appears in the large corpus of texts—scientific, popular, and otherwise—that are available as scans within Google. Basically, Ngrams provide a rough sketch of how common a particular word is during a particular period of time.[1] Figure 7 shows the frequency of the words *andrology* or *andrologist* between 1800 and 2008.[2] There are occasional appearances of the term starting in the mid-nineteenth century and a small blip in the 1890s, which reflects the efforts of Dr. Keyes and his colleagues (chronicled in chapter 1). But the most significant shift occurs around 1970, when there is an exponential increase in the prevalence of the term *andrology*. The spike lasts until 1990 and then levels off. Likewise, as shown in figure 8, a search for the more general terms *men's reproductive health* or *men's reproduction* (and their cognates *male reproductive health*

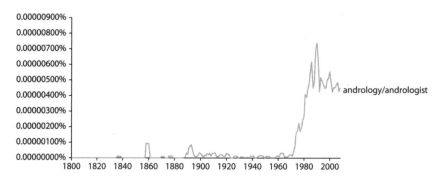

Figure 7. Google Ngram for "andrology or andrologist," 1800–2008.

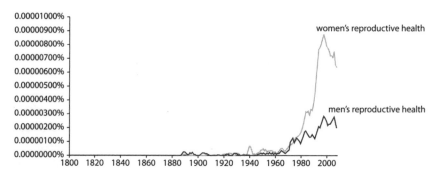

Figure 8. Google Ngram for "women's reproductive health" and "men's reproductive health," 1800–2008.

or *male reproduction*) reveal a similar inflection point around 1970, followed by a steady increase through 2008.[3]

The increasing attention to men's reproductive health was not lost on researchers at the time. The prominent cell biologist Don W. Fawcett, known for his anatomical characterization of human sperm,[4] wrote in 1976:

> There is no doubt that in the more balanced perspective of future generations, the decades from 1960 to 1980 will be considered a golden era in the progress of basic understanding of reproductive biology of the male.[5]

And Emil Steinberger, who served as the first president of the American Society of Andrology (described in chapter 2), noted in his 1981 address to

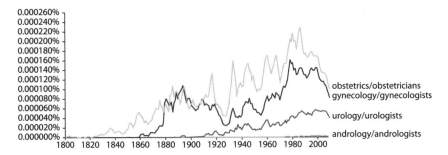

Figure 9. Google Ngram for "obstetrics," "gynecology," "urology," and "andrology," 1800–2008.

the International Congress of Andrology that the "1970s witnessed a true explosion of knowledge in male reproductive physiology."[6]

Yet, even as the topic of men's reproductive health lifted off the x-axis and began to receive some notice, it came nowhere near the high level of attention given to women's reproductive health. This dynamic is clear whether one uses the general search term *women's reproductive health* and cognates (as in figure 8) or compares the relative number of mentions garnered by medical specialties attending to women's versus men's reproductive bodies. Figure 9 shows increasing mentions of *obstetrics* and *gynecology* from the middle of the nineteenth century onward.[7] In contrast, *urology* does not enter the lexicon until the 1910s. Although there is a steady increase over the course of the twentieth century, it never rises to the level of either obstetrics or gynecology. And the comparison to andrology is especially revealing: relative to the first three specialties, *andrology* barely registers on the chart.

In what follows, I look more closely at a subset of these mentions: biomedical studies about how a man's age, behaviors, and exposures can affect sperm and, in turn, his children's health. Collectively referred to as "paternal effects," this research is related to but distinct from the topic of male infertility. Twentieth-century clinicians seeking to assess the fertility or "quality" of sperm relied on aspects of these cells that were easily visible through a microscope: the number of sperm in a semen sample (count), their movement (motility), and their shape (morphology). It was clear that issues with any of these measures could cause male infertility—via low or zero sperm count, sluggish sperm, or misshapen sperm.[8] But, in general, scientists and clinicians operated on the assumption that if sperm were present and could fertilize an egg, then they were healthy.[9] It was not until the late twentieth century that biomedical researchers began to distinguish between the *fertility* of sperm and its *health*. Over the past several decades, there has been a growing realization that some of the same factors that affect sperm count, motility, and morphology—such as a man's age, behaviors, and exposures—might also be causing damage to the genetic material inside sperm, with implications for children's health.

Sifting through the scientific literature, I detail the evidence base for claims about paternal effects in this chapter before turning in the next chapter to the question of whether they are being circulated to the general public. There are several reasons I selected paternal effects as a case within the broader rubric of men's reproductive health to examine questions about the production and circulation of new knowledge. Most important is its "newness." In contrast, most of the topics typically associated with men's reproductive health—male infertility, sexually transmitted infections, and erectile dysfunction—are the very same conditions that preoccupied physicians at the end of the nineteenth century, even though the terminology has been updated (from male sterility, venereal disease, and impotence, respectively). Another twentieth-century newcomer to the list is the male contraceptive pill, but each of these topics has already been the subject of historical and social scientific scholarship.[10] So my analysis of paternal effects excavates one of the newer and lesser-known strands of biomedical research on men's reproductive bodies.

I also chose the topic of paternal effects because it can be compared to the production and circulation of knowledge about maternal effects and, more specifically, to the relatively recent focus of public health officials on "preconception health." Most of the attention and resources in this realm have been directed at women, but the new science of paternal effects suggests that these efforts could be expanded to include men's preconception health.[11] Moreover, these issues extend beyond the clinic and into the domain of law and policy, especially given that women have been incarcerated for their behavior during pregnancy.[12] While men's preconception health cannot be equated exactly to women's preconception health (because pregnancy occurs in women's bodies), there are enough similarities to make possible comparative questions about what is known and what is publicized about paternal effects.

PATERNAL EFFECTS

This section is co-authored with Jenna Healey.

The notion that a father's health might affect his offspring is an ancient one, existing even in Classical Greece.[13] A few millennia later, nineteenth-century campaigns against alcohol and venereal disease raised concerns about how a weakened male constitution might result in "feeble" children or the inability to sire children at all.[14] And since the advent of genetic science, many people are now familiar with the idea that certain diseases "run in families." Examples include Tay-Sachs disease and Huntington's disease, in which a disease-causing mutation in the DNA is passed from parent to offspring.

In recent decades, though, scientists have identified another form of genetic damage in which the chemical compounds that surround DNA are altered, not the DNA itself. Those compounds can then affect whether and how particular genes are (or are not) expressed. Referred to as "epigenetic" modifications, they can arise from things that individuals do or substances to which they are exposed.[15] That is how an individual man's age, behaviors, and the toxins he encounters can damage the genetic material inside his sperm and potentially affect his children's health. In addition to epigenetic effects, these factors can also lead to spontaneous new mutations (called de novo mutations) in the DNA during spermatogenesis. These processes are often grouped together under the umbrella phrase *paternal effects*, but the language is still a bit unsettled. As recently as 2014, scientific researchers were still doing basic definitional work in articles with titles like "What Is a Paternal Effect?"[16]

Resistance to the very idea of paternal effects persisted for so long because there was no obvious way that men mattered for reproductive outcomes over and above providing half the DNA.[17] And the entity through which DNA is transmitted—sperm—was believed to be endlessly "new" because it is constantly being replenished. But now that epigenetics offers a mechanism through which sperm can be damaged and yet still manage to fertilize an egg, there are new questions about when and how men's bodily health can affect sperm and ultimately the resulting child.

In examining paternal effects, biomedical researchers have focused on three factors: (1) men's age; (2) their "behaviors"—namely, what they consume via diet, drinking, smoking, and taking drugs, legal or otherwise; and (3) their exposures to toxins at home, work, and in the environment. A crucial period during which sperm can suffer epigenetic damage is the 2.5 months *before* conception; it takes about that long for sperm cells to develop and mature in the male body. But even before this months-long window, scientists have learned that men's exposures earlier in life, even back to their days as a fetus, can affect the health of their sperm for decades to come.[18] As the evidence has accumulated, particularly during the past fifteen years or so, it has revealed that a man's age and bodily health can influence not only pregnancy outcomes, such as miscarriage and birthweight, but also birth defects,[19] childhood diseases such as autism, and even adult-onset conditions like schizophrenia.[20]

In terms of data, paternal effects researchers typically conduct genetic studies, epidemiological studies, or animal studies. According to the authors of these reports, genetic evidence is considered the most robust because it points to a specific pathway through which variation in fathers' bodily health can be passed to their offspring, even if that variation cannot always be linked to specific disease outcomes. In contrast, epidemiological studies are usually limited to observing a correlation between specific paternal characteristics (such as age or exposures) and pathological effects in children. As anyone who has ever taken an introductory statistics class can explain, correlation is not causation.[21] Finally, animal studies—typically experiments on rodents—allow for the systematic testing of paternal effects in a laboratory setting, after which researchers can follow offspring for several generations. But there are always open questions about whether and how the results of animal research translate to humans.[22]

What follows is an overview of major findings from all three kinds of studies as they pertain to the effects of a man's age, behaviors, and exposures.[23] Of these, paternal age is the most thoroughly documented: numerous genetic and epidemiological studies published in top scientific journals have found that children of older fathers are at higher risk for various diseases. In contrast, research about men's behaviors and exposures tend to appear in smaller specialty journals on developmental toxicology. There is solid evidence for the negative effects of paternal smoking, with animal studies, epidemiological studies, and a handful of human genetic studies showing germ-line mutations being passed to future generations. Research on the effects of a man's diet, body mass index (BMI), and exercise have appeared more recently and rely mostly on animal studies and a few epidemiological studies.[24] As for the magnitude of risk posed by various occupational and environmental exposures, the jury is still out; research on rats and mice indicate a high likelihood of what researchers refer to as "male-mediated developmental toxicity," but it is hard to isolate particular exposures in humans in order to produce convincing genetic evidence.

Paternal Age

It is now common knowledge that advanced *maternal* age is associated with the risk of having a child with Down syndrome, but most people are not as familiar with the ramifications of advanced *paternal* age.[25] Yet, scientists have been investigating the potential problems posed by older men's sperm for more than a century. One of the first such articles appeared in 1912 and was authored by Wilhelm Weinberg, a physician and "canny statistician" from Stuttgart who was a leading German authority on medical genetics; his name is preserved in the Hardy-Weinberg equilibrium still in use by population geneticists.[26] In one of his many investigations into heredity, Weinberg observed that achondroplasia, a form of dwarfism, was more often found in the last-born child within families, and he hypothesized that the father's advancing age might be a factor. Four decades later, Lionel Penrose, a geneticist and professor of eugenics at the University of London, used data from three countries to provide further substantiation of the link between paternal age and achondroplasia in *The Lancet*. Penrose noted that certain conditions did appear to be more closely associated with maternal age, such as Down syndrome (called "Mongolism" in his day), but he pointed to his results on dwarfism to argue that it was crucial to take into account *both* maternal and paternal age. He concluded there needed to be "accurate and comprehensive inquiry in this field."[27]

However, such a comprehensive inquiry appears to have been stymied by the lack of a clear association between paternal age and chromosomal anomalies.[28] The addition or subtraction of entire chromosomes (the technical term is *chromosomal aneuploidies*) as occurs in Down syndrome, in which there are three copies of chromosome 21 instead of two, is clearly linked to maternal age. In contrast, advanced paternal age was initially associated with specific mutations of specific genes on particular chromosomes, making it difficult to establish a clear link between a man's age and his offspring's health prior to the development of detailed genetic analyses. As the precision of genetic testing continued to improve, several studies conducted in the 1970s and '80s found associations between a man's age and rare genetic conditions caused by autosomal dominant mutations (as occurs in achondroplasia), such as Marfan syndrome, Crouzon syndrome, and Pfeiffer syndrome.[29] Now called "paternal age effect disorders," they have been traced to a cluster of mutations in human growth factor genes.[30]

Based on this emerging evidence, sperm banks began imposing age limits on male donors as early as 1984, when the first standards issued by the American Association of Tissue Banks stated that sperm donors should be younger than thirty-six to minimize the chances of aging-related "genetic abnormalities."[31] A few years later, the American Fertility Society (now the American Society for Reproductive Medicine) raised the maximum age for sperm donors to fifty but then quickly revised it to forty when a new review appeared in 1991 with "compelling evidence" that the risk of serious, nonchromosomal birth disorders increased with paternal age.[32] However, as I detail in the next chapter, these early warnings about the potential consequences of advanced paternal age did not spread much beyond the walls of biomedical research labs and sperm banks.

It was not until the early 2000s that researchers began establishing connections between the sperm of older fathers and more common diseases, such as cancer and autism, as well as psychological conditions like schizophrenia and bipolar disorder.[33] Epidemiological studies suggested that children of older fathers were at increased risk of developing leukemia and retinoblastoma, as well as early-onset breast cancer.[34] Initial findings that advanced paternal age was associated with schizophrenia and autism have since been corroborated numerous times.[35] A 2012 article in *Nature* made the front page of the *New York Times* with the astounding claim that the rate of new mutations in the sperm of older men is now believed to be responsible for the same proportion of developmental disorders as chromosomal aneuploidies in older women.[36]

Although scientists are still in the early stages of specifying the exact levels of risk associated with older fatherhood, there are a few statistics that demonstrate just how significant the numbers can be. Compared to fathers under the age of thirty, fathers in their forties have a 1.78-fold increased risk of having a child with autism spectrum disorder; men over fifty have a 2.46-fold increased risk.[37] Men older than forty-five at the time of conception are 3.6 times more likely to have a child who develops schizophrenia later in life.[38] In fact, researchers estimate that 15 percent of all cases of schizophrenia could be related to men having children after the age of thirty.[39] Frans and colleagues found that the children of fathers fifty-five years and older are 1.37 times more likely to be diagnosed with bipolar disorder than those with fathers in their early twenties.[40] A more recent study suggests the relationship between paternal age and the risk of major depressive disorders is actually a U curve, with increased risk both earlier and later in reproductive life.[41]

In addition to developing serious diseases in childhood and beyond, some studies have suggested that the offspring of older fathers are more likely to be born with birth defects. One retrospective cohort analysis of around 5 million births in the United States demonstrated that paternal age over fifty was associated with a 15 percent increased risk of birth defects.[42] Another recent cohort study followed 1.5 million children born to fathers older than forty and found they have a greater risk of dying before age five, due to the higher incidence of birth defects and other malignancies in this population.[43]

As the risks of advanced paternal age come into focus, and as more men become fathers later in life,[44] researchers and clinicians continue to debate whether men should even be informed of these risks. As early as 1981, the geneticist Jan M. Freidman argued that *all* men should be warned about paternal age, noting that "if all men fathered all their children before they reached age 40, a significant reduction in the frequency of disease due to a new mutation would be expected." Thus, "it is good public health policy to recommend that both men and women complete their family before age 40, if possible."[45] In contrast, the American College of Medical Genetics statement about counseling for advanced paternal age in 2008 begins: "There is no clearly accepted definition of advanced paternal age." It goes on to list various risks that may be "minimally increased" with paternal age, but notes that there are no specific "screening or diagnostic test panels" available, so couples should just receive "individualized genetic counseling to address specific concerns."[46]

Indeed, some point to the relatively low levels of baseline risk for autism, schizophrenia, and other disorders to argue that even a "doubling" of the risk for older fathers is not that concerning, at least for individual men. Dolores Malaspina, one of the scientists responsible for quantifying the effect of paternal age, explained in *JAMA:* "I wouldn't discourage a man from having children because the risk is quite small for an individual, but it's quite meaningful at the population level."[47] And in research articles on the question of "how old is too old," there are also admonitions to weigh the health consequences of advancing paternal age alongside its benefits, such as the possibility that older fathers are "more likely to have progressed in their career and achieved financial security."[48] Other scientists and clinicians wonder whether it is *"reasonable* to ask potential fathers to make . . . lifestyle changes" given that the evidence remains "thin."[49] It is worth noting that one would be unlikely to encounter these particular sentiments when it comes to educating women about the risks of advanced maternal age. I return to this issue in the next chapter, where my analysis of news reports reveals that journalists too downplay risks and raise concerns that publicizing the effects of paternal age might cause "panic."

Paternal Behaviors and Exposures

It was also in the 1970s, alongside a growing environmental movement and the establishment of federal agencies to address occupational safety and health[50] that researchers intensified their efforts to understand the effects of chemicals on men's reproductive bodies. In addition to exposures at work and home, developmental toxicologists also examined the effects of substances consumed by individual men, such as through smoking cigarettes or drinking alcohol. While the evidence base is less robust than that for paternal age, scientists' efforts in this arena have been reinvigorated by the advent of epigenetics, which provides a mechanism through which men's exposures can be passed to future generations.[51] Researchers in this field now agree that "a large body of evidence in rodents unequivocally shows that paternal exposure to a variety of chemicals induces embryonic lethality and other abnormal reproductive outcomes." However, the link between paternal exposures and negative reproductive outcomes in *humans* is much less established, a fact that should be attributed to the "huge methodological challenges in demonstrating effects" and not necessarily the nonexistence of male-mediated developmental toxicity.[52]

SMOKING, DRINKING, DRUGS, AND DIET

Initial studies about the reproductive effects of men's smoking, drinking, and drug use appeared in the 1970s and peaked alongside attention to maternal substance abuse, such as the racialized moral panic that erupted around pregnant women smoking crack cocaine in the 1980s.[53] But while there was a great deal of research about the consequences of paternal behaviors on sperm, including its count, motility, and morphology, it was more difficult to pinpoint implications for particular reproductive outcomes, such as miscarriage and children's health.

There is now enough evidence for scientists to state unequivocally that paternal cigarette smoking prior to conception poses a serious risk to children.[54] It not only impedes male fertility; it also increases the risk of genetic damage in sperm.[55] In particular, fathers who smoke are more likely to develop what are called "germ-line mutations," which are then passed not only to their own children but also to their descendants.[56] There is also scientific consensus that men who smoke cigarettes before conception increase the chances their children will develop cancer. In 2009, the International Agency for Research on Cancer concluded that paternal smoking was associated with an increased risk of childhood leukemia and hepatoblastoma.[57] In 2012, Milne and colleagues confirmed these findings and recommended that "both men and women should be informed of these risks, and men should be strongly encouraged to cease smoking, particularly when planning to start a family."[58]

In contrast, there is much less consensus about the relationship between paternal alcohol consumption and reproductive outcomes.[59] Research on rodents suggests it can result in a variety of negative effects in offspring, such as low birth weight, congenital malformations, and behavioral abnormalities, but the results for humans have been inconsistent.[60] Initial research suggested that children of alcoholic fathers were more likely to develop attention deficit hyperactivity disorder (ADHD), but a more recent study refuted that connection.[61] Two large studies in humans also found no relationship between moderate alcohol consumption and male fertility, but both sets of authors acknowledged their null results contradicted previous studies and concluded that the effects of alcohol on men's reproductive health is still an open question.[62]

As with alcohol, research on the effects of illegal drugs, such as marijuana and cocaine, has more often been conducted with animals than humans for both technological and ethical reasons. Rodents demonstrate learning difficulties and other behavioral disturbances following paternal exposure to such substances, but just two epidemiological studies in humans have linked men's marijuana use to an increased incidence of congenital heart conditions.[63] Questions about the effects of drugs on sperm are being renewed in the face of the opioid crisis.[64]

When it comes to a man's diet, both human and animal studies are providing increasing evidence that the quantity and quality of what fathers eat can influence the metabolic health of their children.[65] Research on men from Överkalix, Sweden, revealed that those who had had an ample supply of food between the ages of eight and twelve had grandsons (but not granddaughters) with elevated risks of diabetes and cardiovascular disease.[66] In a second study on humans, researchers found that men in Taiwan who ate betel nuts, which are associated with a risk for metabolic syndrome, were more likely to have children who developed metabolic syndrome, even if those children never ate the nuts themselves.[67] Turning to research on rats, males whose diet was restricted in utero but were otherwise fed normally had offspring with reduced birth weight and impaired glucose tolerance.[68] Those deprived of food for just twenty-four hours prior to conception had offspring with lower serum glucose levels.[69] On the flip side, when male rats are fed a high-fat diet, a study in *Nature* demonstrated their daughters develop a diabetes-like condition of impaired glucose tolerance and insulin secretion in adulthood.[70]

OCCUPATIONAL AND ENVIRONMENTAL EXPOSURES

For much of the twentieth century, "protective" labor laws existed to safeguard (some) women from dangerous working conditions. While scholars have noted that such regulations enshrined problematic notions of feminine delicacy,[71] these laws also reflected assumptions about the invulnerability of male workers, who were not perceived as needing similar protections. Those assumptions began to change in the 1970s, as a trickle of scientific research coalesced with high-profile cases of workplace toxicity to sound an alarm about the reproductive effects of chemicals on men.[72] One important moment in this history occurred in 1977, when a group of male workers at a California factory began talking over lunch about how several of them were having difficulties conceiving children. Their union called in the National Institute for Occupational Safety and Health, which determined that Dow Chemical's pesticide dibromochloropropane (DBCP) was to blame for widespread male infertility at the plant.[73] By that point, there had already been two decades of rodent research clearly establishing the reproductive hazards posed by DBCP, but those risks were never communicated to workers.[74] In 1979, following national media attention,[75] the United States enacted a full ban of DBCP, excepting only pineapple groves in Hawaii (use there too was eventually banned in 1985). However, the pesticide continued to be used widely for years in Latin America, the Philippines, and some African countries.[76] Its toxic effects on agricultural workers was the subject of a 2009 documentary titled *Bananas!*

It was not only among agricultural laborers that scientists were investigating the possibility of male-mediated developmental toxicity in the 1970s. One study suggested that men's occupational exposures to hydrocarbons—such as those encountered by mechanics, miners, and painters—raised their children's risks of developing cancer.[77] And lead exposure was the issue in a 1979 legal case that eventually reached the Supreme Court in 1991, *United Autoworkers Union v. Johnson Controls Inc.* While the case centered on women who were refused employment at a battery manufacturer because of the possibility they might become pregnant and face lead exposure, the union's case actually made the argument that such exposures also posed risks to *men's* reproductive health.[78] In addition to widespread media coverage, this proposition inspired a presentation on paternal effects at the annual meeting of the American Association for the Advancement of Science in 1991.[79]

Workplace toxicity is not limited to low-wage jobs.[80] Male laboratory scientists working with carcinogens are slightly more likely to have children born with "major malformations."[81] Male dentists and doctors' repeated exposures to anesthetics such as laughing gas appear to increase the risk of miscarriage and low birth weight.[82] In addition to specific chemicals used in specific occupations, researchers have also searched for paternal effects among those exposed to radiation, as in the Chernobyl disaster of 1986 or a cancer cluster that developed among children of workers at a nuclear plant in Sellafield, England.[83] However, the precise risks remain unclear.[84] Scientists have also examined men's exposures on the battlefield, including to Agent Orange during the Vietnam War and the indeterminate group of substances that caused a variety of afflictions among Gulf War veterans.[85]

In terms of other environmental exposures, there has been a great deal of attention to endocrine-disrupting chemicals, especially the question of whether they are contributing to a global drop in sperm count.[86] However, that debate typically focuses on questions of fertility (in the form of sperm count, motility, and morphology) and less often takes up the potential effects on children's health, so I do not discuss it in detail here.

In sum, whether it is men's exposures at home, work, or in the broader environment, it remains very difficult for researchers to establish precisely which substances individuals are exposed to and in what concentrations. As a result, scientists concede that "strong evidence" linking paternal exposures to disease "is still limited."[87] And as the power of unions to protect workers continues to decline and environmental regulations are further eviscerated,[88] the lack of clarity is likely to continue.

ADDING MEN TO THE REPRODUCTIVE EQUATION

As this brief review of the scientific literature makes clear, a man's age and what he ingests and is exposed to during the preconception period, as well as earlier in life, have the potential to affect sperm cells and the genetic material they contain. Now that scientific studies of paternal effects are beginning to pile up, it is important to recognize that early researchers in this arena faced numerous challenges in establishing the legitimacy of their inquiries. The political scientist Cynthia Daniels interviewed several scholars who were among the first to begin studying how men's bodily health mattered for reproductive outcomes, such as Gladys Friedler, Barbara Hales, and Bernard Robaire. Amid stories of skeptical advisers, incredulous colleagues, and denial after denial of funding requests, these and other scientists scraped together the time and money to pursue research programs that others perceived as "completely implausible," in part due to the belief that sperm is "forever young."[89] Daniels concluded that in "reproductive medicine, assumptions about masculinity affect not only the questions asked by scientific researchers but also what counts as an acceptable answer."[90] These challenges persist to this day; for example, epidemiologists interested in the developmental origins of health and disease (DOHaD) have issued calls in recent years to stop ignoring paternal effects.[91]

It is also worth noting that many of these scientists are women, a product of the surge in coeducation in the 1960s and '70s, who stayed in academia and earned PhDs.[92] In addition to Friedler and Hales, other prominent women studying paternal effects include the epidemiologist Devra Lee Davis and the psychiatrist Dolores Malaspina. It is probably not a coincidence that women entering scientific fields long dominated by men who had almost exclusively focused on women's reproductive bodies began to ask new questions about paternal effects. The phenomenon has not been lost on those in the field; in a recent *New York Times* article about sperm research, the reproductive biologist Janice L. Bailey noted, "Oddly enough there's a lot of women in the field. We sometimes call ourselves Gals for Guys."[93]

But even as scientists and clinicians attend more assiduously to men's reproductive health, individual studies tend to focus on one or another aspect of paternal effects, such as a man's age at conception, the number of cigarettes smoked, or the effects of a particular chemical. To offer a full assessment of how men matter for reproductive outcomes, one needs solid evidence of not only how much risk is conferred by men's age, behaviors, and exposures but also how each of these factors interact, as well as the potential interplay between paternal and maternal effects.[94] One way of visualizing the kinds of knowledge about men's bodies that would be necessary to generate a cumulative risk assessment is the "reproductive equation" portrayed in figure 10.[95] At the moment, scientists can produce risk estimates for particular aspects of this equation, such as a man's age and his child's risk of autism. However, the varying levels of evidence for each of these factors, as well as the almost complete dearth of information about how they interact with maternal factors, make it impossible to generate a cumulative, personalized risk assessment for any individual man.

Put simply, an enormous amount of work remains to be done to elucidate the precise relationship between men's reproductive health and the

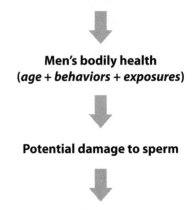

Social conditions as fundamental causes of disease

Men's bodily health
(*age + behaviors + exposures*)

Potential damage to sperm

Potential risks to children's health

Figure 10. Reproductive Equation.

health of their children. But even as scientists struggle to secure the funding, time, and space to fill in the details of this equation, their initial results suggest that men's age and bodily health does have significant consequences for their children. This information could be of use to individuals as they consider parenthood and to clinicians as they discuss reproductive plans with their patients. I turn to this issue in the next chapter, where I examine the extent to which scientific evidence about paternal effects is being publicized to a broader public.

THE RELATIONSHIP BETWEEN MEDICAL SPECIALIZATION AND KNOWLEDGE-MAKING

Here, I return to the question of the relationship between medical specialization and the making of new knowledge. Detailing the inability of andrologists to launch a broad specialty in the 1890s, the emergence again of a specialty named andrology in the 1960s, and the increasing—though still scant—production of biomedical knowledge about men's reproductive health since the 1970s, my analysis underlines the importance of the biomedical infrastructure that accompanies medical specialization for the production of new knowledge. By biomedical infrastructure, I mean the organizational entities such as professional associations, scientific meetings, and journals that bring together biomedical researchers and allow for the exchange and accretion of ideas, knowledge, and technologies. In short, I argue that the lack of such infrastructure resulting from the failure of andrology at the end of the nineteenth century reverberates to this day in the lackluster level of attention given to the reproductive health of men, even though they constitute fully half the population.

The development of andrology in the 1960s began to offer some of the biomedical infrastructure through which researchers interested in topics like paternal effects could begin to share and amplify their work. Some of the scientific studies discussed in this chapter were presented at andrological meetings or published in andrological journals, but the field of andrology remains small and virtually unknown in the United States, even to many physicians. And the production of knowledge about men's reproductive bodies since the 1970s has hardly been limited to those who self-identify as andrologists. Yet there is still no broad, large, well-known specialty that serves as a gathering hub for all those interested in various aspects of men's reproductive health, a topic that goes far beyond paternal effects to include contraception, infertility, sexually transmitted infections, and erectile dysfunction. Instead, research has been conducted by a wide variety of specialists and published in a wide range of mostly specialized journals, such as those focused on developmental toxicology or genetics or occupational health, without much cross-talk between disparate clinical and scientific specialties.

So rather than credit the 1960s emergence of andrology as the sole stimulus for increasing biomedical knowledge-making about men's reproductive health, it is more accurate to say that both likely resulted from the shifting cultural and political dynamics of that period. Just as social movements around gender, race, and sexuality had profound influences on the social institutions of work, family, education, and the law, so too did they alter the conceptual ground on which medical knowledge was made and clinical care was practiced. Biomedical understandings of gendered bodies changed just enough to allow researchers, several of them women, to begin posing new questions about how men's bodies mattered for reproductive outcomes.

To return to the metaphor of the photographer in the Introduction, among scientists and clinicians, there is now a weak feedback loop linking the categories of "men" and "reproductive health." In the next chapter, I turn from questions about the relationship between reproductive bodies, biomedical specialization around reproduction, and the making (or not) of new knowledge to questions about whether and how this knowledge is circulating among a broader public. Are reporters covering paternal effects? Do government agencies and professional associations publicize this new knowledge? And do these new developments lead the metaphorical photographer to alter the "images" of men's and women's reproductive bodies?

4 Reproductive Health for Half the Public

Now that biomedical researchers have determined that a man's age, behaviors, and exposures can damage sperm and potentially affect his children's health, the next question is whether any of this information is making its way to the general public. Typically, social scientists have employed a model of knowledge diffusion in which there is a direct line from the mouth (or pages) of science to the broader public. However, the historians Mary Fissell and Roger Cooter have suggested that "circulation" is a more accurate description of this process than "diffusion."[1] Drawing on the empirical example of "natural knowledge" in the eighteenth century, they suggest that rather than a hierarchical, direct transmission from "science" to "society," the circulation of such knowledge through popular and trade publications, personal correspondence and conversations, and even material objects is more akin to the uneven spillage of a runny yolk in an egg cooked sunny-side up.

This memorable metaphor—in which the yolk is "science" and the egg white is "the public"—is useful because rather than assuming that scientific knowledge will inevitably disseminate, it allows for questions about *whether* particular kinds of information are taken up and by which kinds of entities. In this chapter, I examine a number of potential sites where one might expect to find discussions about the science of paternal effects: national newspapers, consumer websites oriented to health and parenting, federal health agencies, and professional medical associations.[2] Generally speaking, this enables a comparison between approaches taken by the news media (newspapers and consumer websites) versus organizations in a position to issue "official statements" about men's reproductive health (federal agencies and professional associations).

Scholars have examined news coverage of paternal effects in two previous studies. Cynthia Daniels searched nine national newspapers from 1985 to 1996 and found just seventeen articles about the relationship between "fathers and fetuses." These reports tended to minimize the potential risks by referring to the uncertainty of the scientific information, even as they portrayed maternal risks as "certain and known."[3] Noting that Daniels's article was published in the late 1990s, Campo-Engelstein and colleagues wondered whether the expansion of the evidence base for paternal effects during the intervening two decades would be reflected in more attention from the news media.[4] They focused specifically on aging, comparing American news articles about women and men from 1978 to 2012 (N = 64). There were far more articles about maternal aging than paternal aging, and reporters were more likely to blame women for preconception harms while offering men "reassurance" by minimizing risks, a finding summed up in the article's title "Bad Moms, Blameless Dads."

In examining news coverage of paternal effects—not only aging but also men's behaviors and toxic exposures—in the *New York Times* over the past fifty years, I found a consistent, albeit low, level of reporting about this aspect of men's reproductive health in the nation's leading newspaper. Moreover, journalists tend to limit their reporting to the potential damage to *sperm*—that is, the effects that a man's age or bodily health can have on sperm count, shape, or motility. Only rarely do they go beyond this to mention the potential effects of men's health on *children*. And such information is routinely laced with humorous allusions to masculinity and statements about scientists' continuing uncertainty in this realm, both of which serve to minimize concerns about paternal risks. Turning to biomedical organizations—namely, federal health agencies and professional medical associations—to see if they too were publicizing new scientific research about how men matter for reproductive outcomes, I found the answer is "not really." This raises a question about why people might encounter such information in the news media but not hear about it from medical organizations charged with improving the public's health.

NEWS MEDIA

New York Times

My first search was designed to enable a broad overview of coverage about men's reproductive health during the past half century, the period of time in which the scientific evidence for paternal effects began to accumulate (see chapter 3) and cultural norms of masculinity and fatherhood shifted to emphasize the significance of men's involvement with their children.[5] I searched the New York Times from 1968 to 2018 for any articles containing the words "sperm* or semen"; the Times is often used in media analyses because it has an outsized influence on the news agenda for other national news outlets as well as local papers. Reading through the headlines, I found that the Times routinely covered issues of male infertility throughout this period, so I focused on the subset of articles that mention paternal effects (even if that specific language was not used): a total of 138 news reports and opinion pieces.[6]

The articles about paternal effects appeared fairly regularly over the past five decades, averaging about three per year (see figure 11).[7] There are two small spikes in coverage, the first in 1977 (N = 10 articles), when the pesticide DBCP was found to be causing male infertility. The second spike, in 1991 (N = 11 articles), involved more heterogeneous topics, including a focus on men's workplace exposures following the Supreme Court's Johnson Controls decision that year, as well as several studies about men's use of drugs or alcohol (see chapter 3). Overall, though, there was a consistently low level of attention to paternal effects in the New York Times, which stands in stark contrast to the rapidly increasing number of scientific articles published on the topic since the 1960s.

To systematically analyze the focus of these news reports, I coded each article based on whether it discussed the effects of men's age, behaviors, and/or exposures only on sperm (such as its count, motility, or morphology) or whether it also discussed the potential risks to children. Figure 11

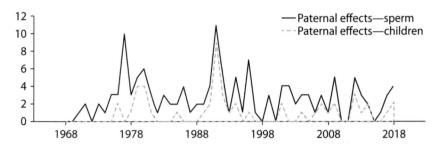

Figure 11. Number of *New York Times* articles discussing paternal effects on sperm versus on children, 1968–2018.

shows that of the 138 articles, a little more than a third specifically mentioned the possibility of risks to children's health.[8]

In terms of the subject matter, there are marked shifts over the fifty-year period. The oldest articles in the sample are from the 1970s and focus on the effects of marijuana and environmental toxins, including DDT, nuclear waste, and Agent Orange. The first article in the sample to mention the possibility that a man's bodily health might have consequences not only for his sperm but also his children appeared in 1976; it is an Associated Press report on a study of vinyl chloride by the National Institute for Occupational Safety and Health. It opens with this sentence: "The wives of men who work with vinyl chloride are twice as likely to have miscarriages or stillbirths, probably because the chemical causes sperm-cell damage in their husbands."[9] In the 1980s and '90s, the most common topic in *New York Times* articles on paternal effects was endocrine-disrupting chemicals, as scientists began to identify and measure the effects of such chemicals on wildlife biology and human reproduction. Other issues covered repeatedly during this time include the harmful effects of steroid use on male fertility and the risks of workplace exposures for men. Occasionally, there were reports of companies looking to profit on such concerns, including a pharmaceutical company marketing a dietary supplement to "improve sperm quality."[10] Starting in the 2000s, as new biomedical research linked the age of older fathers to disease risks for their children, there was a steady drumbeat of articles warning about the consequences of advanced paternal age: schizophrenia, autism, bipolar disorder, and even lower IQ scores.

Some articles contain just a brief reference to paternal effects, as in a spate of reports during the 1990s about the various effects of environmental toxins, one of which was the possibility of "declining sperm counts."[11] In other cases, entire articles or op-eds are devoted to in-depth discussions of how the age or health of men's bodies can affect reproductive outcomes, such as a 1981 article by long-time health reporter Jane Brody titled "Sperm Found Especially Vulnerable to Environment" or a 2012 opinion column by the science editor of the *New Republic* titled "Why Fathers Really Matter."[12] Reflecting the lack of a unified specialty for men's reproductive health, the articles quote a wide variety of experts: epidemiologists, toxicologists, urologists, obstetrician-gynecologists, and endocrinologists. The upshot: the *New York Times* has engaged in a steady level of reporting on paternal effects for decades; such articles are not common, but they are not absent.

Popular Books on Paternal Effects

Next, I looked at news coverage of two books about paternal effects that were written for a popular audience: *The Male Biological Clock* by urologist Harry Fisch published in 2004 and, a decade later, *Do Fathers Matter?* by science journalist Paul Raeburn. Using the Nexis Uni database, I searched major news outlets for two years after each book's publication date, yielding twenty-one news reports about Fisch's book and nineteen about Raeburn's (these figures do not include duplicates—that is, the same article being published in multiple newspapers). While both authors managed to garner national news coverage, the fact that each book was discussed in about twenty reports offers additional evidence that this topic did not gain much more traction in the intervening decade. And like the reports in the *New York Times,* news articles about each book specified paternal effects on *children* in just a fraction of the reports (25 percent).

Consumer Websites

Newspapers are not the only source of news in this day and age, so I also searched consumer websites for discussions of men's reproductive health in general and paternal effects in particular. In March 2015, I visited two leading health websites (WebMD and Mayo Clinic), two leading parenting websites (*Parents,* which is also published as a print magazine, and *What to Expect When You're Expecting,* which is also published as a book), and a website specifically about the health of men (*Men's Health,* which is also published as a print magazine).

These popular websites post articles written for a general audience and represent the kinds of information the public might come across if they were casually searching on the internet. All five sites host pages about male fertility, and some even point out that a man's age, behaviors, and exposures can affect sperm in terms of its count, shape, or motility. These factors are sometimes glossed as "sperm health" or the more eugenic-sounding "sperm quality."[13] For example, the Mayo Clinic's page "Getting Pregnant" includes a discussion of "healthy sperm" and encourages men to "understand how lifestyle factors can affect your sperm and what you can do to improve your fertility."[14] However, unlike the news reports, health and parenting websites almost never go beyond a discussion of sperm to discuss how paternal effects can influence a child's health. There were a few exceptions, and those tended to be about paternal age. In 2006, WebMD published a feature article that was still posted on the website in 2015. The headline read "Men May Have Biological Clocks, Too," and the subhead stated, "Some researchers say a man's age may affect not only his ability to father a child—but the health of his offspring."[15]

GENDER, UNCERTAINTY, AND
THE INDIVIDUALIZATION OF RISK

Reading about paternal effects in these forums, from national newspapers to parenting magazines, I found not only that the news media typically stops with sperm. I also noticed three other trends in my analysis of these materials. First, news reporting on paternal effects is saturated with references to masculinity and gender relations. Second, and in line with previous research, journalists routinely underscore the uncertainty of biomedical claims about paternal effects.[16] And third, news articles often exhibit a default assumption that if there are risks, they should be managed by individuals.

Gender

The persistence of gendered allusions is most clear in the *New York Times* sample. Although the articles span a fifty-year period during which there were enormous social, political, and economic changes, one thing stays the same: reporters' use of gender to frame biomedical debates about men's contributions to reproductive outcomes. Some mobilized gender as a source of humor to introduce the unfamiliar idea of paternal effects, like the joke with which science writer Natalie Angier opened her article: "Heard the one about why it takes 100 million sperm to fertilize an egg? Because none of them will stop to ask for directions."[17] Other reporters and columnists referred to gender in a feminist vein to highlight inequalities, especially in light of the ongoing lack of attention to men in the realm of reproduction. In a co-authored opinion piece titled "Science's Anti-Female Bias," a public health professor and a women's rights activist questioned the then-new warning labels on liquor bottles that were directed only at women:

> Why is the press uninterested in studies showing relationships between chronic drinking in men and abnormal sperm production and testicular atrophy, or behavioral abnormalities that appear in the offspring of male animals fed alcohol?[18]

Likewise, reporter Tamar Lewin pointed to gendered asymmetry in considerations of reproductive hazards. Covering a new study about chemical and electronics companies, she noted that they "restrict women's work options on the ground of potential risk to their reproductive health but most ignored the reproductive hazards faced by men."[19]

Thirteen years later, Lewin broached the topic again in an article about "the fruit of aging loins." The focus of the article was Dolores Malaspina's groundbreaking research, and Lewin wrote that "it may seem puzzling that the correlation [between older fathers and offspring with schizophrenia] was not noticed long ago. But what scientists find depends on what they look for." She underscored the "irony" that a disease once thought to be caused by "bad mothers" may have something to do with men's age.[20] Angier also began an article on paternal aging by pointing to the gendered history of reproductive blame:

When it comes to parceling out blame for birth defects and genetic disorders, women have historically shouldered most of the burden. . . . By contrast, men have been seen as eternally fertile, able to father healthy children well into their dotage.[21]

Even the scientists quoted in news articles sometimes point to gendered cultural biases when discussing their work on paternal effects. For example, Roni Caryn Rabin quotes Malaspina in an article about the relationship between paternal age and children's lower IQ scores: "I think there has been a bit of a cultural bias against even looking at this issue [of paternal age effects], but finally people are willing to entertain this."[22] A decade later, this sentiment was echoed by Shanna Swan, a physician at Mount Sinai, who discussed her research on sperm counts in an article by Nellie Bowles: "The NIH has been focused on males for so long, but reproduction was never considered a male problem." Swan concludes that the research community does not "want to know what they're going to find."[23]

Just as biomedical research on paternal effects may have been spurred by the entry of women into science (see chapter 2), it is probably not a coincidence that many of the news articles about paternal effects have been written by women. As professional women working in a culture where maternal blame remains rampant, female journalists may have been especially intrigued by new research showing the consequences of men's age and bodily health for reproductive outcomes. Indeed, even as men continue to outnumber women in newsrooms,[24] of the thirty-nine bylined articles in the *New York Times* sample that point to the possible effects on *children,* 64 percent were written by women.[25]

On health and parenting websites, both the headlines and the fine print are also suffused with references to masculinity but delivered in more casual, attention-grabbing language. For example, the Mayo Clinic's page on healthy sperm begins with the question "Do your sperm pass muster?" before providing tips "to help your sperm become top performers."[26] Similar sentiments are evoked in the titles of various *Men's Health* articles:

"4 Ways to Make Your Sperm Stronger, Faster, and More Fertile"[27]

"Strengthen Your Sperm in an Hour"[28]

"7 Signs You've Got Healthy Semen"[29]

This language of performance and strength is undergirded by contemporary notions of masculinity associated with the workplace and sports, transposed here onto tiny reproductive cells.

Although consumer websites do use the terms *sperm* or *semen*, they are far more likely than newspapers to employ slang, presumably in an attempt to appeal to a general audience. Sperm become "swimmers" or "boys," and occasionally a man's reproductive system is referred to euphemistically as "your junk." For example, *Men's Health* articles include the lines "Are your swimmers paddling up to par?" and "Too much boozing could put your swimmers in danger."[30] *What to Expect*'s article "Fertility Foods for Women and Men" includes details about how to "keep men's little swimmers healthy."[31]

It is on parenting websites in particular that one finds yet another gendered assumption guiding the reporting: several articles about paternal effects are actually written to women. The *Parents* article "10 Ways He Can Have Better Baby-Making Sperm" is explicitly directed at women with the expectation they will pass the information on to their male partners.[32] The first paragraph advises "To keep his boys in tip-top shape, he should make these changes," which is followed by a bullet-pointed list of specific suggestions, such as "To give his swimmers a boost, your guy should stop smoking." In a *What to Expect* Q&A titled "Folic Acid and Male Fertility," author Heidi Murkoff embeds archaic notions of women as homemakers with advice to "dish your man up a hearty salad" to help "safeguard his boys."[33]

Yet even as reporters routinely make gendered jokes and refer to gendered norms and biases, there is almost no discussion of the intersections of masculinity with race, class, or sexuality. Just a handful of newspaper articles mention these issues, and all do so only briefly, such as an article positing racial differences in sperm count or an op-ed pointing to the potential role of "poverty and powerlessness" in paternal effects.[34] Such references are even more rare on consumer websites.[35]

Uncertainty

Another clear trend in reporting on paternal effects is the emphasis, both by reporters and the experts they are quoting, on the continuing lack of certainty plaguing the field. To some extent, this is a vestige of the traditional approach to any issue in the news, in which the goal of avoiding bias manifests in an attempt to present multiple perspectives. To avoid bias in reports on scientific research, reporters typically identify experts who support whatever finding is being announced as well as experts who question its validity. However, as Daniels found in her analysis of news reports in the 1980s and '90s, it is striking how intensely journalists emphasize how "limited" the research on paternal effects is, particularly in comparison with how maternal effects are discussed.[36]

Certainly, in the early days, the studies of paternal effects were few and far between, so even the scientists themselves would occasionally label their results "speculative," as did one author of a 1991 epidemiological study finding that paternal smoking increased the risk of childhood cancers.[37] Likewise, a report issued by the National Research Council on endocrine-disrupting chemicals was discussed under the headline "Experts Unsure of Effects of a Type of Contaminant" before quoting the chair of the panel as stating, "This field is rife with uncertainty."[38] On very rare occasions, scientists did make the point that even if research is sparse or inconclusive, it does not mean that paternal effects are not real. Devra Lee Davis, a leading environmental epidemiologist, penned an op-ed in 1991 following the *Johnson Controls* decision noting, "The absence of research detailing how the exposure of fathers affects their future babies does not mean that no such effects occur."[39]

But as time went on and the studies began to stack up, reporters would still find experts who questioned the magnitude of such effects and wondered whether the risks were really worth mentioning, given that they might "worry" men or even cause them to "panic." In one recent article, a physician expressed concern that his research on sperm counts would cause "male hysteria,"[40] an old-fashioned term that usually refers to *women's* out-of-control emotions being rooted in their reproductive tracts—in their "wandering wombs."[41] The fusion of gender and uncertainty evident in this quote is possibly a result of the perceived feminization of men that occurs when their reproductivity is both probed and questioned.

Indeed, such dynamics are brought to the surface in another article about sperm counts and male panic that made the headlines as I was drafting this chapter. Written by Nellie Bowles, the *New York Times* article reported on a scientific meta-analysis (a systematic review of a large number of research studies) under the headline "Men Are Freaking Out about Their Low Sperm Counts." The next day, the same article was retitled "Manosphere in a Panic: Are Your Swimmers in Peril?"[42] True to form, the article did point to some "skeptical" experts, but it also quoted a leading men's health physician who hoped to turn "sperm panic" into a "tool for preventive public health." Bowles also spoke to a number of men's rights activists who participate in what they call the "manosphere." They articulated concerns about how "modern society was weakening men," an echo of debates at the end of the nineteenth century (see chapter 1).

The intertwined themes of gender, uncertainty, and panic are particularly evident in media reports focused on paternal aging. Now fairly well-documented, the potential reproductive significance of a father's age raised eyebrows when it began getting more attention in the early 2000s. For example, one of Malaspina's early studies about the relationship between paternal age and schizophrenia was discussed in a *New York Times* article that labeled other scientists as "skeptical."[43] Just a few years later, the urologist Harry Fisch published his book on the male biological clock, harnessing a temporal metaphor that had long been associated with women's bodies.[44] For his efforts, he was thoroughly denounced in newspapers around the country. A New York *Newsday* article labeled the book "provocative" and described it as flying "in the face of social convention and scientific consensus." It quoted Larry Lipshultz, past president of the American Society for Reproductive Medicine (ASRM), describing the book as "dangerous" because it raises "red flags that aren't warranted." Moreover, Lipshultz was concerned the book would result in "a lot of very anxious guys running to the doctor" based on "information that is totally untrue."[45] Likewise, a *USA Today* article cited general "others" who called Fisch "an alarmist relying on sketchy research" before quoting the current president of ASRM as reassuringly stating that "plenty of men have children later in life."[46]

Indeed, just as Campo-Engelstein and colleagues found that articles on paternal aging were twice as likely to involve "reassurance" as articles on maternal aging, there are numerous examples of reporters and scientists seeking to assuage men's potential worries.[47] This often takes the form of lists of famous "old dads"—such as the singer Paul McCartney, the actor Michael Douglas, the comedian Dave Letterman, and the writer Saul

Bellow—to underscore the point that men can father healthy children later in life.[48] Likewise, scientists downplay even some of the more dire findings on paternal age, as in the front-page *New York Times* article about the Kong study in *Nature*, which found an association between new mutations in aging sperm and the development of autism and schizophrenia in offspring.[49] It concludes with a quote from a genomicist at the University of Washington: "You have to understand that the vast majority of these mutations have no consequences, and there are tons of guys in their 50s who have healthy children."[50] Some reporters even took pains to elaborate the *advantages* of older fatherhood, noting that men with more life experience might be better able to handle the pressures of raising small children, not to mention the extra time they had to attain career success and financial stability.[51]

The accumulating research on paternal age has led some reporters to hypothesize a shift in the "gender conversation," as when Lisa Belkin wondered whether the new biomedical findings might usher in a different world in which men too would begin to think about the timing of parenthood.[52] Others are not so convinced: Charles McGrath's meditation on the possibility of panic about paternal age argues that men are actually "inclined" to "take things easy" and perhaps women should draw some "inspiration" from them.[53] But in effect, suggestions that men should take it easy and not worry too much serve to downplay the risk and minimize the potential significance of paternal effects. Paul Raeburn, the prominent science journalist and author of *Do Fathers Matter?*, which includes several chapters on paternal effects, challenged just this mentality. In a detailed analysis of news reports about studies showing an increased risk of bipolar disorder and attention deficit disorder among children of older fathers, Raeburn wonders why reporters at the Associated Press and the *New York Times* buried the risk percentages in their articles. He writes, "The numbers are far higher than what's been found in other studies, and they should be prominently featured near the top of every story."[54]

Individualization of Risk

Even as the media underscore the uncertainty associated with research on paternal effects, reporters routinely offer advice about what men might do in light of the *potential* risk. Just as in articles about women's reproductive health, news reports and consumer websites offer infographics and listicles to encourage men to eat different food, exercise more, stop smoking, avoid drugs, and steer clear of chemicals. There is quite a lot of variation in which bits of advice are included, but almost all of it exhibits an implicit assumption that men have all the time and money in the world to modify their lives. For example, when *Men's Health* advises "guys" to eat more beef and hit the gym,[55] there is no discussion of the resources necessary to enact such advice.

Moreover, nearly all the suggestions focus on individual actions and not on structural or environmental contributors to paternal effects. For example, governments and other institutions can reduce health risks for the entire population; the EPA could work to ensure that the air and water is clean, and OSHA could systematically evaluate and ban harmful chemicals at work.[56] Even when it comes to health behaviors, which are typically perceived as individual-level choices, regulatory and organizational efforts can have quite an impact. As just two examples, they can enable access to affordable, healthy foods and make possible widespread usage of programs to treat addiction. These kinds of structural approaches have been adopted when it comes to women's reproductive bodies, such as the 1998 federal requirement adding folic acid to commonly consumed grain products (e.g., cereal, bread, pasta) in an effort to reduce the risk of certain birth disorders. And the 2010 Affordable Care Act included coverage for women's preconception health appointments; it did not cover such appointments for men.

But of the hundreds of news reports I reviewed, only a tiny fraction referred to the notion that institutional and organizational approaches to paternal effects might even be possible. This is not unrelated to the theme of uncertainty: if the data on paternal effects were deemed more certain, then the responsibility of health officials and government agencies to act would be more clearly defined. So the repeated insistence on uncertainty contributes to the devolving of responsibility to the individual. Put another way, since biomedical researchers cannot be entirely sure of the type and magnitude of various paternal effects, men are left to figure out for themselves what, if any, actions they should take.

OFFICIAL STATEMENTS

Pivoting from the news media to federal health agencies and professional medical associations, I examine whether they too are working to bring scientific research on paternal effects to a broader audience. Are they posting official statements on their websites about how a man's age, behaviors, and exposures can damage sperm and affect his children's health? Do they generate patient-friendly fact sheets in accessible language? The answer is usually no. Governmental and professional organizations, whether oriented generally to issues of health and medicine or specifically to the topic of reproductive health, devote relatively little attention to paternal effects.

Federal Agencies

The primary federal agency responsible for medical research in the United States, the National Institutes of Health, has a budget exceeding $30 billion and an entire department—an "office" in NIH lingo—oriented to research on women's health. This is a legacy of the important efforts made by feminist health activists to ensure that women be included in biomedical research and clinical trials.[57] Yet, contemporary scientists and clinicians lament the ongoing lack of funding for research on men's reproductive health, especially when compared to the high levels of funding for women's reproductive health.[58] And it is not just the NIH. Sarah Vij, a physician specializing in male infertility at the Cleveland Clinic, recently noted in the *New York Times*, "There's no funding. . . . There just are not a lot of foundations out there looking to fund male fertility projects."[59]

The lack of funding is matched by a lack of official information posted on the NIH website. Searching "men's health" on the homepage will bring the reader to particular pages on aging or specific diseases, but there are only a few pages on the topic of "men's reproductive health." They are further subdivided into just three research areas: "contraception, avoiding sexually transmitted diseases, and infertility/fertility."[60] For the latter, the NIH lists a number of potential "conditions" that can affect the count or shape of sperm, including chromosomal anomalies, diseases such as diabetes or thyroid problems, and exposures to medications or radiation.[61]

But nowhere in any of these pages is there any mention of how those factors can pose a risk not only to sperm but also to a man's children. Even the article "Aging Changes in the Male Reproductive System" posted on the NIH's National Library of Medicine site focuses only on changes in sperm production and erectile dysfunction, with no mention that advanced paternal age has been linked to an increased risk of several diseases in offspring.[62] Instead the article includes the reassuring sentence: "Some fairly old men can (and do) father children."

Likewise, the Centers for Disease Control and Prevention, the government agency charged with "saving lives and protecting people" according to the tag line on its website, posts extensive information on infertility, most of which is focused on women's bodies and health.[63] In the subsection devoted to men's infertility, it does mention that medical conditions, "unhealthy habits," and environmental toxins can affect the number, shape, and movement of sperm. But it too does not go further to say anything about how such factors can also affect children's health.

The CDC does have a landing page for the topic of men's reproductive health that includes a list of subjects men can click for more information, from broad categories such as sexual health or contraception to more specific issues like bicycle saddles and reproductive health.[64] It is here that men will find a link to a document titled "Preconception Health for Men." An unwieldy phrase that is not part of the popular lexicon, "preconception health and health care" refers to a CDC initiative to improve reproductive outcomes by encouraging people to adopt healthy habits prior to becoming pregnant.[65] However, the bulk of the initiative's efforts have been directed at women, such as a 2013 public health campaign called "Show Your Love" that Miranda Waggoner analyzes in her book *The Zero Trimester*. So perhaps it is not a surprise that to create a page on men's preconception health, the CDC simply copied its advice for women and changed the pronouns (see figure 12). While one might reasonably expect this to be a site that addresses directly the possible paternal risks to children's health, the reader will find only general advice for men about the individual-level actions they can take to prepare for becoming a parent. There are bullet points about the effects of "toxic substances" and other things that can "change" sperm—diseases, pharmaceuticals, age, and so on—but these admonishments do not go beyond sperm to highlight paternal effects on children.

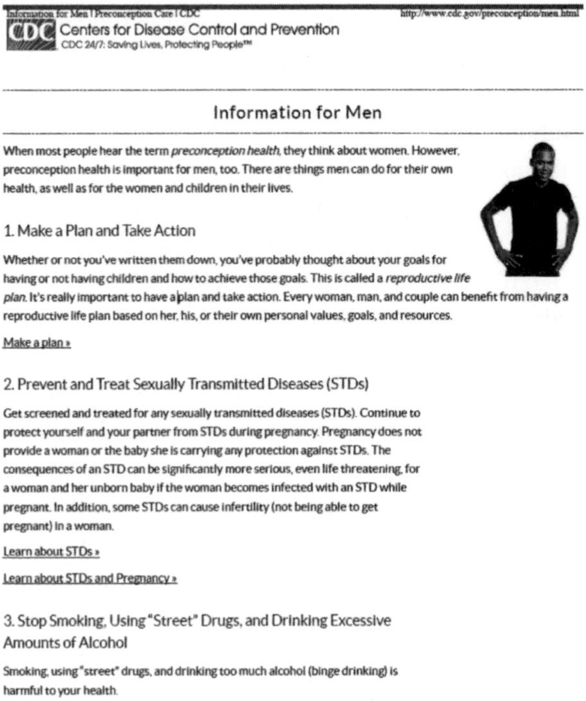

Information for Men | Preconception Care | CDC http://www.cdc.gov/preconception/men.html

CDC Centers for Disease Control and Prevention
CDC 24/7: Saving Lives, Protecting People™

Information for Men

When most people hear the term *preconception health*, they think about women. However, preconception health is important for men, too. There are things men can do for their own health, as well as for the women and children in their lives.

1. Make a Plan and Take Action

Whether or not you've written them down, you've probably thought about your goals for having or not having children and how to achieve those goals. This is called a *reproductive life plan*. It's really important to have a plan and take action. Every woman, man, and couple can benefit from having a reproductive life plan based on her, his, or their own personal values, goals, and resources.

Make a plan »

2. Prevent and Treat Sexually Transmitted Diseases (STDs)

Get screened and treated for any sexually transmitted diseases (STDs). Continue to protect yourself and your partner from STDs during pregnancy. Pregnancy does not provide a woman or the baby she is carrying any protection against STDs. The consequences of an STD can be significantly more serious, even life threatening, for a woman and her unborn baby if the woman becomes infected with an STD while pregnant. In addition, some STDs can cause infertility (not being able to get pregnant) in a woman.

Learn about STDs »

Learn about STDs and Pregnancy »

3. Stop Smoking, Using "Street" Drugs, and Drinking Excessive Amounts of Alcohol

Smoking, using "street" drugs, and drinking too much alcohol (binge drinking) is harmful to your health.

Figure 12. Screenshot of CDC website on men's preconception health, 2015.

In 2010, a few years after the launch of the preconception health initiative, the CDC did convene its first-ever meeting about men's reproductive health. It began as a brown-bag lunch, but as more scientists and clinicians heard about it, it quickly grew to a day-long event with over one hundred presenters and attendees, many of whom financed their own travel.[66] Even though there were several talks by researchers who had published on paternal effects, such as Dolores Lamb, the forty-two-page report summarizing the day's activities includes just *one* mention of the subject. Stanton Honig, a urologist, reviews research about how men's use of steroids, tobacco, alcohol, and cocaine can affect the production of sperm and its shape but does not discuss the potential effects on children's health.[67] Most of the rest of the report discusses the usual topics of contraception, STIs, and infertility.

There are other federal agencies one might expect to issue official statements about paternal effects. Perhaps the Environmental Protection Agency (EPA) warns men about the dangers of environmental exposures? No. Perhaps the Occupational Safety and Health Administration (OSHA) warns men about the potential effects of chemicals in the workplace? Yes! In a fact sheet titled "Reproductive Hazards" dated more than two decades ago, OSHA includes a warning that substances at work "may affect the reproductive health of women or men or the ability of couples to have healthy children."[68] The reference to "healthy children" marks this site as one of the only places in all the federal agencies to draw a direct link between a man's exposures and the health of his children.[69]

Yet, even as OSHA points to the potential reproductive consequences of chemical exposures, it stresses the profound lack of data about what precisely these risks might entail. Here, though, the agency is not referring to uncertainty to minimize the risk. Quite the opposite. That same fact sheet goes on to cite the preamble of the National Occupational Research Agenda Statement on Reproductive Hazards, which notes that of the millions of chemicals in commercial use, only a fraction have been tested.

> Physical and biological agents in the workplace that may affect fertility and pregnancy outcomes are *practically unstudied*. The inadequacy of current knowledge coupled with the ever-growing variety of workplace exposures *pose a potentially serious public health problem*.[70]

Not only is OSHA one of the only federal websites to mention paternal effects on children, it is one of the few to take seriously the risks. In stark contrast, the Department of Defense (DoD) website posts various press releases from the 1990s discounting the potential effects of chemical exposures on the battlefield, such as Agent Orange during the Vietnam War and the toxic stew faced by soldiers fighting in the Gulf War. The DoD statements emphasize the lack of "concrete evidence" linking such exposures to pregnancy outcomes, even as research continues.[71]

Professional Organizations

The websites of professional medical associations reveal a similar story: they post almost no information about paternal effects. Searching the

American Medical Association's website for "sperm" or "men's reproductive health" produces zero results about paternal effects. There is an "Atlas of the Human Body," but it lists only the "female reproductive system" and not the "male reproductive system."

Perhaps organizations representing specialists in reproduction, such as the American College of Obstetrics and Gynecology (ACOG) or the American Society for Reproductive Medicine (ASRM), have posted resources about paternal effects? No. On both sites, information is limited to male infertility and occasional references to "sperm quality," defined as count, motility, and morphology.[72] ACOG's "Preconception Care Guide" discusses only women's bodies, and while it does publish a "Father's Guide to Pregnancy," it contains no references to paternal effects.[73] In all of the many pages on ACOG's and ASRM's websites, the only direct mention of possible effects from men's age, behaviors, or exposures on children is in ASRM's short statement on alcohol and drug use.[74] Here it is in its entirety:

> Drugs such as steroids, cigarettes, marijuana, and alcohol can negatively impact your health in many ways, including greatly affecting testicular function, leading to abnormally shaped sperm, decreased sperm motility and/or decreased sperm production and they have well-documented effects on the developing fetus.

Yet, even here, ASRM does not specify exactly what the effects on the fetus are or how they might affect offspring even into adulthood.

Searching through the websites of many other professional medical organizations, I reviewed hundreds of pages of materials only to demonstrate a lack, a profound absence of material on men's reproductive health in general and paternal effects in particular. The American College of Medical Genetics has nothing on men's reproductive health. The American Academy of Family Physicians (AAFP) and the American Urological Association (AUA) each have a few pages on male infertility but no mention of paternal effects. There is a Society for the Study of Male Reproduction that holds meetings alongside the AUA, and a separate Society for Male Reproduction and Urology that is affiliated with ASRM, but both focus on male infertility. As for international medical organizations, such as the World Health Organization, there are occasional mentions of the damage that can be wrought by chemicals at work and in the environment.[75] But typically when the topic of men is raised during discussions of reproductive health, these organizations are working to position "men as partners" who will be supportive of the women in their lives, with the ultimate goals of fostering gender equity and reducing intimate partner violence.[76] In these documents, there is no mention of men's own age and bodily health and how they might affect reproductive outcomes.

·   ·   ·   ·   ·

Cataloguing the paucity of materials produced by federal agencies and professional organizations suggests yet another legacy of how medical specialization around reproduction has unfolded over the past century: with no unified, cohesive specialty oriented to men's reproductive health, there is little formal infrastructure in place to publicize new knowledge about paternal effects. Of those sites that do have pages on men's reproductive health, many of the materials have not been updated in years, even as biomedical researchers have published major studies about the potential reproductive significance of men's age, behaviors, and exposures.

THE EXCEPTION TO THE RULE: A NATIONAL PUBLIC HEALTH CAMPAIGN ON PATERNAL EFFECTS

Even as government agencies and professional associations largely ignored the issue of paternal effects, there was one nonprofit organization that did spotlight—albeit briefly—the risks associated with men's age and bodily health: the March of Dimes. Founded in 1938 by President Franklin Delano Roosevelt to eradicate polio, today it is best known for working to promote healthy pregnancies. Its efforts are largely focused on women's reproductive health; their current slogan is "Healthy Moms. Strong Babies." Yet, for a short time in the early 1990s, the March of Dimes ran a national public health campaign called "Men Have Babies Too." It included television ads, radio spots, and a brochure with detailed information about how the "father factor" can lead to miscarriages and affect a baby's health (see figure 13).

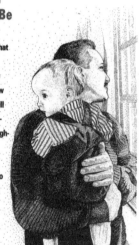

March of Dimes

Men Have Babies Too

A Guide for Fathers-to-Be

Dad, did you know that your diet, habits, lifestyle and attitude can play a part in how healthy your baby will be? Even before conception and all throughout pregnancy, an expectant father can take positive steps to help his partner have a healthy baby.

Figure 13. March of Dimes brochure for Men Have Babies Too campaign, 1993.

To find out how the March of Dimes came to develop what I believe to be the only public health campaign in the United States ever to focus on paternal effects, I drove an hour down Highway 95 to visit their meticulously kept archives in White Plains, New York. Leafing through the internal files related to media relations, I learned that the Men Have Babies Too campaign actually originated with the Greater New York chapter in the late 1980s. That chapter's director, Jennifer Howse, would go on to

The Father Factor

Every year in America, approximately 560,000 infant deaths, miscarriages and stillbirths occur. Among couples who want to have a child, an estimated 2.3 million (or 7.9 percent) find out they are infertile. About 150,000 infants are born with birth defects annually; in 60 to 70 percent of these cases, the cause is unknown.

Many people think that a man's contribution to making babies begins and ends at the moment of conception, but today there is a growing body of scientific evidence that suggests fathers have a larger impact on the reproductive process and on the health of their unborn babies.

In fact, the father's influence on the unborn baby may begin long before conception. Scientists used to think that infertility, miscarriage or genetic damage to the fetus might occur only if the *mother* smoked cigarettes, drank alcohol, took non-prescribed drugs before or during pregnancy, or if she was exposed to toxic chemicals in the environment or workplace. But some researchers now suspect reproduction and fetal development may be affected also, if a biological *father* has been exposed to any of these lifestyle or occupational hazards. And during a mother's pregnancy, the father's lifestyle and emotional support of his partner can affect her behavior and even her level of psychological stress – some experts believe maternal stress may influence the baby's health.

No More "Macho" Sperm

Scientists used to believe that if sperm were damaged they could not fertilize an egg; therefore, only the "fittest" sperm would carry on the species – some call this the "macho sperm" theory. Research now shows sperm are vulnerable and that even when damaged, they may still fertilize an egg. Some toxins may alter the sperm's chromosomes, which carry genetic information. If this happens, the results may range from infertility and miscarriage to stillbirth, birth defects, learning disabilities and even childhood leukemia and kidney cancer.

Throughout this brochure, when we say that a substance is "suspected" to influence or "may cause" a certain problem, we mean some studies show harmful effects, but more research is needed to substantiate the findings. Yet there is enough evidence to warrant concern now. The National Institute for Occupational Safety and Health (NIOSH) states: "There is no biological basis for assuming that either the embryo/fetus or the female is more susceptible [to toxic damage] than the male."

It is therefore wise for expectant fathers and men thinking about fatherhood to change unhealthy lifestyle habits and, when possible, protect themselves from toxins in the environment and workplace. Sperm develop over a three-month period; even if a man quits smoking, drinking, using drugs or if he removes himself from other toxins, some experts advise waiting three months before trying to conceive a child.

With the above in mind, this brochure answers some important questions that expectant fathers ask, and offers guidelines on how men can contribute to a healthy birth.

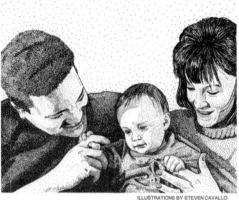

ILLUSTRATIONS BY STEVEN CAVALLO

serve as the president of the March of Dimes from 1990 to 2016. In an interview, she described to me how the New York chapter decided "men's reproductive health would be one of our priority areas":

> There was science emerging in the mid to late '80s on the quality of sperm and its relationship to pregnancy outcomes. We had a scientific advisory group, and we would ask them, "What's new, what's breaking?" And it was

in a meeting where somebody said, "There's emerging data on the quality of sperm that we should really be paying attention to." Interest was sparked, and more research was done. At some point, the weight of the evidence was there. We were sitting in a room, talking about what's the simplest message you can boil all this down to. We had this discussion: it's not all on women. Someone from the staff said, "Men have babies too." Men need to think actively that they're having the baby too, and that's where it came from.[77]

Following her transition to the presidency of the March of Dimes in 1990, Howse took part in the New York chapter's Male Role Press Conference in December 1991 alongside the president of ACOG and Frank Gifford, a celebrity sports commentator. After playing two new public service announcements designed to air as television commercials, they encouraged the assembled reporters to write stories about the possibility of what they called "paternally transmitted birth defects." Labeling the campaign's focus on men as "unprecedented," the assembled officials expressed pride at being "the first health organization to launch a comprehensive program to educate the public about the important role men must play in ensuring the health of their children."[78]

Just a few days later, the national March of Dimes hosted a related editorial luncheon at the Lincoln Center in New York City. Titled "Real Men Do Get Pregnant: The Father's Role in Creating a Healthy Pregnancy," it was moderated by CBS News health reporter Dr. Robert Arnot and featured scientists studying paternal effects. Staff at the March of Dimes tracked media coverage from both of these events, clipping numerous articles in newspapers and magazines, including Jane Brody's "Personal Health" column in the *New York Times* on Christmas Day, 1991, which was reprinted in local papers all over the country.

With public service announcements running locally for much of 1992, the Greater New York chapter of the March of Dimes received hundreds of calls and quickly decided to develop a new brochure it could distribute.[79] The national office had been printing a single-panel brochure titled "Dad, It's Your Baby Too" for at least a decade, but it focused on how men could "support" their partner during pregnancy and did not include any information about paternal effects.[80] As is clear in figure 13, the Greater New York chapter used a similar title—"Men Have Babies Too"—but expanded the brochure to five panels with markedly different content. Showing several heterosexual couples, some with an infant, the text invokes norms of masculinity to argue against the notion of "macho sperm," and it signals the importance of individual behaviors when asking men whether they are aware their "diet, habits, lifestyle and attitude can play a part in how healthy your baby will be." Quantifying the number of miscarriages, infant deaths, and birth defects in the United States, it then states:

> Many people think that a man's contribution to making babies begins and ends at conception, but today there is a growing body of scientific evidence that suggests fathers have a larger impact on the reproductive process and on the health of their unborn babies.

While the brochure notes that some of the findings are uncertain and "more research is needed," it specifically mentions the potential risks to children from paternal smoking and drug use, as well as men's exposures to hazardous chemicals at home and work.

To announce the new brochure, the Greater New York chapter issued a press release and mailed copies to media outlets in time for Father's Day 1992.[81] The Men Have Babies Too campaign was such a success that the national office decided to take it countrywide the following year. Again pinning the launch to Father's Day, the national March of Dimes staff spent the first part of the year developing press materials and encouraging all its local chapters to take part in the new campaign by hosting events, submitting op-eds, and contacting their local media to run public service announcements on television and radio. One local chapter partnered with a tie shop while another worked with tire stores to stock the Men Have Babies Too brochures. For its part, the national office's media relations team issued a press release and personally followed up with reporters from dozens of national newspapers and magazines, including those focused on health and parenting as well as what they called "male-oriented magazines" such as *Sports Illustrated* and *Playboy*.[82] Staffers would occasionally use the shorthand "male responsibility PSA" in their memos to each other as they worked to develop the campaign and assiduously track the media coverage and chapter activities.[83] In recalling the reactions to the campaign at the time, Howse remembers there being "a lot of enthusiasm for this particular message among March of Dimes volunteers around the country" and "a pretty good media uptake" because "men had not really been given the information they needed to make the best choices about parenthood."[84]

Even with all this activity, the Men Have Babies Too campaign was miniscule compared to the effort and resources put into March of Dimes' campaigns about women's reproductive health before and after, such as the Campaign for Healthier Babies (launched in 1989) and the National Folic Acid Campaign (launched in 1998).[85] The national office did start a new campaign on pre-pregnancy health in 1995 called "Think Ahead: Is There a Baby in Your Future?" However, internal memos and campaign materials, including a videocassette and accompanying booklet, make it clear that women's preconception health is the primary focus.[86] In the forty-six-page booklet, there are just two pages about men's preconception health, and the information about paternal effects is much less detailed than it was in the original Men Have Babies Too brochure. The March of Dimes did continue to print a brochure with that title until the mid-2000s, but it toned down the focus on paternal effects. Their newest brochure for men, "Becoming a Dad," contains no mention of paternal effects at all.

So while the Men Have Babies Too campaign from the early 1990s does represent one instance in which a national medical organization worked to publicize how men matter for reproductive outcomes, it was the exception that proves the rule. And it offers further evidence of just how difficult it is to institutionalize a mechanism for circulating information about men's reproductive health to the public. Even as there was a moment that a storied nonprofit dedicated to promoting infant health did spotlight men, both the institution and its public education materials quickly returned the primary focus to women and reproductive health.

CIRCULATING MESSAGES ABOUT MEN'S REPRODUCTIVE HEALTH

Surveying the landscape of messages about men's reproductive health, it is not uncommon for the general public to encounter discussions of male fertility. But such messages are almost always limited to sperm—its count, its shape, its motility—while the potential ramifications of paternal age, behaviors, and exposures for children's health are rarely acknowledged. So even as consumer websites or federal health officials use the language of "sperm health" or "sperm quality," the way these phrases are deployed makes it appear to be "just" a matter of fertility and not longer-term effects on the next generation.

As chapter 3 makes clear, questions about those longer-term effects have been posed since the beginning of the last century, and the evidence base has grown enormously in the past few decades. Yet, the topic of paternal effects barely registers on the radar screen of public health priorities; it is only mentioned in the margins by governmental agencies, professional associations, and websites devoted to health and parenting. The surprising finding that the national news media has been covering paternal effects on a consistent basis for the past half century reveals it is not impossible for this kind of knowledge to circulate beyond the small community of scientists producing it. And it leads one to wonder why these messages are found primarily in news reports and not in official statements. The very presence of such messages in newspapers makes it clear that the answer to this question has nothing to do with the information itself.

Instead, the lack of attention to paternal effects in governmental and professional websites can be explained by the argument I have been developing thus far in the book: just as there has been little biomedical infrastructure for producing new knowledge about men's reproductive health, there has been little biomedical infrastructure for publicizing that knowledge once it is produced. It is left to individual reporters (often women) reading individual articles written by individual scientists (often women) to generate discussion about how men matter for reproductive outcomes. The result is that new knowledge about paternal effects rarely makes its way to a broader public, and the feedback loop linking women's bodies and reproduction continues almost wholly unimpeded, loop upon loop.

In the remaining chapters of the book, I turn from questions about the production and circulation of biomedical knowledge to its reception. Drawing on a series of interviews with individual men and women from the general public, I begin with a broad analysis of how they conceptualize a man's role in reproduction before turning to specific questions about paternal effects. Have they encountered some of these messages? If not, how do they react to learning for the first time that a man's age, behaviors, and exposures can affect his children's health?

PART III　Men's Views of Reproduction

5 Sex, Sperm, and Fatherhood

There are no medical specialties devoted solely to men's reproductive health, the researchers who study it are few and far between, the media rarely run stories, and health officials hardly mention it. Given these gaps in the production and circulation of biomedical knowledge about men's reproductive bodies, this lack of attention, how does the general public think about a man's involvement in reproduction? To what extent do biological and social processes factor into their definitions of how men matter for reproduction?

Social scientists have conducted a fair amount of research on fathers and fatherhood, but they are usually interested in questions about men's relationships with children once they are born, such as whether and how fathers care for their children and their willingness (and ability) to offer financial support if they live elsewhere.[1] Historians point to significant shifts in these kinds of expectations during the latter part of the twentieth century, as changing beliefs around gender led to new norms for fathers becoming much more involved with their children.[2] However, there is little research about how men think about the process through which they become fathers—namely, reproduction. Certainly, demographers and others survey men about particular reproductive topics, such as their contraceptive use or experiences with infertility, but I could find no previous study that asked men broad, open-ended questions about how they understand their involvement in reproduction.[3]

As one of the first qualitative inquiries into this topic, I sought to recruit interviewees from a wide range of backgrounds. I wanted to find men in the general population who were not drawn solely from medical offices or sites of reproductive significance, such as fertility clinics or sperm banks, where the issue of men's involvement in reproduction is unusually foregrounded. I posted flyers around a small Northeastern city and in online forums (such as Craigslist and local Facebook pages) that indicated the study's focus was on men's life experiences; the ads said nothing about reproduction or fatherhood because I did not want respondents who were particularly interested in those topics. To maximize variation in men's backgrounds, I screened potential respondents based on their age, race/ethnicity, educational level, occupation, and whether they were fathers.

In the end, I interviewed a total of forty men ranging in age from eighteen to forty-nine. About half were fathers, and one was a grandfather. Half were of lower socioeconomic status (SES), a category that included homeless men and the unemployed, as well as those eking out an existence with meager pay from low-wage jobs, such as a forklift driver and hotel janitor. The other half had higher SES, including college students, middle-class suburbanites, and an international businessman. Twenty-one men identified as White, eleven as Black or African American, five as Asian, and three as Hispanic or Latino. Nine identified as either gay or as "men who have sex with men" (MSM). See table A for the respondents' demographic characteristics.[4] (I discuss my interviews with women later in this chapter. More details about the interviews and respondents can be found in the appendices.)

After spending about twenty minutes talking with each man about his past, including childhood experiences, work history, and family life, I asked a series of questions to elicit his views about reproduction in general and sperm in particular. Given that so much research has focused on the social aspects of fatherhood, such as breadwinning and caregiving, I was especially interested in how biological processes might figure into men's narratives about reproduction. As a result, rather than ask general questions about "having children" or "fathering," I decided to use the biologically tinged word *reproduction* in asking each man, "How would you

Table A Demographic characteristics of interviewees

	Men n = 40	Women n = 15
Age	Mean: 34	Mean: 31
	(18–49)	(21–39)
Race/Ethnicity		
White	53%	53%
Black/AfAm	28%	27%
Latinx	8%	13%
Asian	13%	7%
Education		
High school or less	28%	20%
Some college	25%	40%
College degree	25%	27%
Graduate degree	23%	13%
Occupation		
High-wage job	30%	20%
Low-wage job	28%	33%
Unemployed	25%	33%
Student	18%	13%
Socioeconomic Status		
Lower	45%	47%
Higher	55%	53%
In a Relationship	48%	40%
Parent	43%	53%
Gay/MSM	23%	7%

NOTE: *Totals may be more than 100% due to rounding error.*

describe a man's role in reproduction?"[5] Almost all responded by discussing the importance of providing both financially and emotionally for their
families, which are well-established cultural norms, but I was surprised
when many also defined a man's involvement as having sex and providing
sperm. In analyzing men's descriptions of sex, sperm, and fatherhood in
this chapter, I keep a close eye on when and how they root their claims in
biology. I conclude by discussing how these kinds of biological stories can

be enormously consequential, not only for how individuals think about their bodies but for gender politics more broadly.

DEFINING A MAN'S ROLE IN REPRODUCTION

As I prepared to interview men about reproduction, I was in the unusual position of having almost no idea what they would say. My uncertainty was a direct result of the lack of biomedical and social scientific attention to this topic, and it also affected the men I interviewed. When asked how they would describe a man's role in reproduction, men would often pause as they thought through how to respond to the question. Nathan, a thirty-one-year-old, unemployed high school graduate, was among the most flummoxed:

> A man's role in reproduction? [*pause*] Wow. [*pause*] A man's role. [*pause*] I never thought about that before. [*pause*] Really, I don't think it would be too much different from a woman's role. [*pause*] A man's role. What would my role be? [*long pause*] I guess [*long pause*]. Can you rephrase the question?

Here, I take pauses as a form of data, a gap in speech indicating the lack of a readily available cultural script for a question one has never before considered. For some men, like Nathan, the pauses arise because they are truly at a loss for how to even begin describing a man's role in reproduction.[6]

For others, though, the pauses result from uncertainty about what I mean by the term *reproduction*, and men would often laugh as they tried to clarify whether I meant the "obvious" or something more general about having children. For example, Neeraj, a forty-five-year-old Indian American who had just been released from prison after serving more than twenty years for murder, replied by asking, "I assume you mean more than the [*laughs*] simplest biological act?" Likewise, Bobby, a thirty-five-year-old Italian American and father of three who works at a nonprofit organization, chuckled and said,

> Well, I mean, I guess that [*pause*] because you phrased it as reproduction, I think of that as meaning the biological, sexual aspect of it. And so my answer is kind of skewed towards that biological, sexual answer, where, you know, in the classic textbook sense, the male provides a sperm, and a female provides an egg, and so on and so on.

Like Neeraj and Bobby, about two-thirds of the men I interviewed began their answers to my question by talking about what they called the "biological" or "physical" aspects of a man's involvement in reproduction. But most did not stop there, quickly referring to sex or sperm before elaborating on the significance of a man's role as "provider." In contrast to the pauses and chuckles that marked their initial reactions, there was no hesitation in defining what it means to be a good father. Gary, a forty-one-year-old African American forklift driver who lives in a hotel room with his girlfriend and four of their seven children, first confirmed that I meant "reproduction as in bringing forth life" before stating:

> I think he should be the provider. I think he should be the caretaker of the mother *and* the new life that they're bringing in. The supporter. I think he should be everything that a woman and a baby need to make sure that the baby is safe, safeguarded. I think that's what a man should do. I mean, I'm following my own principles, but I think that's what every man needs to do in order to secure their family.

Even as some men described their own fathers as absent or narrated difficulties "being there" or providing financially for their own children,[7] nearly every single man voiced a similarly idealized vision of contemporary fatherhood at some point in the interview.

While actions such as emotional caretaking and protective safeguarding do appear in many men's definitions of being a provider, the core element of this role is the provision of money. Deshawn is a thirty-two-year-old high school graduate with a seven-year-old son. He occasionally works as a security guard at a nightclub but has long been looking for more stable employment. Reflecting the cultural norm of men as breadwinners,[8] Deshawn explains:

> As a father, you got to have finances to follow suit. If you are going to reproduce, that's just my belief. You know, the baby is going to need somewhere to rest his head, going to need Pampers, a lot of Enfamil, going to need clothes and all of that.[9]

Men who fail to fulfill their responsibilities as providers, especially those who have children and leave, are subject to criticism. In a technological update to the old phrase "deadbeat dad," several interviewees referred to these men as "sperm donors." They had contributed cells to the creation of a child but did not truly "father" those children.

The idealized image of father as provider is so powerful that it crosses lines not only of race, class, and nationality but also sexuality. Tom, a thirty-three-year-old gay man who had contemplated hiring a surrogate to have a child with his new husband, answered my question in a way that was very similar to the straight men I interviewed.

> TOM: Um [*pause*]. What do you mean in terms of reproduction? [*laughs*] Obviously—
>
> RENE: What comes to mind?
>
> TOM: Obviously, there's the standard of they have sex and impregnate a woman, but I mean I think there's more than that. I think a guy should be there for the woman while she's pregnant and the child is growing. A man should be there to help and support. The father should be there to support the mother while she's pregnant, helping her do whatever she needs to do so it doesn't put stress on her or the baby. But I think the role is bigger than just having sex to make a child.

Tom's description of a man's involvement in reproduction reflects neither his own experiences nor his future plans. Instead, it is rooted in a generic heteronormative portrayal of a man and woman having sex, the woman becoming pregnant, and then the man supporting her and the baby. Although I do not have enough interviews with gay men and MSM to draw strong conclusions, this kind of narrative was surprisingly common among them and reflects the persistence of deep-seated assumptions about reproduction, even as the number and variety of family forms continues to flourish in the United States.[10]

These descriptions of men as providers do not come as any surprise. They reflect widely documented cultural norms around fatherhood, which naturalize men and women as different kinds of parents who offer different kinds of care to their children. I include these quotes primarily because of the stark contrast they offer to men's halting descriptions of their "biological" involvement in reproduction. Men's references to being a provider roll right off the tongue without pause or laughter, and the ease and smoothness with which these idealized portrayals are delivered suggests just how powerful, commonly held, and well-known the cultural script for fatherhood is.

THE "BIOLOGICAL" IN MEN'S DISCUSSIONS
OF REPRODUCTION

Men's responses also reveal their propensity to dichotomize men's involvement in reproduction into "biological" and "social" components. Such a
categorization reflects a broader cultural distinction between biological
parenthood and social parenthood, one that appears in discussions of
adoption, stepparenting, and the use of assisted reproductive technologies,
such as egg donation, sperm donation, and surrogacy.[11] Indeed, scholars
working on these topics have devoted a great deal of attention to the question of precisely how individuals define and value biology. Classic anthropological studies of kinship pointed to the use of "biological ties" as one
way of defining familial relationships.[12] More recently, social scientists
studying assisted reproduction have documented the wide variety of meanings given to biological and genetic relationships, depending in part on the
intentions of those using such technologies.[13] For example, an egg donor
who provides the biogenetic material for an embryo but does not carry the
pregnancy or parent the child can argue that she is "not the mother"
because all she gave was "just an egg."[14] Likewise, surrogates who carry a
pregnancy but do not provide the egg or plan to raise the child can also
distance themselves from the label of "mother" by contending that all they
provided was a "tummy."[15] However, as these two examples suggest, the
focus—at least when it comes to research on reproductive technologies—
has generally been on women's narratives, and in particular, on how they
mobilize biology (or do not) in defining familial relationships.[16]

Given the novelty of asking men from the general public about reproduction, I devote the remainder of this chapter to examining a connected
but slightly different question about whether and when and how men discuss *biology* in describing their involvement in reproduction. My focus is
less on *relatedness* (which the men I interviewed tended to assume) and
more on how men conceptualized the embodied and biological processes
through which they become fathers: in their words, "having sex" and "providing sperm." In describing these two aspects of their role, it is intriguing
that men see them as "obvious" and yet are uncertain about exactly what
to say. For example, Rob, a forty-nine-year-old high-school graduate who
was in recovery after a long history of using illegal drugs, employed a

slightly questioning tone and sought reassurance at several points during his articulation of a man's role in reproduction.

ROB: Well, [*laughing*] first you have to have sex. A man's role. That's—that's—that's an interesting question. I don't know quite how to answer that.

RENE: It's whatever comes to mind. It's one of these very open questions.

ROB: Okay. Well, the man has the semen and fertilizes the egg in the female. So that would be a role of the man, correct?

RENE: Okay. Mm-hmm.

ROB: In reproduction [*pause*]. I think that would be it, right?

RENE: It's up to you. I mean, everybody has a different way of answering the question.

ROB: Well, in the question of reproduction, I think that about covers it.

Rob is one of just four men who responded to the question by talking only about sex and sperm without going on to discuss some of the more social aspects of fatherhood, such as providing.

However, Rob's response is similar to others in that it includes both hesitation and laughter. One might be tempted to attribute his uncertainty to his lack of higher education; perhaps he was genuinely unsure about the basics of conception. However, men with college degrees responded in very similar ways. For example, Travis, a thirty-three-year-old college graduate married to a doctor, had just moved to town and was looking for work. He had majored in zoology before working in real estate and volunteering as a youth minister for his church.

RENE: How would you describe a man's role in reproduction?

TRAVIS: [*pause*] That's a very interesting question [*laughs*]. Can you elaborate at all? Like, how?

RENE: It's really whatever comes to mind.

TRAVIS: What is a man's role in reproduction? Well, on a physical, I think it's pretty obvious. It's pretty—but [*pause*]. Well, I guess if you don't mind me going more into the spiritual aspects and the theology?

Like Rob and Travis, Chad appears surprised by the question and unsure how to answer, even though the twenty-six-year-old had a master's degree in psychology, worked as an EMT, and was in the process of submitting applications to medical schools.

RENE: So if somebody asked you to describe men's role in reproduction—

CHAD: Oh!

RENE: —how would you describe that?

CHAD: Okay. Um, so men's role in reproduction. Are we talking biological, I would imagine?

RENE: However you'd like to answer that.

CHAD: Okay. Well, boy, I think [*pause*]. Wow, that's a difficult one. I mean, biologically, I feel like we have the easier time as far as reproduction, because it's just the implantation [*laughs*], the implanting of sperm, and then that's pretty much it.

In the end, about 80 percent of the men referred to "biological" or "physical" processes in answering the question, either obliquely (like Travis) or by specifically mentioning sex and/or sperm. Thus, seeming uncertainty about what exactly they should say is paired with remarkable consistency. In contrast to the easy articulation of fathers as providers, though, the pauses indicate the lack of a ready-made cultural script for men's *bodily* involvement in reproduction. Indeed, several men noted they had never thought about the question, and certainly none had ever been asked to say it out loud. At the same time, men considered the answer to be "obvious," in some cases so obvious as to require no further elaboration. Moreover, this obviousness is often accompanied by slight discomfort and embarrassment, as evidenced by the nervous laughter punctuating men's discussions of sex and sperm. In both the pauses and the snickers, one can discern the historical lack of attention to men in this realm, in which the basic question of how men matter for reproduction has gone unspoken.

WOMEN TALKING REPRODUCTION

As I listened to forty different men try to describe their role in reproduction, I began to wonder how women would answer this question. Given women's greater bodily involvement in pregnancy and birth, I thought it would be surprising if women defined their role as including "having sex" or "providing an egg." I returned to the social scientific literature to see if anyone had ever asked women this kind of open-ended question about how they conceptualize their involvement in reproduction, but I could not find a single study among the decades of published research. Instead, women are interviewed about particular reproductive topics—birth, contraception, abortion—while reproduction itself goes undefined.[17]

So I decided to recruit a small sample of fifteen women to see how they responded to questions about women's and men's involvement in reproduction. I used the same strategies I had with men to find women from the general public who were diverse in terms of age, race, SES, and parenting status (see table A). It turned out that just one woman mentioned sex when describing a woman's role in reproduction, and just one other woman mentioned eggs. (I suspect this is because each of them had just listed these factors when describing a man's role.[18]) However, when asked to describe a *man's* role in reproduction, the women's answers were very similar to those of the men, underscoring men's bodily involvement via sex and sperm, as well as their significance as providers.

WHAT'S MISSING?

Just as important as noticing what people say is what they do not say. And when asked about a man's role in reproduction, it is striking that neither men nor women said a thing about how a man's age or his behaviors and exposures might affect his children's health. In fact, just two men referred to their own age or health in defining a man's involvement in reproduction. Angelo, a thirty-nine-year-old lawyer whose focus is the toxic effects of chemicals, described how he and his wife were having difficulties conceiving a second child. Having visited fertility doctors and acupuncturists alike, Angelo speculated that perhaps his "physical state" or even his age might be playing a role but concluded, "I don't know." The second man to mention his own bodily health was Elijah, a twenty-one-year old Black community college student, who, after much prodding to elaborate on his definition of a man's role in reproduction, mentioned his concern about passing on the "sickle cell trait." Just one woman, Sarah, a twenty-nine-year-old who is married and stays at home with her two-year-old, said she was aware of recommendations that men "not smoke or drink less or be healthier" but noted that "in my experience, that wasn't even necessary for us to conceive."

Since so little effort is being made to publicize research about how men matter for reproductive outcomes (as demonstrated in chapter 4), it is understandable that just three of the fifty-five interviewees brought up anything related to men's age or bodily health. But I was surprised that so few people mentioned genetics when defining men's involvement in reproduction. Just a couple of the men (and none of the women) talked about "DNA" or "genes" in referring to men's contributions to the embryo. However, my next question about sperm and eggs did elicit more biological references to genetics.

SPERM TALES

To probe further about how people think about men's involvement in reproduction, I next asked interviewees a more specific question: "How would you describe the relationship between the sperm and the egg?" Since the previous question about a man's role in reproduction was broad and focused solely on men, this question was intended to train their attention on one aspect of men's and women's bodily involvement in reproduction. In using the word *relationship*, I hoped that respondents would reflect on both kinds of cells and not discuss them as stand-alone entities.

While I had no clear hypotheses about how men would describe their role in reproduction, there has been enough research on people's views of sperm and eggs that I could reasonably expect them to imbue these tiny cells with stereotypically masculine and feminine characteristics.[19] In particular, cultural beliefs about sperm as "active" and eggs as "passive" are so deeply held that they affect even biologists who study conception. As Emily Martin documents, scientists expecting to find evidence for the standard biological tale of active-sperm-penetrates-passive-egg could not see what was happening right before their very eyes in the lab.[20] In fact, sperm swim in aimless circles while muscles inside the female reproductive tract move them toward the fallopian tubes, at which point the egg's chemical signal begins to draw them in.[21] Nevertheless, the narrative of active sperm and passive egg continues to be told and retold in medical textbooks, biology classes, popular documentaries like the BBC's *Great Sperm Race*, and videos on YouTube.[22]

Would men parrot this same old story about sperm, portraying it as prolific and active and penetrating while the egg passively waits around? Or would they tell some other tale about these cells? In the end, nearly every one of the thirty-three men asked this question did narrate some version of the active sperm, passive egg story.[23] Some versions were more elaborate than others, but the basic plot elements of sperm racing, competing, and entering the egg were all there. Unexpectedly, though, about half the men also told another kind of biological story about these cells, a more egalitarian narrative where the egg and sperm "come together" as "equal parts" or "two halves of a whole." In what follows, I examine how these stories are told and who tells which one.

Sperm Tale #1: Active Sperm, Passive Egg

More than 90 percent of the men told some version of the active sperm, passive egg story, an inherently asymmetrical conceptualization of reproduction. In telling this tale, some kept to the barest of details. For example, Avi, a twenty-three-year-old graduate student from Israel, stated succinctly, "Well, the sperm goes in the egg, and then they blow up and become a baby." Others were more expansive, drawing on metaphors of racing, swimming, or fighting to generate colorful descriptions of large numbers of sperm competing before the winner triumphantly enters the awaiting egg. Here is an example from Bruce, a thirty-eight-year-old working as a janitor at a hotel and raising his teenage son by himself.

> I would describe [sperm] as multiple busybodies in a race, and it's more or less like "Let's see who can get there first." Everybody's just pushing each other out of the way, just to get to the egg, and that's that golden prize, so to speak. It's just like whoever's the fastest, the most intelligent one. I know it's not necessarily like that, but it's like that's the one that wins the race.

Like Bruce, about a quarter of the men underscore the importance of numbers, noting the large quantity of sperm men make and pointing out that just one will "win the race." As Emily Martin finds in medical text-books, references to "millions" of sperm position the male body as a powerful and prolific producer of reproductive cells in relation to the female body, which manages to release just one egg every month.[24]

It is the large quantity of sperm that leads to competition, a core plot element of the active sperm, passive egg story. For example, Angelo, the environmental lawyer, draws on his experiences growing up in Italy to describe the "fight" between sperm as similar to men on a dance floor:

> The relationship between egg and sperm is pretty much like the relationship between man and woman. It's like a dance floor in an Italian club. The man-and-woman ratio in a club is three to one, but on the dance floor is like maybe seven to one. So I guess that's whatever you have, like, limited resources: a woman. The men are fighting to get there.

Similarly, a twenty-four-year-old graduate student in biology named Wei tells a "scientific" version of the story that is thoroughly driven by the dynamics of competition.

WEI: During fertilization, there is many sperm competing to get one egg. [*pause*] So the process of fertilization is a very harsh competition, but there is a lot of preselection before the sperm could even reach the egg. So there might be only a few sperm that might reach the egg in the end, and then it's about which one reaches first.

RENE: When you say preselection, what kinds of things are you thinking about?

WEI: As the sperm enters the vagina and then uterus, there are already a lot of harsh environments that kill most of them, and many of them don't have motility to reach the egg. So only a few can climb up those chemical signals, can sense the chemical signals and then reach the end. There's already a lot of competition there.

At the end of the interview, the issue of competition came up again as I debriefed him about the study. I mentioned I was intrigued by the different kinds of stories men were telling about sperm, and he replied:

WEI: My education in biology does give me more of a materialistic or objective view of what's going on. I don't think of them as active agents or live agents or anything. I don't give them any personalities.

RENE: Except that they're competitive. [*chuckles*]

WEI: That's a descriptive word. If I tried to study the outcome using mathematics, that's just a descriptive word.

As is clear below, where I analyze the second, more egalitarian sperm tale, other "descriptive" words can just as accurately capture the dynamics between sperm and egg. When people—scientists, journalists, or the general public—anthropomorphize sperm as competing, they draw on cultural notions of masculinity to tell a particular kind of biological story, one that places the male cell as an antagonistic protagonist.

Not only does sperm drive the action, its vibrant agency stands in vivid contrast to the egg, which is portrayed as just waiting around ready to be fertilized. This kind of depiction is present in Aaron's response. A forty-three-year-old gay man married to Tom, he is currently taking classes toward a nursing degree.

RENE: If you were going to describe the relationship between the sperm and the egg, how would you describe that?

AARON: Well, I think that [*pause*]. I never really thought about this. I think it's kind of in the DNA of each—the sperm and the egg—as this is your purpose. Okay, sperm, go in there and just fertilize. Then the egg is just, okay, here-I-am type of thing, I guess. I've never thought about it. [*laughs*]

A slightly more violent version appears in a stream-of-consciousness answer from Craig, a forty-six-year-old working-class man who described himself as bisexual: "Sperm: intruder, barbarian, break into the gates, divide and conquer. It's pretty much how I would portray it."

The most extreme version of the egg's passivity I heard came from Tony, a forty-five-year-old with a college degree working as a sound tech; he was in the midst of his second divorce. In his rendering, the egg is not alive in the same way as sperm, which he imbues with full responsibility for the offspring with the repeated refrain "You come from your father."

An egg is not a live breathing thing. It's a cell. Your father's sperm is a live breathing tadpole. It eats. It breathes. It moves. It swims. It's a live breathing organism, whereas your mother's egg, it's a shell. Your father's sperm— you would still be born if your father had sex with the nurse at the hospital. You won't have your mother's traits. You won't have your mother's eyes. You might not have your mother's nose. This is not my—these are just facts. If you really pay attention, you think about biology, the truth, you come from your father. That's where your genetic—When they test for your DNA, when they test you to see if a child is yours or not, they're looking for—and I get it confused—they're looking for the X or the Y. They're looking for that gene because there's the old saying, "Mother's baby, father's maybe." Okay? You come from your father. You came swimming out of him.

Tony's response is unusual for being so inconsistent with contemporary biological knowledge. In fact, his version of the active sperm, passive egg story actually harkens back to an earlier understanding of conception known as the doctrine of "preformation." Eighteenth-century scientists were convinced there was a tiny, preformed human (called a homunculus) inside each reproductive cell, although they debated whether it resided in the egg or the sperm.[25] Rob, too, refers to this centuries-old theory but melds it with a metaphor from the genomic age, in which DNA is the "map of life."[26]

ROB: Well, I would describe it as the sperm being the seed of creation and the egg being the host. I think all the DNA and all the map of a human being is in the sperm, right? I think? [*laughing*] And that fertilizes the egg in the female, and I guess it's hit or miss whether it's male or female. I don't think it's preconceived. I don't know.

RENE: Expand on that idea of the host a little bit.

ROB: Well, the female would, in my mind, nurture the child as it develops: feeding it, just giving it life, and sustaining the life to grow.

This portrayal of women—and their eggs—as a "host" (or "shell" in Tony's telling) positions women literally as vessels for male reproductive material. It is rooted in a truly ancient understanding of conception; Aristotle wrote about the male as seed and the female as soil.[27] This view of women's bodies has been criticized by contemporary feminist scholars who see it echoed in modern-day reproductive politics, particularly around abortion.[28]

The expectation that eggs/women will nurture the incipient life sparked by men occupies the final scene in the active sperm, passive egg narrative. In this example, Will, an eighteen-year-old freshman interested in the biological sciences, describes the egg as nourishing the sperm's genetic material:

The sperm goes into the egg and leaves its genetic material there. And then it just kind of goes away or is absorbed into the egg. Meanwhile, the egg's the thing that has to take in nutrients and divide and go through all these developmental changes to eventually become a baby or a fetus.

Antoine, a thirty-six-year-old father of two with a high school diploma who works as a roofer, brings together metaphors of building and racing to articulate a similar distinction between the sperm as instigator and egg as recipient.

> Okay, an egg is like, um [*pause*]. Let me see. The sperm is what, um [*pause*]. The sperm is like a traveler, and the egg is like the recipient, the holder. So the egg part is just to build. It's to make a foundation, but the sperm is more like the—. You know how when you run track and the person hands you the baton? So the sperm is handing you a baton, and once you get the baton, the egg is [*slaps hands to illustrate the egg taking off down the track*]. That's how I can describe it.

Old notions of masculinity associated with active production and femininity with caring nurturance—here written into the body at the level of cells—clearly persist into the present day, animating individual beliefs about how men matter for reproduction.

Indeed, it is notable that not a single person placed the egg in charge of conception or ascribed it responsibility for creating life. The only person who came close is David, a forty-eight-year-old, single White man on disability, who at one point in the interview engaged in a long diatribe about how the "male's role today is extremely emasculated by society."

> The egg is singular. The sperm is multiple, thousands knocking on the door. There's only one door, only one egg. In nature's own way, it has a special way of weeding out the lessers. The dog, there's always a runt, fighting for that teat to get milk. Sperm, very much the same way. The stronger sperm get there, and the stronger sperm usually gets in. Very similar to a lot of animals on the planet, the stronger one survives, and the female chooses the stronger one. And the egg is the egg. That's the baby basket. That's the start of everything. And the control usually is with the egg. Usually, females control in a lot of situations, as to where the male wishes he could control, but can't. And that's just the way things are, male-female-wise.

David's narrative is unusual in emphasizing the egg's "choice" of sperm and the "control" it exerts, but it is still sperm that initiates fertilization.

And his description is not at all unusual in its references to nature and animals. A nonexhaustive list of the animal analogies used by men to describe their role in reproduction includes birds, lions, tadpoles, pigs, and seahorses, another form of biological storytelling that positions men and their involvement in reproduction as outside the realm of human sociality.[29]

In essence, the active sperm, passive egg story renders men the active agent in establishing a pregnancy, as the *cause* of pregnancy. As Nathan puts it, "Sperm is what makes the baby. Without that, you have nothing." This understanding of conception is deeply woven into cultural representations of how men and women are involved in reproduction; think of the colloquialisms "he got her pregnant" or, more crudely, "he knocked her up." However, taking a step back, the notion that men alone produce a pregnancy becomes strange. One could just as easily say, "The egg is what makes the baby. Without that, you have nothing." But the biological story told by nearly every man I interviewed places the male cell as protagonist, driving the action and producing the results.

Sperm Tale #2: Sperm and Egg as Two Halves of a Whole

The active sperm, passive egg story was told by just about everybody: younger men and older men, men who had children and those who did not, those with a little education and those with a lot, men just scraping by and men with higher-paying jobs. But about half the men also told a different tale, a more egalitarian biological story in which the egg and sperm "meet" and "come together." In this second version, the two cells are "equal parts" that form a "combined unison." Patrick is a twenty-five-year-old who attended a few semesters in college and was now working in retail. He responds by laughing and saying:

> I would describe the relationship between the egg and sperm like, let's see, how do I say it? Like two necessary components that need to come together to create something much larger.

Likewise, Luke, a twenty-eight-year-old college graduate who maintained hiking trails, also draws on language from the hardware store to describe how the egg and sperm come together.

LUKE: [*pause*] It's like two-part epoxy, where there's two strips, and they're each a different color. Mix the strips together, and then you've actually got epoxy that will harden and form a seal on whatever you want.

RENE: [*laughs*] I've never heard of that.

LUKE: All right. Well, sperm's not doing anything on its own, and the egg's not doing anything on its own. So those two things have to combine for a child to exist.

In contrast to the active sperm, passive egg story, there is no race, no penetration. There is no competition, just "combination." And perhaps most surprisingly, neither the sperm nor the egg is the active agent in establishing a pregnancy. Both are necessary, and neither is sufficient.

Men telling this second tale commonly did so with a nod to genetics. Seth is a twenty-three-year-old Vietnamese American who had just graduated from art school. His response is succinct: "Sperm and an egg. It's just like they both provide genetic information. That's pretty much it." Mark, a thirty-eight-year-old White nurse also answered the question through the lens of genetics:

> Well, the egg obviously is from the female, and the sperm is from the male. They each have a set of genes, where they come in for fertilization. It's like a 50-50 sharing of genetic information.

Henri, a twenty-eight-year-old, French engineer married to a man, pairs similarly mathematical information with the lyrical phrase "perfect wedding" to describe the relationship between sperm and egg.

> You need like 50 percent of the gene from the sperm and 50 percent from the ovule [egg]. So it's a very sort of sharing relationship where you share halfway. It's like a very perfect wedding, like you're split in half, and half of everything belongs to this one, and half of everything belongs to the other half.

In contrast to the first sperm story, where male cells and female cells are assigned different characteristics and portrayed as doing different things, this second version positions the sperm and egg as similar: they both "come in" for fertilization and each "provides" half the DNA. Things are "50-50." When Miranda Waggoner and I examined how clinicians envision men's involvement in reproduction, we found they were most likely to consider their contributions equal to women's if they were thinking in terms of genetics.[30] Here is evidence that genetic stories are also associated with more egalitarian thinking about these cells in the minds of individual men.

It is important to note that the two sperm tales are not at all mutually exclusive. Of the thirty-three men asked about the relationship between sperm and eggs, almost all (N = 30) told the first active sperm, passive egg story. Then about half of them (N = 14) also told the second, more egalitarian version. Almost everyone who told the second story also told the first; just two men told the second story *without* telling the first. So the two tales coexist easily, despite their very different narratives. Indeed, in some of the interviews, they appear very close together. Kenneth, a forty-nine-year-old office manager at an insurance company, offers a classic version of the active sperm, passive egg story in responding to the first question about a man's role in reproduction before transitioning to the more egalitarian version in answering the sperm-and-egg question.[31]

TODD: How would you describe a man's role in reproduction?

KENNETH: Well, they, the man, the male provides the sperm that has to fertilize the egg. So that's his role.

TODD: Okay, now when you say "provides"—

KENNETH: Yeah [*laughing*]. Well, I mean, that's the only way it's gonna get fertilized is if he provides it. So basically when you're having sex, he ejaculates, the sperm swims, a whole bunch of them—millions—but only usually one fertilizes the egg—usually [*laughing*].

TODD: Okay, so how would you describe the relationship between an egg and a sperm?

KENNETH: Well, let's see, the egg being in the woman has to be fertilized by the sperm from the male, okay. There is no life without both of those two coming together. So basically, they need each other. They're dependent on each other.

Like Kenneth, the women I interviewed would occasionally narrate both stories, but about a third of the women told *only* the second, more egalitarian version. This is an interesting gender difference in the kinds of biological stories men and women tell about reproductive cells, particularly given that women largely echoed men's responses to the "man's role in reproduction" question. Women also used different metaphors in defining the relationship between eggs and sperm; three of them described it as "romantic" and one used the word *dangerous*. Neither of these terms was mentioned by any of the men.

Biological stories are powerful. They both reflect and produce our collective understandings of our bodies and ourselves, and I began to wonder if men who thought in more egalitarian ways about gender relations were more likely to tell the second story. To answer this question, my research assistant Dana Hayward and I both reread each interview in full and separately coded each man as "more egalitarian" or "less egalitarian" based on their descriptions of women in general, as well as their relationships with particular women.[32] (To avoid circularity, we did not include their discussions of eggs and sperm in our coding.) Most men were easy to categorize as either "more egalitarian" (e.g., those stating that women and men are similar or emphasizing the importance of men sharing household and child-rearing responsibilities) or "less egalitarian" (e.g., those noting that women and men are different kinds of people who inhabit separate spheres of work and home or stating explicitly that men should be in charge). A few men were deeply misogynistic, asserting that women are less intelligent than men or that domestic violence is understandable. Some of the men, however, fell in between more and less egalitarian, requiring judgment calls.[33] In the end, I categorized twelve of the men as more gender-egalitarian and fourteen as less gender-egalitarian. For the remaining seven men, there was not enough relevant talk to ascertain their views.

It turns out that views of gender *are* associated with which sperm story men tell: men who are more egalitarian are more than twice as likely to tell the second tale, in which sperm and egg are two halves of a whole (see figure 14).[34] They also tend to be younger and have higher levels of education, which is consistent with national surveys showing more Americans adopting more gender-egalitarian attitudes over time.[35]

In sum, men tell two different kinds of tales about sperm and eggs, with the second, more egalitarian story being narrated by a distinct subgroup of men who are younger and more educated. Moreover, it does appear as though men's views of these biological entities are deeply associated with their broader beliefs about gender relations. Such variation underscores

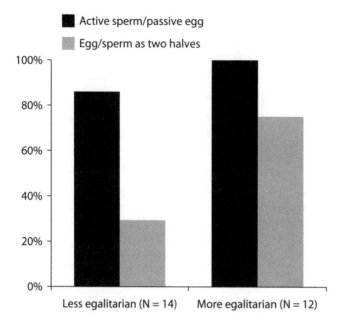

Figure 14. Men with more gender-egalitarian views are more likely to tell second sperm story.

just how malleable biology can be as a substrate for social meaning: men are using the exact same cells to illustrate opposing beliefs about gender.[36] It is not eggs and sperm that are more or less egalitarian; it is the biological stories we tell about them that are.

BIOLOGICAL STORIES

Biology is the study of the living world, a science that seeks to understand the plants and animals that populate the planet. At the same time, it provides a rich trove of metaphors that one of those species—humans— mobilizes to make sense of themselves and one another. Blood ties. Maternal instinct. Monkey business. Men are dogs. Biological stories are powerful because they root human experience in something seemingly primal and asocial. They can be used to render a condition more or less "natural," one's behavior more or less volitional.

Social scientists also tell biological stories. The economist Thomas Schelling famously compared the complexity of our economic system to an ant colony, noting that no one ant is in charge but the system is nevertheless "full of patterns and regularities and balanced proportions."[37] Second-wave, liberal feminists argued that biological sex differences did not matter and should not be used to bar women from full participation in schools and workplaces.[38] Scientists searched for a "gay gene" to shore up the argument that people were simply "born that way."[39] As these examples suggest, biological stories are often profoundly political and can do nearly invisible work in justifying people's beliefs.

At the same time, it is important to reiterate the point that biological knowledge—and the ways it permeates everyday life to inform people's understandings of bodies and behaviors—is hardly immune from the inequality-riven social world in which it is created.[40] As this book has demonstrated, beliefs about women's reproductivity continually edged out a full investigation of men's contributions to reproductive outcomes, a gap in biomedical knowledge that has profound implications for how individuals from the general population conceptualize reproduction. To extend the metaphor of the photographer from the Introduction: with the image of men so blurry, it is difficult for men to articulate just how they are involved in the process of reproduction.

Indeed, the effects of biomedical non-knowledge can be detected clearly in how men talk about reproduction: they tell *biological* stories but not *biomedical* stories. They pause and search for words, but even when pressed they are almost uniformly unaware of how their own age, behaviors, and exposures matter for their children's health. They narrate scenes in which a male protagonist cell actively produces life with no risk posed by the male's own body, while the leading lady cell waits patiently in the shadows, ready to receive his spark and give all the nourishment it needs to grow into a baby. Masculine metaphors and animal analogies are operating not only in the minds of biologists and in the pages of medical textbooks but in the talk of men.

However, along with changing notions of gender and genetics, another tale about conception exists, one in which both sperm and egg are stars who contribute equally to the action by combining to create life. Even as most respondents offer traditional narratives about men as providers and sperm as the spark of life, there is another vision of gender relations peeking through in the more egalitarian descriptions of eggs and sperm, which suggests that increasing interest in gender equity is influencing biological stories about reproduction.

In the next chapter, I draw on recent biomedical research about paternal effects (reviewed in chapter 3) to challenge one part of the dominant narrative—that sperm is invulnerable—and examine how men react. Does learning this new information change how men talk about their involvement in reproduction?

6 Healthy Sperm?

The historical lack of attention to men's reproductive health offers an unusual opportunity to analyze what happens when people encounter the rarely linked terms *healthy* and *sperm* in the same phrase. Americans are certainly used to reading headlines about the latest in biomedical research, and they hear all kinds of advice from health officials. But in contrast to many of the enduring debates in health and medicine—Can exercise stave off Alzheimer's? Is eating eggs good for you or not?—the emerging evidence about how men's bodies matter for reproductive outcomes is surprising. As I described in chapter 3, researchers have been working to document what they call "paternal effects," or the ways a man's age, behaviors, and exposures can damage sperm and affect children's health. It is not only that this knowledge is relatively new and mostly unfamiliar to the general public. It also fundamentally challenges deeply held and widely accepted beliefs about the overwhelming significance of *women's* bodies for reproductive outcomes. How would individual men respond to hearing this kind of health information, possibly for the first time?

I looked for a patient-friendly brochure about paternal effects but found only the single page on the CDC website about men's preconception health (discussed in chapter 4), and it did not include detailed informa-

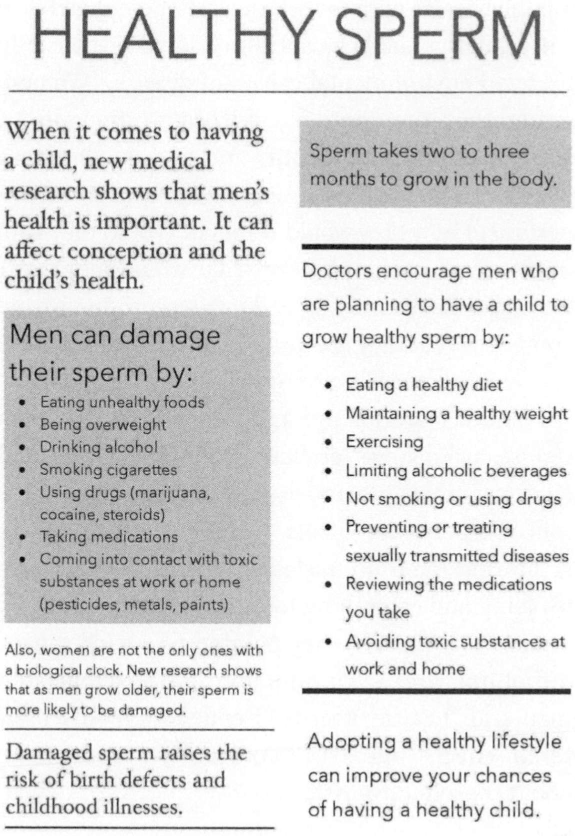

HEALTHY SPERM

When it comes to having a child, new medical research shows that men's health is important. It can affect conception and the child's health.

Sperm takes two to three months to grow in the body.

Men can damage their sperm by:

- Eating unhealthy foods
- Being overweight
- Drinking alcohol
- Smoking cigarettes
- Using drugs (marijuana, cocaine, steroids)
- Taking medications
- Coming into contact with toxic substances at work or home (pesticides, metals, paints)

Also, women are not the only ones with a biological clock. New research shows that as men grow older, their sperm is more likely to be damaged.

Damaged sperm raises the risk of birth defects and childhood illnesses.

Doctors encourage men who are planning to have a child to grow healthy sperm by:

- Eating a healthy diet
- Maintaining a healthy weight
- Exercising
- Limiting alcoholic beverages
- Not smoking or using drugs
- Preventing or treating sexually transmitted diseases
- Reviewing the medications you take
- Avoiding toxic substances at work and home

Adopting a healthy lifestyle can improve your chances of having a healthy child.

Figure 15. "Healthy Sperm" leaflet.

tion about how damage to sperm can pose risks to children. So I designed my own leaflet. Drawing on the biomedical literature and echoing language used in public health campaigns, I created a one-page information sheet and titled it "Healthy Sperm." The bullet-pointed text is pegged to a tenth-grade reading level and spells out the significance of men's own bodily health for reproductive outcomes. Specifically, it notes that "damaged sperm raises the risk of birth defects and childhood illnesses" and underscores the conclusion that "adopting a healthy lifestyle can improve your chances of having a healthy child" (see figure 15). I asked each interviewee to read it and then walk me through their reactions.

Typical of public health approaches, the leaflet emphasizes individuals—individual bodies, individual behaviors, individual responsibilities—rather than structural and environmental causes of disease.[1] Women are used to hearing individualized prescriptions and proscriptions like these, all of which index a broader duty to identify and personally manage potential reproductive risks.[2] But the novelty of directing such messages to men raises the question of how they would respond. Would they willingly accept the leaflet's message and its implications? Or would men express disbelief that their own bodies have anything to do with reproductive outcomes?

Men's responses reveal they are quite familiar with reproductive health messages . . . about women. Unprompted, many men discussed in detail the risks of advanced maternal age and the need for pregnant women to eat right, exercise, avoid stress, eschew alcohol and drugs, and steer clear of toxins. However, men are much less familiar with recent medical research about the potential effects of their own age and health. After learning this information from the leaflet, men stated their ready willingness to do anything and everything to improve their children's chances in life. At the same time, though, they pointed to a wide range of cultural, economic, structural, and environmental barriers that stand between individual men and "healthy sperm." I conclude by discussing how the case of "paternal effects" offers an opportunity to rethink public health messaging about reproductive risk.

MOTHERS MATTER

Continuing a long tradition of locating reproductive risk primarily within women's bodies, men from the general public are well-versed in contemporary public health messages about the significance of maternal bodies for reproductive outcomes.[3] Even though I did not ask a single question about women's reproductive health, the topic peppers my interview transcripts, with men of all educational levels mentioning the importance of women's age, health, and exposures for their children's health. Indeed, in a question designed to ascertain whether men knew anything about paternal effects before I gave them the leaflet—"If a couple is planning to have a child, do you know of anything *the man* can do to increase the chances the baby will be healthy?"—more than 70 percent said that what men can do is make sure that *women* are healthy.

Nearly half the men mentioned risks associated with women's age, and about a third talked about the importance of being supportive of their pregnant partners, echoing the provider narrative discussed in the last chapter. Support included everything from being present and "stable" to "going out at 2 a.m. to grab peanut butter and Slim Jims." In particular, several men discussed the need to minimize women's stress during pregnancy, lest it affect the baby. As Bobby put it, "The environment that the partner supports or creates or promotes positively or negatively impacts the health of the baby." Some men, though, understood *support* more in terms of enforcement, especially when it came to diet and exercise or avoiding alcohol and drugs. Josh, a thirty-three-year-old Southeast Asian businessman and father of two, could not think of anything he would do to change his own behavior prior to conception but said that "during the pregnancy, maybe I will *push her* to relax more, have more exercise, not stress too much" (emphasis added). Likewise, Matt, a forty-year-old who had lost his children to the state after struggling with drugs and homelessness, recalled being "very protective" during his ex-wife's pregnancy more than a decade before: "I made sure she was healthy. I made sure she didn't smoke cigarettes or be around cigarettes. Um, eating the right foods. I didn't argue with her—no stress on the baby."

Occasionally, men would extend this responsibility for healthy living to themselves, noting their potential "influence" on their pregnant partners. For example, Craig, who did not have children, described the relationship between a man's and a woman's "lifestyle":

> The woman is eating for two. Whatever you put in your body affects the fetus, but I also believe that the man is such an influence. I mean, I can't tell you to stop drinking if I drink. Am I going to smoke a cigarette next to you while you are not smoking? I am not directly affecting the body or the baby. I am affecting your environment or your emotions—I mean, you can put a woman through mental hell for nine months. What stress does that put on the fetus?

However, even as Craig pointed to the possible effects of men's behaviors, he never articulated a direct effect; the woman's body was still situated as the vector through which men's actions could affect the fetus.

A few men took individualized public health messages to their logical conclusion, explicitly blaming women for children's health problems. For example, Tony, who earlier defined the woman's egg as a "shell" filled by a man's sperm, described a hypothetical situation in which a child is born with Down syndrome (a genetic condition that, according to the NIH, does not appear to be linked to maternal or paternal behaviors):

> The mother is drinking, smoking, doing drugs during pregnancy. Now the kid comes out with Down syndrome. [*Mimics mother whimpering to baby:*] "Oh, how did this happen? It's not my fault. I love you." But, realistically, what were you doing during pregnancy? That's why the child has Down syndrome, because you weren't taking care of yourself.

In these unprompted discussions, men reveal that it is difficult for them to talk about reproduction *without* talking about women, a legacy of biomedical knowledge-making about reproductive risk focused on women's bodies. Next, I turn to the question of whether men have encountered any of the newer messages about the importance of *paternal* age, behaviors, and exposures.

FATHERS MATTER?

Even as they expressed a great deal of certainty about the importance of women's health, some men did respond to my question about whether there was "anything men could do to increase the chances of having a healthy baby" by venturing guesses about the importance of their own behaviors. It was almost as if they heard the word *health* and began rattling off all the standard advice they had ever been given. For example, Deshawn listed the following: "I would say no nicotine, no alcohol, no tobacco, gotta be healthy, you know, make sure you are eating right. Get a lot of exercise, so stuff like that." Paul, who like Deshawn is a high school graduate and father of one, summed up his answer with the slogan-like statement: "A healthy father gives birth to a healthy son."[4]

Table B summarizes the long list of actions men believed might increase their chances of having a healthy child.[5] As detailed in chapter 4, the media does occasionally offer sperm-specific advice, such as avoiding hot tubs,

Table B   Proportion of men mentioning actions they could
take to increase the chances of having a healthy child

	% Men Mentioning (n = 34*)
Avoiding alcohol	56%
Eating healthy foods	53%
Healthy lifestyle	47%
Not smoking	44%
Not using drugs	32%
Exercising	29%
Taking genetic test	24%
Preparing mentally	21%
Sleeping	21%
Avoiding toxins	15%

*Of the 39 men asked this question, 5 answered there was nothing men could do. Hence, the percentages in this table are based on an N of 34. I do not include actions mentioned by fewer than 15% of the men.

tight underwear, and bicycle seats because heat can decrease sperm count. However, each of those factors was mentioned just once (by three different people). Consistent with the individualizing tendencies of public health approaches, every single man described *individual* health behaviors. Just 15 percent referred to environmental toxins or other supra-individual factors that might influence a man's chances of having a healthy child.

These answers might suggest that men have a deep familiarity with recent biomedical research about paternal effects, but their subsequent responses and reactions to the leaflet made it clear that most were simply guessing and not stating known facts about sperm damage. For example, Mark, the nurse, finished reading the leaflet, laughed, and exclaimed, "Hey, I was right with a lot of it!" Indeed, many of the men explicitly communicated uncertainty even as they answered the question. For example, Patrick speculated about what men can do but was "not too sure" about it.

Well, if a man wanted to have a healthy baby, I don't know of anything else other than—because he's not carrying the baby. But I would say, definitely something I'd recommend is, you know, eliminate certain drug use or drinking, even though I'm not so sure if that would be a deciding factor on whether or not you'd have a healthy baby. I'm not too sure about what a man can do. I guess stay healthy. But then again, he's not carrying the baby. So that's kind of tricky to me.

Given how little effort has gone into circulating messages about paternal effects, it is not at all surprising that men are largely unaware of how their own health might affect their children's health. At the time of the interviews, though, research on advanced paternal age and arguments about a "male biological clock" had been making headlines for at least a decade. So I followed up the general question about "anything men can do" with a specific question about men's age: "There are studies that show that older women are more likely to give birth to children with Down syndrome. Do you think a man's age has any effect on the health of a child?"

Most men were not familiar with the potential risks of paternal age, and in contrast to the previous question, they were less likely to speculate that it mattered. Instead, about a third pointed out that even very elderly men could have children, resonating with media coverage of celebrities such as Mick Jagger who become fathers at advanced ages (see chapter 4). Rob explains:

I have heard that men as old as seventy have gotten a woman pregnant. I think the age of a man is not as important as the age of a woman. I think as long as the man is healthy and can produce enough sperm, I don't think age really matters that much.

Some men did express worries about being an "older dad," but these concerns were about playing with and caring for small children. Twenty-three-year-old Daniel wanted to be able to pick up his future child "with full strength, as opposed to a bad back." Thirty-three-year-old Tom was unsure whether he and his new husband "want a kid," but if they do, he would "like to have one sooner than later because I want to be able to do things with it and not be older, not be able to go out and play catch because my arthritis is bothering me or something."

Several of the African American respondents defined *old* as men becoming fathers in their 30s and 40s, a decade or two before some of the other respondents considered men to be "old dads." For example, Bruce responded to the question about paternal age by explaining it was not a problem in his community:

> Unfortunately, where I come from, everybody has kids as teenagers until their twenties. One of the guys I work with—I think he's forty-four—we were just talking about kids and stuff. He just had a daughter, and he was joking, "Man, I didn't even expect to have none. I've been going all this long without having no kids." He was like, "When I found out my girl was pregnant, no disrespect, but I had to ask her whose was it, because I'm just so used to shooting blanks. Man, I'm forty-something years old, I'm sitting here having a kid.

Bruce was not currently in a relationship, but he had thought about the possibility of having another child. He continued: "Now I'm thirty-eight, so I feel as though my time is ticking, ticking, ticking. I don't want to be like sixty years old with a five-year-old son!" The metaphor of the biological clock has long been applied to women's reproductive aging,[6] but Bruce was the only man I interviewed to use it in reference to men's bodies. However, unlike the clinicians who are mobilizing this metaphor to raise awareness of paternal aging,[7] Bruce was not concerned about fertility or sperm damage. After all, he envisioned a (male) child being born and becoming a presumably active five-year-old. His concerns were about keeping up with a young son at such an advanced age. Regardless of differences in how men defined "old" fathers, though, few incorporated a consideration of aging sperm into their definitions.

However, there were a few men—about a fifth of the sample—who *had* encountered messages about paternal age, behaviors, and exposures posing risks to children's health. In keeping with a well-documented association between education and health knowledge,[8] seven of these nine men had college degrees or graduate degrees. About half of them came across this information while undergoing fertility testing in a medical clinic, one of the few sites where men might hear from clinicians about sperm. The others had come across the information incidentally, as had Chad, who worked as an EMT and was applying to medical school:

> I've heard recently there are actually some studies that show the man should be younger. I know that for women, there's definitely—you don't want to be past a certain point, because then the likelihood of certain disorders go up. But I guess they have been finding that's really the same with males.[9]

Victor, a self-described "news junkie," is a forty-three-year-old gay man with a master's degree in accounting; he had just emerged from a long bout of depression-induced homelessness. His knowledge of paternal effects was the most extensive of anyone I interviewed:

RENE: If a man wanted to have a child, is planning to have a child, do you know of anything that men can do before the baby is conceived to try to increase the chances the child will be healthy?

VICTOR: I think there might be. Some of the things I've read—maybe certain dietary things to stay away from, maybe physically, maybe certain things that you wouldn't ingest. I know there's things that can damage our means to procreate but also can damage our cells and DNA. So maybe the man himself could refrain or abstain from particular behaviors or particular dietary things that might cause harm. Staying away, keeping themselves away from things that might damage their sperm or reproductive ability.

He pivots to discussing how "there also might be a need for him beforehand to ensure that the mother herself is in a state and condition that she can biologically reproduce without a problem." I redirect him by asking, "Is there anything else you're thinking about for men in particular?"

VICTOR: For the men? Again, I think a lot of it maybe comes down to ingesting alcohol, ingesting harmful things, or ingesting—or not even necessarily ingesting, but maybe putting yourself in a situation that might could cause some cellular or like you hear things about people working in nuclear plants and microwaving-type stuff and how that can damage a man's ability to procreate or even to pass on a damaged mutation or cellular trait that might not have necessarily been there. Medications might could cause these types of things. Trying to restrict those types of activities beforehand probably, whether it's dietary or physical or proximity to something harmful. Risk reduction, I guess, overall.

Victor has a detailed knowledge of paternal effects, as when he refers to epigenetic processes in mentioning the possibilities of a "damaged mutation or cellular trait that might not have necessarily been there." Yet, his answers are still laced with multiple maybes and mights, evincing a sense of uncertainty similar to those who were simply guessing about how their health might matter for reproductive outcomes. Victor's uncertainty is probably related to the relative scarcity of such messages; he had heard them before but does not routinely encounter this kind of information, making him hesitant about both the mechanisms and the outcomes. His discussion is also notable for its insistence on individual-level responsibility, that "risk reduction" involved "the man himself" refraining, abstaining, and generally keeping away "from things that might damage . . . sperm or reproductive ability." But unlike Victor, most men had not heard any of this information before. What happens when they encounter it for the first time?

MEN REACT TO THE NOTION OF HEALTHY SPERM

Given that women are most often the target of reproductive health messages like those in the "Healthy Sperm" leaflet, I faced yet another moment of being unsure about how men would react. On the one hand, social scientists who study health and medicine have pointed to cultural tenets of masculinity, such as risk-taking behavior and disinterest in seeking medical care, as important factors in persistent gender differences in morbidity and mortality: in the United States, men suffer more serious illnesses and die earlier than women, on average.[10] From this perspective, the men I interviewed might be expected to dismiss the leaflet, because it does not fit a cultural narrative of men's bodies as strong and invulnerable.[11]

At the same time, though, shifting cultural norms around fatherhood have led to new expectations that men will invest more time and effort in caring for their children, and not just providing for them.[12] National surveys based on time diaries reveal that men spend more time with their children than they used to (even though the number of hours women spend continues to outpace that of men),[13] and social scientists debate the extent to which men have adopted the tenets of "intensive" parenting.[14] As just one reproduction-specific example, men are now more likely to be found in the birthing room than in the waiting room during a baby's birth.[15] Perhaps men would react to the leaflet by expressing an interest in doing everything possible to optimize their children's chances in life.

To demonstrate how men fulfilled *both* these competing hypotheses, I present extended excerpts from two of my interviews. When speaking about their own reactions, men pronounced themselves ready and willing to do all they could to give their children the best start in life. However, when next asked how "the average man" would respond, they identified a variety of social and structural processes that would make it difficult for men to adhere to the leaflet's advice. The excerpts are from James and Malik, who differ from one another in age, race, SES, and parental status but are similar in how they reacted to the leaflet. Both are representative of my respondents in ways I discuss in more detail below.

James and Malik

James grew up the oldest of three children in the second family of a wealthy older man and his much younger wife. Raised on the Eastern Seaboard with nannies and private schools, James's life of privilege continues at one of the most elite universities in the country, where as a nineteen-year-old White student, he follows in his father's footsteps with interests in public service and politics. He has a "long-term girlfriend" of two and half years. They had talked about the possibility of having children at some point in the far-off future, and he spoke of wanting to be "more involved" than his own father had been. Walking into our interview, he wore a T-shirt and shorts. His answers were thoughtful and earnest, as if he were sitting in a college seminar.

RENE: Now I have something I'd like you to read and then react to in any way you want. There is no right or wrong answer.

JAMES: Healthy sperm. [*pauses while reading*] Is this all true?[16]

RENE: You can take this as something your doctor might hand you.

JAMES: Okay. So, if my doctor gave me something, I would assume it was true. [*pauses while reading*] Great. All the more incentive to get healthier.

RENE: So just walk me through whatever reactions, responses you have.

JAMES: I think it makes sense. I obviously don't know the biology behind it, but it seems like if you work to be healthy, then all the parts of your body are probably healthier, including organs that make the sperm. Reading it, I sort of feel compelled to be healthier and continue my attempts to have a healthy lifestyle because, my goodness, I would want healthy children. And I would want to conceive—I would want my child to be healthy. So, to me, this makes intuitive sense, and this makes me very much want to try to maintain this sort of lifestyle.

RENE: So, you and your girlfriend—let's flash forward ten years in the future. Do you think this would be something difficult for you to do, to manage all of these things for several months before you even start trying to have kids? Or does it not seem that difficult?

JAMES: It doesn't seem incredibly difficult, especially for two or three months, relative to the idea of having a healthy child, especially since you know my partner would have to go through pregnancy, which is sort of an ordeal [*laughs*]. It wouldn't seem to me completely onerous to exercise more and give up alcohol. I don't use drugs or smoke, and I don't plan to. I knew sperm were sort of always growing and regenerating; I didn't know that it took two to three months or that your activities in those two to three months specifically affected the sperm. But assuming it's true, now that I know that, it would seem reasonable for two to three months before I wanted to conceive really trying to follow these even more to the extent than I already do.

RENE: So that's your response. Now think about the average guy out there. How do you think the average guy would respond to this?

JAMES: I think, on average, people tend to be more skeptical than me about medical information they receive. I tend to take doctor things at face value. I know there are a lot of people out there who have conspiracy theories about doctors, and I guess there are a lot of people out there who see men as having less responsibility when it comes to conception and even child-rearing, because of antiquated views about a woman's role. So, I can see men being (a) like skeptical to accept that the science behind this is true and (b) sort of not necessarily as willing to accept they have sort of a moral need to adjust their lifestyle choices to provide for healthy kids.

Malik was born a few miles away from James's college campus and endured a difficult childhood punctuated by trauma. His parents—his father a construction worker until he hurt his back, and his mother a waitress, receptionist, and whatever else would pay the bills—went through an "awful divorce" that made Malik feel like a "yo-yo" going back and forth; he is no longer in touch with the man he calls his "biological father." When he was just five years old, Malik and a seven-year-old friend accidentally hit a baseball into a windshield; the owner of the car came raging out of his house and shot Malik's friend dead in the street. These early experiences resulted in struggles with depression; at the age of "eleven or twelve," he was admitted to a hospital for being suicidal. At thirteen, he joined a gang and was kicked out of high school after high school before finally getting his diploma. At that point, his mother had remarried and moved south; Malik joined the Army and did a two-year tour in Afghanistan.

Walking into our interview, Malik was a twenty-seven-year-old Black father of three, wearing a black knit cap over a short ponytail and smelling of cigarette smoke. Belying the difficult stories he was about to tell, he exuded a calm kindness, and his answers were laced with humor as he carefully considered the questions. He was in the midst of a divorce from the mother of his seven-year-old daughter, and he lived with his girlfriend and their three-year-old twins; they had started talking about having another child. He dreamed of a position designing video games but was unemployed after several stints in various low-wage jobs.

RENE: So I have something I'd like you to read and then just react in any way you want. There are no right answers, wrong answers.

MALIK: Healthy sperm. [*short pause while reading first part*] Oh, that's pretty much everything I just said. That's interesting. [Tells anecdote about his stepfather thinking he was "too old" to have a child in his late thirties.] [*long pause while reading*] So yeah, I've definitely heard it. It's just surprising to actually see it though. I just said eating right, maintaining a healthy weight. You got to exercise. Alcohol, drugs, preventing and treating sexually transmitted diseases. But "avoiding toxic substances at work and home," that's new. Because I wouldn't know how to avoid toxic substances if they're already in your home. So like you're using bleach to wash your clothes or any types of disinfectants that hold all types of other chemicals. So yeah, you got to avoid them, but I wouldn't say it's major. But at work, I've had people say there's lead, and what else? When I was working at [a shipping company], they would ship these huge barrels of toxic chemicals. And there has been spills, and you pretty much have no choice but to contain the substance that's in it—which is higher than my pay grade, I'm going to tell you that. Because there was a couple instances where that happened to me, where this huge container—it had to be like half my height, at least one hundred, maybe two hundred pounds of stuff [*laughs*]. I don't know what was in it, but it began leaking, and my supervisor wanted me to touch it. I'm like, "I'm not touching that stuff. I don't care what you say. You can send me home now." But other people say, "Oh well, we got to get it out, we got another truck to do and da-da-da." Dude, I'm not touching that stuff, man. I don't care what you say. I'll go on another truck; I'm not touching it. But yeah, that is hard to do, to avoid it at work, at times. It depends on what you do, obviously.

RENE: And so when you say it's surprising to actually see it, how is that so?

MALIK: Because you don't really see stuff. Well, in my life, because I rarely go to the hospital. I'm deathly afraid of the hospital. [*laughs*] I have a little phobia. I don't care for needles or anything like that. It's just like the whole garb thing with the masks. It's like, "Oh God, please no." [*laughs*] The last time I seen something like this was like in health class. We talked about stuff like that, but I haven't seen it for years.

RENE: So if you brought this home, and you and your girlfriend said, "Okay, twins aren't enough, we want more kids"—

MALIK: Oh yeah, 'cause we actually already talked about that stuff right now. She would say, "Okay, we got to stop smoking cigarettes." We already had this discussion, 'cause I want to stop. I'm better at stopping than she is. But yeah, we already discussed having another one, 'cause she wants—honestly, I want another one as well, but she doesn't think I want another one. But anyway, we already said that we need to stop smoking cigarettes. We don't use drugs. We don't drink literally at all. It's like really, really, really rare occasions that we drink. Like a holiday or a special occasion, we get a bottle of wine, or I get a little half pint of liquor. We don't do it every day like everybody else does. Well, not everybody else, but people that we know. But yeah, eating unhealthy foods, I don't have a sweet tooth. She does. I mean we do eat three times a day, obviously, 'cause we have kids. I make sure they have breakfast. We have lunch at home, and then they come home at around 3:00. I got to go get them around 2:30, 3:00, and then they have another lunch on top of their lunch. So they eat good. My kids love all types of vegetables and all types of fruit, and we do too; that's how we eat. So I wouldn't say eating unhealthy, but my girlfriend on the other hand, she loves, loves ice cream. I'll sit down, and I'll have a couple spoonfuls and okay, I'm good. This Halloween that just passed, we still have candy, and she's sitting here snacking on their candy. But we don't eat really crazy unhealthy. We don't order out that much. Some days—everybody's got those lazy days— you know what, I'm going to order a pizza or Chinese food. But it's rare.

RENE: So that's how you would respond. Now if you were going to imagine the average guy you know—

MALIK: [*laughs*]

RENE: How do you think the average guy you know would react to this?

MALIK: The average guy I know? Whew! He'd be like, "Okay, well, I got to stop eating. I got to stop drinking." [*laughs*] It's a lot of stuff. My brother-in-law, he's pretty bad off. He's the only guy I could really relate to in this situation. He has heavy use of drugs. He's in a methadone clinic. He smokes cigarettes. He drinks like a fish. He's just really, really unhealthy, and he's talking about another kid. So it's like, "Dude, really?" But for him to react to that, or any of my other friends, it's like [*laughs*] they got to do a lot of stuff to actually be healthy. And it's not going to work overnight, definitely not with all this stuff. So their reaction is going to be like, "Okay, well, how am I going to do all this in less than nine months?" You know, it's not going to happen. And it would have to change their entire lifestyle, and it's not going to work like that. People have to be mentally set for stuff like this. If it's not going to work, it's just not going to work.

Individual Intentions and Barriers to Health

Reacting to health messages about the effects of individual behavior on sperm, James and Malik exemplify a common pattern amongst my respondents: a sharp disjuncture between what men themselves say they would do versus how they imagine the average man's reaction. Far from dismissing the leaflet, nearly every man in this very diverse sample made it clear that if they were in the position of trying to have a child, then "of course" they would do everything possible to reduce the risks to their children's health. Like Malik, several of the other men took a checklist approach, ticking through their lives to identify problem behaviors in need of modification. And like James, about half laced their discussions with intonations of morality, designating those who would "take heed" of such advice "good fathers" and underscoring men's "duty" to their future children. Putting these same sentiments in more colorful terms, Nick, a thirty-three-year-old, single gay man, explained he would try to follow the recommendations because "I don't half-ass things. So I would not half-ass being a parent if and when I was going to be a parent. Not doing this would be half-assing it."

Shortly after we discussed the leaflet, I did a debrief with each interviewee, alerting them that some of the bullet points had a stronger evidence base than others (see the "Interview Guide" in Appendix A). Then I asked whether this sort of uncertainty would change their response. Just four men said it would. For example, Wei explained, "If there's uncertainty,

I think it's less compelling for me or for anybody to try to avoid a birth defect in, for example, choosing a diet." However, the majority of men said the precise levels of risk did not matter and stated, like Travis, that they would "err on the side of caution." Daniel, a twenty-three-year-old who planned to have children someday, noted, "I don't know how bad the numbers are, but I mean if there's any way to increase the probability of having a healthy child, then by all means take all necessary precautions."

Now, one of the most well-documented findings in the health literature is the gulf between what people say they will do and what they actually do. Entire models have been elaborated on the disconnect between health beliefs, health intentions, and actual health behaviors.[17] Aware of these dynamics, several respondents underlined the difference between what they saw as "basic" health advice in the leaflet—what David called the "life code," and Michael the "hallmarks of healthy living"—and the actions men could reasonably be expected to take. Neeraj, who had been incarcerated for most of his adult life, put it this way:

> Everybody knows to be healthy and eat healthy. These aren't groundbreaking things, right? These are fundamental whether you want healthy sperm or not. You should be healthy and maintain healthy weight and exercise and not smoke. But what we know and what we do are two completely different things in this life.

Thus, men's professed willingness to comply with health maxims about sperm is just that: talk. It cannot be taken as an indication of what they would actually do in their everyday lives.

Nevertheless, men's initial responses will not come as any surprise to Foucaultian-inspired scholars of biopolitics, who document the nearly mandatory response of acquiescence in the face of health information, all in the service of demonstrating that one is a modern, responsible individual.[18] As James put it, reading through the leaflet made him "feel *compelled* to be healthier" (emphasis added). Indeed, men's descriptions of how they themselves would react reflect the intertwining processes of individualization and moralization, in which health becomes a function primarily of individual behavior and not broader forces.

But stopping there would offer only a partial read of men's responses, because more than half did go on to identify a range of barriers—personal, structural, economic, environmental—standing between individual men and "healthy sperm." That they did so in the context of answering a question about *other* men suggests their initial reactions might be tinged by "social desirability bias," a common phenomenon in research, where people strive to present themselves in the best possible light, offering more socially acceptable answers while displacing their actual beliefs onto others.

Sometimes I asked about the average guy "out there," and other times I asked about the "average guy you know"; both queries yielded an array of reasons why men would be likely to "blow off" the advice or find it difficult to follow even if they were interested in doing so. For example, James pointed to widespread skepticism of science and medical expertise[19] and to "antiquated" beliefs about gender that could preclude men from taking the leaflet seriously. Malik might have been obliquely referring to a long history of medical abuse toward people of color in describing his fear of clinicians.[20] He also underscored the difficulty of avoiding chemicals at home and work, which is true not only for those in low-wage jobs but also for people in professions such as dentistry and laboratory research (see chapter 3). And he laughed as he contemplated the preposterous proposition that the average guy he knows would undertake the complete lifestyle overhaul outlined in the leaflet, repeating, "It's just not going to work."

Likewise, many of the other reasons men gave were rooted in their own personal circumstances, while also casting a critical light on broader processes that powerfully shaped those circumstances. Here are some examples.

- Those taking medications for physical or mental health pointed to the necessity of prioritizing their current well-being over the possibility of future sperm damage:

  I am taking antidepressants [for depression and social anxiety, which are] medications [for my] immediate health. . . . I would really like to enforce [the leaflet] on myself: to have a healthy diet, try to be more active than I am, and I guess for mental health, kind of also treat my mental health just as important.
  Seth, 23

- Gay men familiar with the demands of heteronormative masculinity referred to the cultural belief in male invulnerability:

Even if you told them, I don't think guys would think about [healthy sperm]. "Oh, my sperm is fine. It's good. I have super sperm." That's what they would say. [*laughs*] I think that people, mostly men, think that they're immortal and that nothing can hurt them.

Aaron, 43

- African American men who had experienced the harmful effects of racism resisted a long history of social control over Black people's reproduction[21] by questioning medical authority in this realm:

[The average men I know would respond] very immaturely. They would sit here and look at this list and be like, "Oh well, so what? I'm fat, and I eat cheeseburgers everyday, and yeah, I drink alcohol and smoke and everything else, but all of my kids, they're fine, so this is just a bunch of BS. How are *they* going to tell me how to have kids?"

Bruce, 38

- Men living in poverty lamented the many structural health inequalities built into the American system, from the lack of access to quality care to the need for copious amounts of time and money to "eat right" and exercise:

If you're born into a low-income situation, the culture is entirely different than if you're born into a healthy and wealthy family. If you're born into a wealthy family you have better health care, you have a better nutritional model to learn from. If you're poor, you can't afford healthy food.[22]

Paul, 29

- Those who had struggled with homelessness and drug addiction indicted economic and political systems that place profit over protecting the vulnerable:

I think that people don't take care of themselves as well as they should. I think there are more things on the market that's sold that are bad for you today then there was years ago, and people get addicted to these things, whether it be food that's bad for you or drugs and alcohol.

Rob, 49

- And for everyone, the environmental hazards encountered every day as one breathes air, drinks water, and eats food:

> Avoiding toxic substances is impossible.
>
> Angelo, 39

In each instance, men are making clear that an individual's health is not solely a matter of that individual's choices. Instead, the health of any one body is the outcome of complex interactions between biological, cultural, economic, structural, and historical processes; think back to the nested dolls in the Introduction. This argument has been made by those working in a variety of academic fields, such as medical sociology and social epidemiology.[23] However, it has yet to garner the organizational and financial clout of the more traditional public health focus on individual volition. I conclude the chapter by considering what it would mean to take this perspective seriously and how it would shift public health messaging on reproductive risk and responsibility.

EQUALIZING REPRODUCTIVE RISK AND RESPONSIBILITY

In addition to trenchant critiques of the over emphasis on individual culpability, another curious dynamic emerged during the latter part of many interviews. At some point after reviewing the leaflet, more than half the men took a moment to reflect on how it had shifted their perceptions of women's and men's responsibility for reproductive outcomes. As we were wrapping up the interview, Matt said he thought this would be important information to share with his friends:

> It's not just the woman. It's the man too. And I never really thought about that. But you're right, it is the man's responsibility to eat healthy and stuff to have a healthy child. It's not just the woman. It's both.

Elijah, the twenty-one-year-old who had talked about children with his girlfriend, adapted the leaflet's advice to tell a new version of the old story about men causing pregnancy:

> I was going to say it mostly has to do with the women, but no, it's really us because we carry the sperm. Without us, there would be no baby, so I mean we play a huge factor in having kids. I thought it was just always women have to be tiptop, but no, we have to be.

And Chad returned to what he learned as a pre-med to revise some of those lessons in light of this new information about paternal effects:

CHAD: Women's reproductive systems seem to be always talked about as being far more complex, whereas with men it's—. My physiology teacher, she was explaining the whole parasympathetic and sympathetic, how it all plays into reproduction. "With men, it's simple. Remember it's just point and shoot." Erection and ejaculation; so it's simplified in those terms. [But now that you ask me to pick three words to describe the topic of men's reproduction] I guess I am trying to think of a way to say like *deceptively simplified*, because no matter what everybody—. The smallest thing in our bodies is so complex. So yeah, I'd say that it appears to be simple where it can be somewhat complex.

RENE: So what is complex about men's reproduction?

CHAD: With men, I think it has to do with where it all starts: with sperm production itself. You start at these little cells, the spermatogenesis. It goes through all those different phases, and then it becomes sperm. Then it has to travel through a very sort of complex system of tubes and loops. Then that's finally deposited into the woman. I think that's kind of what I meant as far as complexity. It's not as simple as just "point and shoot." There's a lot more that goes into it.

With these comments, men are incorporating information they had just learned from a one-page leaflet to tell a new biological story about the surprising significance of men's health for reproductive outcomes. Moreover, it was not only those who already held more gender-egalitarian beliefs or told the second sperm story (as discussed in chapter 5) who articulated this sense of equalization when considering women's and men's contributions to reproductive risk. This is consistent with what Kate Reed found about genetic screening during pregnancy: men become more interested in how their genes affect fetal outcomes when they too are offered prenatal testing alongside their female partners.[24] In this case, that such a brief introduction to paternal effects could shift the tales men tell about sperm suggests that publicizing this information more widely could have ramifications not only for gendered beliefs about reproductive health but for reproductive politics more broadly. I return to this point in the Conclusion of the book.

RETHINKING REPRODUCTIVE HEALTH MESSAGING

Given the historical lack of attention to the health of men's reproductive bodies, there is no reason to expect men would spontaneously draw connections between the terms *healthy* and *sperm*. While men do tend to perceive their bodily involvement as crucial to reproduction—recall from the last chapter that most men conceptualize sperm as the active agent in establishing a pregnancy—the significance of this bodily involvement does not currently extend to a consideration of their own age and bodily health. It is the "surprise" of this information being applied to male bodies that offers an opportunity to think anew about the well-worn messages everyone is used to hearing about women's reproductive health. Here, I consider what might happen if there was a sustained effort to forge such a cognitive link between *health* and *sperm*, of using public health messages to draw attention to the significance of men's age, behaviors, and exposures for reproductive outcomes.

On the most basic level, to frame any issue as a matter of health immediately trains one's attention at the level of individual bodies and away from structural and environmental causes of disease. This has long been recognized as a key feature of "medicalization," in which issues that may previously have been considered a matter of morality or criminality are reinterpreted as medical conditions to be treated by clinicians. Classic examples include infertility (redefined from a matter of God's will to a biological condition) and alcoholism (redefined from a moral failing to a disease).[25] One reason the social process of medicalization tends to result in the further individualization of conditions is that diseases afflict some bodies and not others, and so those who are sick must be (individually) treated. However, it is almost never the case that any one condition is solely the result of individual-level processes. Because individual bodies are nested within families and neighborhoods and nations in particular times and places, the powerful confluence of cultural, structural, and environmental processes should not be ignored.[26]

It is not only that the significance of these broader forces are ignored (or downplayed) in most approaches to health and medicine; the focus on individuals easily slides into an expectation of personal responsibility for wellness. This dynamic is manifest in the following quote from Hong, a twenty-nine-year-old scientist from China, who explains how his wife's first pregnancy ended in miscarriage. Afterwards, they both underwent fertility testing in the hospital, and after coming across research on paternal effects, his wife asked Hong to change some of his behaviors as they attempted to have a child.

> In China, the air and water is heavily polluted. So you have to do everything to be careful to have a baby before you are trying to make your wife pregnant. So I and my wife, she required me to do everything to be cautious. So I don't drink at that time when we were trying to have a baby. About for half a year, even with a party with friends, I never drink. And I try—I don't eat unhealthy food. And also I don't smoke. No drugs. We do everything trying to be cautious.

In contrast to James and Malik, Hong was not at all representative of my respondents. Not only was he already familiar with much of the advice in the "Healthy Sperm" leaflet, he had actually attempted to enact much of it. This may be due to Hong's origins in China, where there has been more publicity about the effects of pollution and smoking on sperm.[27] But his quote reveals that even as he pointed to the importance of environmental pollution, his efforts were concentrated on his own individual actions: what he eats and drinks. Norah MacKendrick finds a similar dynamic among women who attempt to manage "chemical body burdens"—the accumulation of everyday toxins in bodily tissue—through careful consumption: buying organic food, avoiding baby bottles made with BPA, and the like. MacKendrick notes that these kinds of approaches place the onus on individual women and fail to address the larger, collective problem that is pollution.[28] Hong's experience suggests that men are not immune from these sorts of pressures, even as he describes a traditional gendered dynamic in which the person responsible for finding the information and encouraging him to follow it is his wife.

Social scientists have long noted that an individual's failure to achieve health can result in blame and stigmatization, not to mention feelings of anxiety and guilt.[29] Certainly, these various pitfalls are well-known to contemporary women, who continue to shoulder the bulk of responsibility for reproductive outcomes.[30] In the Conclusion, I return to John, the imaginary man living in the imaginary world, with whom I opened the book, to consider more fully how the "newness" of knowledge about paternal effects can be mobilized to rethink reproductive health messages. How can men be brought more fully into focus when talking about reproductive health while avoiding the individualization of damaged sperm, with its tendency to stigmatize those who are already socially disadvantaged?

Conclusion

THE POLITICS OF MEN'S REPRODUCTIVE HEALTH

It turns out that it is no small task to argue there is a missing science of men's reproductive health. Taking on the hegemony of biomedical knowledge about bodies and sifting through historical records and contemporary conversations, I have sought to establish how the conceptualization of the male body as not reproductive has influenced which knowledge is made, whether it circulates, and how it permeates the thinking of everyday Americans.

This research is both necessary and urgent, and it is made more so by the social and political exigencies of the contemporary United States, where inequalities of all sorts intersect to afflict reproductive politics. In what follows, I summarize the main argument of the book before drawing out its implications for scholarly debates about gender and medical knowledge. Then turning to the question of what's next, I offer potential paths forward for those in the general public, biomedical research, health care, and public health.

NON-KNOWLEDGE ABOUT MEN'S REPRODUCTIVE
HEALTH HAS CONSEQUENCES

Age-old assumptions about gender—namely, that women's biological and social capacities are rooted in reproduction, while men's lives are defined in more expansive terms—infused the initial development of medical specialties in the late nineteenth century. Many of those early specialties and some of their assumptions are still with us, in part because the initial infrastructure offered by professional societies and medical journals created an institutionalized space for the production and accretion of knowledge. However, even with the expanding base of biomedical knowledge, there was no sustained attention to how men's health matters for reproduction. Certainly, a variety of experts took interest in various aspects of male reproductive bodies: life scientists studying embryology, eugenicists advocating reproductive fitness, endocrinologists characterizing hormones, fertility doctors assessing sperm. But their efforts did not cohere into a singular, organized realm of biomedical inquiry, much less a specialty. Instead, founded on cultural conceptions of sex as a binary, attempts to create a formal entity called "andrology" that would parallel gynecology repeatedly fell flat. Thus, there has been little professional infrastructure to support the production of knowledge about men's reproductive health. To this day, andrologists in the United States are few and far between, and their purview tends to be restricted to the technical aspects of sperm. And while the topic of men's reproductive health certainly hovers around the edge of multiple specialties—urology, sexual health, infertility, endocrinology—it does not serve as the focus of any specialty in particular. It is a form of medical specialization that has not occurred.

This lack of a biomedical specialty and, more generally, the *in*attention to men's reproductive bodies reverberated throughout the twentieth century and into the present, affecting the production, circulation, and reception of knowledge about men's reproductive health. For much of this period, questions about how men's bodies might affect reproductive outcomes were hardly thinkable, so they went unasked. Even in reproductive medicine, many twentieth-century physicians did not consider doing a simple sperm analysis even as they simultaneously subjected female patients to endless tests and procedures. When a few scientists and clinicians did begin to conduct research on paternal effects, they faced unusually strong opposition to their hypotheses. Several described difficulties securing the funding necessary to collect data and then endured disbelief from colleagues even when they achieved noteworthy results.

Without the biomedical infrastructure that accompanies a developed specialty, the little knowledge that has been produced is hardly publicized. There are no federal health agencies devoted to men's reproductive health issuing official statements or professional medical organizations trumpeting the latest findings, and it is left to individual reporters to track down studies and write the occasional news article. Even then, the focus is typically limited to how men's age, behaviors, and exposures can harm sperm; only rarely do they mention that these factors can also affect children's health.

Non-knowledge about men's reproductive health also shapes the thinking of individual men and women. Given how little effort has been made to produce and then circulate such knowledge, it is hardly surprising that when people try to define a man's role in reproduction, they stumble and pause. Eventually, they settle on a trinity that includes having sex, producing sperm, and being a provider, but they almost never mention the potential effects of a man's age or his bodily health. When asked specifically about sperm and eggs, their biological stories are profoundly shaped by cultural conceptions of gender and genetics. Almost all of the men narrate a traditional tale of active sperm competing to penetrate the passive egg, but the younger and more-educated also tell a different, more egalitarian story in which these cells are two halves of a whole that come together. Men's reactions to learning about paternal effects and the prospect of "healthy sperm" only underscore the possibility that new stories can be told about men's reproductive health. Expressing both surprise and curiosity that their own health might affect their children's health, men wanted to share this information with their family and friends, even as they pointed to the pitfalls of individually oriented solutions in this realm.

In examining the historical and contemporary processes through which men's reproductive health has come to be overlooked, this study makes empirical contributions to social scientific research on gendered bodies, medical specialization, and knowledge-making. Of particular note, it is the first in-depth analysis of efforts to establish andrology as a specialty in the 1890s and the 1970s, as well as one of the first open-ended interview studies with men from the general public about their views regarding reproduction. A number of theoretical and policy implications flow from these results.

CULTURAL BELIEFS ABOUT GENDER SHAPE THE MAKING OF NON-KNOWLEDGE

The central theoretical argument of the book is that cultural beliefs about gender influence both the making and non-making of biomedical knowledge about reproduction. Specifically, it is the relationality of gender, undergirded by a historical belief in sex as two (and only two) dichotomous categories, that has enabled the long-standing association between women's bodies and reproductive health and the just as long-standing *non*-association between men's bodies and reproductive health. Crucially, these associations are related to one another, as illustrated by the photographer metaphor in the Introduction. It is because of the relationality of gender that the association of women and reproduction inhibits a focus on men and reproduction.

Moreover, as I have documented in this book, these associations (of women and reproduction and of men and non-reproduction) are maintained and reinforced over time by a feedback loop consisting of intertwining biological, cultural, and organizational processes. Cultural beliefs about the biological significance of sex differences—namely, that men and women each contribute biological material to conception but that pregnancy and birth occur primarily in women's bodies—come together with cultural beliefs about the invulnerability of male bodies to stymie the development of biomedical infrastructure oriented to men's reproductive health, with enormous implications for both the production and circulation of knowledge as well as how individuals conceptualize reproduction. Rather than asking *what* the relationship between gender and reproductive health is, which presumes a static answer, emphasizing the relationality and temporality of feedback loops allows for a theorization of the *process* through which reproductive health has become associated with women's bodies and not men's.

Indeed, none of this is written in stone. While the associations between gendered bodies and biomedical knowledge-making about reproduction have persisted for more than a century, one reason I chose the metaphor of feedback loops is that they allow for the possibility of change. Any shifts in the relevant biological, cultural, or organizational processes have the potential to influence the photographer's gaze and alter the resulting "images"— that is, biomedical knowledge, official statements, news reports, or individual beliefs. For example, the increasing visibility of trans scholarship and activism has already begun to shift the conceptual ground on which sex and gender binaries have been constructed.[1] Some reproductive health care providers have started referring to "pregnant people" (rather than pregnant *women*) in an effort to unsettle the gender binary and be inclusive of transmasculine and gender-nonconforming individuals who may seek contraception, an abortion, or prenatal care.[2] If efforts to reimagine gender as fluid or as a spectrum become widely adopted, then such shifts in cultural beliefs could affect everything from how biomedical scientists categorize subjects and pose research questions, who visits which kinds of health care providers, how those clinician-patient interactions unfold, as well as how individuals experience their own reproductive bodies.

This book also offers a new analytical approach for scholars interested in the production of non-knowledge, or the making of ignorance. Certainly, paternal effects is a case of non-knowledge that can be characterized in terms of typologies such as Croissant's.[3] It is not just a few facts that need to be clarified but a broad domain of knowledge that was missing, caused not by intentional obfuscation but by the interaction of biological, organizational, and cultural processes that rendered questions about damaged sperm un-thinkable. That is, until the 1970s, at a moment when social change from sources as disparate as the feminist movement and biological research on genetics set the stage for scientists to begin asking new questions about how men's age, behaviors, and exposures might affect sperm and, in turn, their children's health.

This crucial element of temporality makes it possible for present-day observers to "see" non-knowledge, to point to knowledge that now exists but that previously did not. And it is here that my adaptation of a rubric from the sociology of culture can extend the standard approach to non-knowledge by formulating an additional set of questions about what happens when knowledge goes from unmade to made. Sociologists of culture have long emphasized the importance of attending not only to the production of cultural objects—defined as anything from a song or a painting to legal regulations and scientific claims—but also to their circulation and reception.[4] By transposing this three-part framework of production, circulation, and reception from the broad realm of culture to the specific realm of non-knowledge, one can move beyond the question of whether or not knowledge exists to inquire about what happens when it begins to be produced. To what extent does it circulate, and how is it received?

When it comes to men's reproductive health, the answers to these questions shine new light on the relationship between medical specialization and non-knowledge in the United States. The first part of this book reveals the significance of biomedical infrastructure in the form of professional societies, annual meetings, and journals for the production and accretion of knowledge. The second part of this book demonstrates that even as new knowledge about paternal effects begins to be produced, the lack of a cohesive medical specialty focused on men's reproductive health means there are few organizational entities to publicize it, dramatically limiting its circulation. As a result, the American public remains generally unaware of new information about how a man's bodily health can affect his children's health.

While scholars have raised concerns about medical specialization fragmenting the body and precluding a holistic approach to the "whole person,"[5] this book illustrates some of the consequences that can stem from a *lack* of specialization. It also underscores crucial questions to ask as the medical profession carves up the body into particular specialties: what are scientists and clinicians paying attention to, and what are they ignoring? How does the process of grouping certain body parts and excluding others, or associating particular kinds of knowledge with particular kinds of bodies, affect which knowledge is made and which is not made?

WHAT'S NEXT?

The overarching recommendation that flows from the analysis in this book is for people to pay more attention to men's reproductive health, especially those people who are biomedical researchers, health care providers, and public health policy makers. By focusing on men's reproductive bodies, experts are in a position to create new knowledge and circulate it to the general public. And as more detailed information is available, particularly about how men's age, behaviors, and exposures affect children's health, this will likely influence how individuals think about reproductive risk and reproductive responsibility.

New knowledge about men's reproductive health could also reshape gender politics in surprising ways. That pregnancy and birth occur in women's bodies has long figured centrally in gendered expectations and gendered inequalities, such as assumptions that women with children are less committed to their jobs, resulting in reluctance to hiring mothers and paying them less.[6] New ways of thinking about whose bodies are reproductive may have ripple effects into broader social processes around gender.

But just *how* to pay more attention to men's reproductive health is not at all obvious. There are a number of complexities to consider, many of which are rooted in the historical relationship between gender and medical knowledge-making. First, there is the question of how to bring men's reproductive bodies into focus without replicating the problematic aspects of typical approaches to reproductive health. In the past, such messages have usually concentrated on individual women's bodies and behaviors, which tends to moralize the issue of health and stigmatize those who cannot achieve it. It can even result in medical surveillance, the pernicious effects of which are especially damaging to people who are already marginalized, such as racial minorities and the poor. For example, in hundreds of cases, women have actually been incarcerated for their behavior during pregnancy.[7] Rather than just adding men to the list of those who can be blamed, clinicians and public health officials could use the "newness" of information about paternal effects as an opportunity to rethink the usual approach to reproductive health information. How might these messages minimize individualization, avoid blame, and assuage anxiety and guilt?

One possibility would be to provide information about *both* women's and men's age and bodily health while *simultaneously* emphasizing the significance of structural and environmental factors for reproductive outcomes. To illustrate, think back to the vignette about John from the

Introduction, a hypothetical scenario in which a man tries to follow all of the advice about how to grow healthy sperm. To be sure, there are men like John in the world, who could work with their female partners to plan conception carefully and spend time and money preparing months in advance. And it is even likely that John's actions will mitigate reproductive risk to some as-yet-to-be-determined extent (see chapter 3). However, his approach is fundamentally individualist and consumerist: he finds books and magazines to read, purchases specific household products, and buys expensive organic food. What John is not able to control, what no individual can fully control, are the broader structural and environmental processes that can also damage sperm and pose risks to children's health.

Reframing reproductive health as not just about women and not just about individuals would entail nothing less than a paradigm shift. What if *all* bodies—female, male, trans, gender nonconforming, intersex, and so on—were conceptualized as (potentially) reproductive? And what if structural and environmental sources of risk were emphasized alongside individual factors? How might these twin developments shift our understandings of reproductive responsibility? Rather than placing the onus on individual women to eat right and avoid toxins, would officials redouble their efforts to ensure that *everyone* has access to healthy food and that *nobody* is exposed to harmful chemicals?

At the same time, there is reason to be cautious: many people have no interest in having children, and categorizing all bodies as potentially reproductive could easily be mobilized to justify various forms of social control, whether through informal norms or even government regulation. One need only think of Romania during the latter part of the twentieth century, where the dictator Nicolae Ceauşescu sought to build the population of future workers by banning abortion and conducting regular pregnancy tests on the factory floor, ensuring that women who became pregnant stayed that way.[8] Margaret Atwood has cited this history as one of the inspirations for her classic novel, *The Handmaid's Tale*.

In the end, though, addressing structural and environmental contributors to disease would benefit *all* bodies, whether they are reproducing or not. Actions such as increasing access to quality health care, reducing racial and economic inequalities, and adopting more stringent regulations to protect the air and water would also address another crucial social fact about reproduction: about half of all pregnancies in the United States are not planned.[9] Unlike John, millions of people every year become pregnant without a fully realized, intentional plan to do so. As such, they would not be in a position to take any of the individual-level measures enumerated in the "Healthy Sperm" brochure (chapter 6, figure 15). Consequently, for those who are not necessarily "trying" to have a child, a higher baseline level of bodily health that is only possible through structural interventions would likely reduce some amount of reproductive risk.

I do worry that emphasizing a man's involvement in reproduction will somehow be used by those advocating for "men's rights" to further erode women's already fragile reproductive rights in this country. Over the past several decades in the United States, access to safe and legal abortion has come under increasing threat from conservative activists and legislators, the effects of which are particularly dire for women with few financial resources.[10] It is not difficult to imagine these activists arguing that men should be given even more authority over women's bodies based on the newfound significance of sperm. So let me put it as bluntly as possible for an even-toned academic book: the person whose body is pregnant should be the only one with final say over whether a pregnancy continues.

It is with these all complexities in mind that I now turn to some specific recommendations for biomedical researchers, health care providers, and public health policy makers, suggesting ways they can pay more attention to men's reproductive health and how it is shaped by individual, structural, and environmental processes.

Biomedical Research

Biomedical research about men's reproductive health in general and paternal effects in particular has been garnering more attention than ever before, but women are still the primary (and often exclusive) focus of research in this realm. A Google Scholar search in 2018 for "maternal effects" yields 83,000 results, compared to just 6,400 results for "paternal effects."[11] Even the National Institutes of Health has taken notice of the gap, stating on its website: "Reproductive health is an important component of men's overall health and well-being. Too often, males have been overlooked in discussions of reproductive health."[12]

So the recommendation here is clear: biomedical researchers should stop thinking about women's bodies as the sole vector of reproductive risk and expand their sights to include the potential effects of men's age, behaviors, and exposures. As illustrated in the "reproductive equation" I sketched at the end of chapter 3 (figure 10), there is a great deal of work to be done to identify the various kinds of risks posed by men's bodily health, including how their health is the result not only of individual-level processes but also structural and environmental processes. Researchers need to quantify the amount of risk posed by each of these factors, as well as their cumulative impact and how paternal factors interact with maternal factors. Such data are crucial because as long as the focus remains primarily on women's bodies, researchers will be missing some unknown amount of risk that emanates from men's bodies.

The question is who will do that research. As I document, there is no cohesive biomedical specialty for men's reproductive health. One approach would be to advocate for the creation of such a specialty, or perhaps the expansion of andrology, to serve as a broad umbrella for the various scientists and clinicians who study and treat male reproductive bodies. However, such a move to institute men's reproductive health as a separate entity from women's reproductive health would echo previous attempts to create a "parallel" specialty, and it would just end up reifying the gender binary. By that, I mean it would reinforce the cultural belief that humans are categorizable as just one of two completely separate and "opposite" sexes: male or female. If the subject of reproduction, which is now implicitly associated with women, were to be explicitly bifurcated into women's reproduction versus men's reproduction, it might increase attention to the importance of men's reproductive health, but it would simultaneously serve to biologically ground (problematic) claims about sex and gender difference. Thus, for both logistical and theoretical reasons, I believe the topic of men's reproductive health should be more deeply incorporated into *preexisting* biomedical infrastructure.

Indeed, there are various mechanisms that could be mobilized to spur more research on men's reproductive health. During the past decade, a handful of articles in medical journals have offered a range of suggestions, many of which have yet to be enacted.[13] For example, medical schools, nursing schools, and programs in the biological sciences could incorporate material on men's reproductive health into the curriculum, and they could establish training programs, such as postdoctoral fellowships, for those interested in paternal effects. Medical training programs, especially in family medicine and internal medicine but also in specialties such as urology, ob-gyn, pediatrics, reproductive endocrinology, maternal/fetal medicine, sexual health, and genetics, could ensure that residents learn about the significance of men's age and health for children's health. Federal agencies could emphasize men's reproductive health and earmark funds for innovative research on this topic. Philanthropic organizations, including those devoted generally to health or reproduction as well as foundations focused on particular diseases linked to paternal effects, could work to help financially support this emerging area of research. Professional medical associations could issue statements about the need for additional research about men's reproductive health and develop clinical policy guidelines for those in a position to advise patients about paternal effects. At present, there are offices in federal agencies, departments in medical schools, and professional associations that focus on "reproductive health" and "reproductive medicine." These technically gender-neutral terms could be intentionally expanded to include the reproductivity not only of women's bodies but also of men's, trans, and nonbinary bodies.

Individual researchers, too, have a role to play. In making decisions about how to study reproductive risk, they can be sure to integrate an analysis of paternal factors. Such factors can be systematically incorporated into preexisting research frameworks, such as the developmental origins of health and disease (DOHaD), which has historically focused on maternal factors.[14] Questions about men's reproductive health could also be added to national surveys about fertility and health. One commentator in *Pediatrics* points out, "*No* existing data set is dedicated to fathers in the perinatal period, and few comprehensively follow fathers over time."[15]

As researchers turn their attention to men's reproductive health, they will need to avoid making a priori assumptions about how male and female bodies are different. Social scientists have pointed to a persistent lack of precision in just how *sex* is defined and operationalized in health research.[16] Beliefs about sex difference are all too often built into the research design instead of actually being investigated. This is particularly prevalent in "gender-specific medicine," an approach that is rooted in biological essentialism and has resulted in an endless parade of findings that tautologically confirm the "realness" of biological sex.[17]

Finally, it may be necessary for institutional review boards (IRBs), which are charged with the protection of human subjects enrolled in biomedical research projects, to begin considering the possibility of reproductive risks to men. At present, research with pregnant women receives extra scrutiny from IRBs to ensure that any risks to offspring are minimal. For clinical studies involving the use of substances that might damage sperm (e.g., chemicals and pharmaceuticals), IRBs could pivot to a gender-neutral question, asking researchers to request information about the reproductive plans of all their subjects. The goal would be to incorporate an analysis of reproductive risk for men as part of the broader evaluation of potential risks and benefits for each study.

Health Care

Turning from the realm of biomedical research to the clinic, where new knowledge can be put into practice, health care providers need to begin routinely raising the topic of reproductive health with men. Currently, those conversations are not happening. In my interviews with men, they reported picking up bits and pieces of information from a wide range of sources, such as social media and blogs; conversations with family and friends; television dramas and documentaries; classes in high school and college on topics such as sex education, biology, and physiology; and magazines and books.[18] But the men almost never mentioned receiving information from a health care provider. The few surveys on this topic concur, revealing that men are extremely unlikely to hear about paternal effects or preconception health from clinicians.[19]

In part, this is because men rarely go to the doctor.[20] Unlike women, who are encouraged to have their reproductive organs examined on a regular basis throughout adulthood, men could jump from a late-adolescent physical to their first colonoscopy at age fifty without ever seeking preventive health care.[21] When men do go to the doctor, their visits are typically shorter than women's and less likely to include preventive health information.[22]

So what is the medical profession to do? There is some low-hanging fruit in the form of preconception care appointments, which are designed to enable people who are already planning to become pregnant to assess whether there is anything they can do to increase the chances of a healthy child. Currently, the advice typically dispensed in those appointments is directed exclusively at women, but it would be very easy to include a discussion about how men's age, behaviors, and exposures can affect reproductive outcomes. Even as the precise amount of risk remains uncertain, the available evidence suggests that individual men may be in a position to reduce some amount of that risk, such as by decreasing their consumption of various substances and considering the chemicals they encounter at home and work. Likewise, in fertility clinics, when heterosexual couples have already walked in the door seeking assistance with conception, clinicians can take the time to evaluate and advise male partners about how their reproductive health can influence the success of fertility treatments.

It is less clear how clinicians might reach men who are not already seeking reproductive health information. Certainly, most men do find themselves visiting a health care provider for one reason or another during their adult years, such as a physical required for a job, routine screening for blood pressure or cholesterol, or sickness. Indeed, primary care clinicians have begun making the argument they are best positioned to address men's preconception health, with the American Academy of Family Physicians stating in a position paper that "male reproductive health issues should be an integral part of *every* wellness visit."[23] One approach would be to inquire about a man's reproductive plans, the equivalent of the "one key question" already routinely asked of women.[24] If the man indicated the possibility of having children, then the clinician could offer advice about paternal effects. Another potential venue is the pediatrician's office, where the parents of small children may mention they are trying to have another child. To prepare clinicians for such conversations, the topic of men's reproductive health could be added to continuing education requirements for those in family medicine, internal medicine, and pediatrics. Part of that continuing education will likely need to address the possibility of embarrassment not only on the part of patients but also clinicians, who may not be used to discussing men's reproductive bodies. In settings where "men's health" or "sexual health" is already a focus,[25] clinicians can work to ensure that some amount of attention is given to the reproductive health of men and to paternal effects in particular.

Another potential way of reaching men is through women who make regular visits to an ob-gyn or reproductive health clinic, such as Planned Parenthood. Already, reproductive health care providers are encouraged to ask women about their reproductive plans during each visit; if women indicate an interest in becoming pregnant, then the clinician could provide information about preconception health not only for women but also for men. While many of their patients will be coupled with men, this information would be just as useful to single women or lesbian couples who are seeking sperm from donors. There is much to like about the logistics of this strategy; many women already regularly visit a reproductive health care provider, and if they are thinking about becoming pregnant, they will likely be interested in learning that a man's age, behaviors, and exposures can matter for children's health. However, this approach does reinforce the notion that reproduction is women's responsibility, putting the onus on them to manage not only their own health but that of men.

Public Health

Ultimately, the infrequency of men's interactions with clinicians suggests that more generalized public health messages may be a more effective way of circulating information about men's reproductive health. At the moment, very little effort is being made to do so (see chapter 4). So here too the recommendation is clear: public health officials should devote more resources to publicizing the significance of men's reproductive health, how it is shaped not only by individual-level factors but also by structural and environmental processes and how damage to sperm can affect the next generation. They could develop new fact sheets and patient brochures to be distributed to local health departments and primary care providers, posted on health websites, and shared on social media. Likewise, nonprofit organizations that focus on reproductive health, such as Planned Parenthood and the March of Dimes, could work to publicize the significance of paternal effects. Government officials could consider requiring warning labels on alcoholic beverages, cigarettes, and pharmaceuticals, as well as on chemicals used in homes and workplaces, notifying men of the potential for harm to sperm. For their part, federal regulators need to dramatically expand their efforts to assess and regulate chemicals and other pollutants.[26]

Given how few Americans are aware of paternal effects, public health officials may also want to develop a national campaign to introduce the general public to basic facts about how a man's age, behaviors, and exposures can affect not only sperm but the health of his children. My qualitative interviews with men about their reactions to this information provide a starting point for such efforts, and public health scholars have called for just this type of data to better inform preconception healthcare and messaging.[27] Information about paternal effects is likely to be of most interest to those who are currently contemplating children, but it is worth noting that most of the men I spoke with expressed curiosity about the possibility that their health might affect reproductive outcomes. They called it "eye-opening," and several asked for a copy of the "Healthy Sperm" leaflet I created so they could share it with family and friends. However, nearly half the men wanted more detail: How much alcohol is too much? Which medications posed a threat? How old is too old? One man summed it up by asking, "How unhealthy is unhealthy?"

Even without precise answers to these questions, public health officials can communicate the basic fact that men's reproductive health matters. Careful thought—and rigorous pretesting—will be necessary to figure out how best to communicate such messages. In the interviews, the men suggested using humor and playing on beliefs about masculinity. One offered the slogan "Real men grow strong sperm," and another suggested playing off the Army slogan "Be all that you can be." One man recalled the ubiquitous eggs-in-the-frying-pan ad from the 1980s to suggest a series of images, such as "This is your sperm on drugs." While this tongue-in-cheek approach can be quite effective, as in the "Don't mess with Texas" campaign against littering, it does also reinforce traditional notions of manhood.

Health officials could also integrate a focus on men's reproductive health into preexisting initiatives, such as goals related to preconception health in Healthy People 2020.[28] Scholars and activists working on "reproductive justice" have used a human-rights framework to move beyond the focus on individual women to spotlight the importance of healthy communities,[29] a crucial insight that also applies to men's reproductive lives. Environmental advocates concerned about the effects of endocrine disruptors could expand the focus beyond sperm count to argue that such exposures can also damage the DNA inside sperm and affect children's health. Globally, international organizations have sought to "involve" men in reproductive health by advocating a men-as-partners framework.[30] This could easily be expanded beyond the current focus on social support to underscore the significance of men's bodily health to reproductive outcomes.

Beyond the direct purview of public health, educators teaching high school courses on health or sex education can add information about men's reproductive health and paternal effects to the curriculum. Several of the men I interviewed noted that high school was the last time they heard anything about their reproductive systems. A few men mentioned churches and gyms as other sites that could publicize the role of men's health in reproductive outcomes. Additionally, companies offering at-home sperm tests could include information about how men's age, behaviors, and exposures can damage sperm. Similarly, the developers of apps designed for women who are attempting pregnancy, including those that track ovulation and offer general advice (such as What to Expect When You're Expecting), could incorporate messages about the importance of *men's* health for reproductive outcomes, although this raises similar issues to asking ob-gyns to talk to female patients about their male partners (discussed in the previous section). Indeed, it may not take long for entrepreneurs to seize on the moneymaking possibilities of publicizing paternal effects; at least one start-up is already encouraging men who may want children someday to bank their sperm now while they are still young, calling it the "best life investment you'll make."[31]

.   .   .   .   .

As biomedical researchers, health care providers, and public health officials take steps to pay more attention to men's reproductive health, it will be important to consider language. Right now, there is no agreed-upon terminology, with phrases like *paternal effects, male-mediated effects, men's preconception health,* and *healthy sperm* being used interchangeably. It would be helpful to develop consistent language, so that the general public can get used to hearing about this topic and pull together bits of information from different sources.

At the same time, it is necessary to be cognizant of both the long history of eugenics and ongoing discrimination against people with disabilities. Terms such as "sperm quality" echo through this history, and one can imagine the language of "damaged sperm" being invoked to describe "damaged children." Thus, it is crucial to underscore the purpose and limits of improving men's reproductive health: the focus is on *reducing* reproductive risk while understanding that the *elimination* of all such risk is impossible. And these efforts should proceed hand in hand with ongoing work to create a more inclusive society where all kinds of bodies with all kinds of abilities are welcome.

FINAL WORDS

Now, as centuries of scientific inquiry demonstrate, just because knowledge is made does not make it the final word on a subject, or even correct. Recent revelations about men's reproductive health and its influence on the next generation are hardly immune to the iterative, plodding nature of knowledge-making. Five years or ten years from now, there may be new findings and other interpretations. So what is one to do about the current state of knowledge, about the incipient and still-minimal attention to men's reproductive bodies? Indeed, it may seem contradictory to argue in the same book that biomedical conceptualizations of reproduction are socially constructed *and* that we should think about them differently in order to conduct new scientific research, allocate federal dollars, and distribute public health resources.

Here, I take a page from Nancy Tuana's history of knowledge-making about the clitoris, one episode of which includes her comparison of its portrayal in 1970s-era medical textbooks versus the feminist-inspired handbook *Our Bodies, Ourselves*. In the medical texts, cross-sections of female genitalia imaged the clitoris as a small nub or left it out altogether, while *Our Bodies* included large, detailed drawings that distinguished among three structures: the shaft, glans, and crura. As Tuana writes, it is not as though the feminist handbook offered the final "truth" of the clitoris. Instead, she uses its competing "cartography" to spotlight a "politics of knowledge-ignorance" rooted in a long history of controlling and delegiti-mizing women's sexuality and pleasure.[32] Likewise, I argue that non-knowledge about men's reproductive health is a vital element in the poli-tics of reproduction.

Many questions—scientific, social, and political—about men's repro-ductive health have gone unasked and unanswered. The ultimate goal of this book is to stimulate the asking of such questions. Ours is a society in which reproductive risk and reproductive responsibility are located pri-marily in women's bodies. Adjusting the aperture to bring men's repro-ductive bodies into focus not only has the potential to improve men's health and the health of their children. It could also reshape reproductive politics and gendered inequalities.

APPENDIX A   Methods

Although I discuss some methodological specifics throughout the book, the purpose of this appendix is to detail the full process of data collection and analysis so that the reader can evaluate the evidentiary basis of my argument. When I first conceptualized this research project in a grant proposal to the National Science Foundation in 2014, I described the goal as "examining the historical and contemporary processes through which men have come to be overlooked in the realm of reproduction, as well as the social, clinical, and policy consequences that result from this gap in knowledge." I organized data collection around the production, circulation, and reception of biomedical knowledge about men's reproductive contributions from the late nineteenth century to the present, using a range of historical, qualitative, and quantitative methods.

THE PRODUCTION OF BIOMEDICAL KNOWLEDGE

As a starting point for examining when and how knowledge about men's reproductive contributions had been produced, as well as how it had been shaped by changing cultural norms, biological knowledge, and biomedical infrastructure, I began by reading widely in the relevant historical and social scientific literature, including studies about reproductive medicine,[1] hormones,[2] male contraception,[3] sperm,[4] venereology,[5] male circumcision,[6] men's experiences of birth,[7] impotence/erectile dysfunction,[8] and male infertility,[9] as well as research on men's bodies outside the context of the clinic, including in the military and sports.[10]

Taking a cue from historians, who had noted the significance of the latter half of the nineteeth century for both the professionalization and specialization of medicine, I began looking for instances in which the nascent medical profession focused on male reproductive bodies. It was in reading Ornella Moscucci's history of gynecology and Adele Clarke's history of reproductive medicine that I came across brief mentions of an andrological society founded in the late 1800s. This seemed like a promising starting place for my analysis, but I could not find any additional historical studies that discussed this event. I turned to my historian colleagues, spoke with medical history librarians, and searched historical databases and documents for mentions of andrology or its cognates, such as *andrologist* and *andrological* (in, e.g., Google Books, HathiTrust, ArchiveGrid, JSTOR, and the *Index Catalogue of the Library of the Surgeon-General's Office*). I used these same sites to search more broadly for references to men's reproduction, sperm, and related locutions of the time such as "organs of generation."

Building from the results of these searches, I pieced together the emergence of andrology in the late 1800s by tracking down meeting minutes, transactions from medical conferences, articles and letters published in medical journals, medical textbooks, obituaries, and the scant archival material about the key actors, such as personal correspondence, memoirs, and photographs. I analyze these materials in chapter 1, paying attention to how cultural notions of gender shaped the actions of late-nineteenth-century physicians attempting to organize a new medical specialty oriented to male bodies.

Given that so many materials from the twentieth century are now digitized, it was easy to track the occasional mentions of andrology that appeared in the decades following its organizational demise in the United States. As the Ngrams in chapter 3 reveal, though, there was an exponential uptick in mentions of andrology and men's reproductive health at the end of the 1960s. Rather than attempt to systematically analyze the entire twentieth century in terms of medical specialization around male reproductive bodies, I decided to compare and contrast these two key moments: the failed effort to establish andrology in the 1890s with the successful effort in the late 1960s.

For the latter period, I looked first to meeting transactions, obituaries and memoirs, early issues of andrological journals (*Andrologie* in 1969, *International Journal of Andrology* in 1978, and the *Journal of Andrology* in 1980), and websites of professional societies (e.g., International Society of Andrology, American Society of Andrology). I also reviewed the digitized archival materials of the American Society of Andrology, housed at Iowa State University, which includes letters and materials from the organization's founding. I employed research assistants who spoke German, Spanish, and Portuguese to try to track down connections between the various international figures involved in establishing andrology. I supplemented this historical research with qualitative interviews of three andrologists who were around at the time the specialty was being founded.[11] For additional context, I conducted five more interviews with prominent scientists and clinicians who are active researchers now on issues related to men's reproductive health.

There was very little information about some of those involved in andrology in the 1970s. For example, the Argentinean scientist Roberto E. Mancini was a cofounder of the Comité Internacional de Andrología, which became the International Society of Andrology (discussed in chapter 2). One of the few places he appears on the internet is an entry on the bare-bones website NeglectedScience. com, which describes itself as containing "biographical notes of distinct and forgotten scientists from developing countries." In searching for information about Mancini, I came across a profile of Roberto C. Mancini, a physicist at the University of Nevada whose degrees were from the University of Buenos Aires. He kindly responded to my email inquiring if he knew Roberto E. Mancini by identifying himself as his son; he then spent an hour on the phone sharing what he knew of his father's scientific life and sent along various materials I discuss in chapter 2.

THE CIRCULATION OF BIOMEDICAL KNOWLEDGE

Pivoting from biomedical specialization to biomedical knowledge-making, chapter 3 is a scientific literature review of research on paternal effects. Working with Jenna Healey, then a graduate student in Yale's History of Science and Medicine program, we first conducted a cursory review of research on sperm published in *JAMA* (a top medical journal) from its inception in 1883 through 2015.[12] Based on the trends we observed in the *JAMA* articles, we narrowed our attention to the scientific and medical literature on paternal effects published since 1970. Searching PubMed, ScienceDirect, and Google Scholar, we used terms such as "paternal effect*," "male-mediated developmental toxicology," and "advanced paternal age." Once we identified a high-quality review, we used its bibliography to identify additional studies. We excluded studies that were solely about male infertility and included studies about how men's age, health, behaviors, and exposures can affect pregnancy outcomes and children's health.

To examine whether and how new biomedical knowledge about paternal effects was circulating amongst a broader public, I worked with research assistant Celene Reynolds to search for reports and statements produced by federal health agencies, professional medical associations, consumer websites devoted to health and parenting, and the news media. Based on several thousands of pages, the content analysis in chapter 4 still does not include an exhaustive list of every word published about how men matter for reproductive outcomes. Instead, my goal was to capture the kinds of messages men might hear as they go about daily life.

The first search involved American government agencies with missions centered on health and illness (National Institutes of Health, Centers for Disease Control and Prevention, Department of Health and Human Services) or related matters (Environmental Protection Agency, Occupational Safety and Health Administration, and the Department of Defense). I also searched the website of one international organization, the World Health Organization. Since there is no singular medical specialty oriented to men's reproductive health, the second search for statements issued by professional medical associations involved first creating a list of any organizations that focused on reproductive health, men's health, and/or primary care: American Medical Association, American College of Obstetricians and Gynecologists, American Society for Reproductive Medicine, American Academy of Family Physicians, American Urological Association (and its patient site, Urology Care Foundation), Society for the Study of Male Reproduction, American Society for Men's Health, Society of Toxicology, American College of Medical Genetics, and the Academy of Nutrition and Dietetics. In the third search, I reviewed high-traffic consumer websites about health (WebMD, Mayo Clinic, and Men's Health) and parenting (Parents.com and What to Expect When You're Expecting).

In each of these searches, Celene first reviewed the home page for any mentions of men's reproductive health, sperm, conception, preconception, or related topics. Then, she used each site's search function to look for terms such as "reproductive health," "sperm*," "men's health," "reproductive hazard*," and "workplace hazard*." If a site returned scientific or clinical reports, I did not include those in the sample because that information was analyzed in chapter 3. Instead, I sought materials designed to be accessible to the general public. I also worked to ensure the temporal alignment of the scientific research discussed in chapter 3 with that of the publicly available materials discussed in chapter 4; since I conducted the searches for chapter 4 in the first few months of 2015, I restricted most of the analysis in chapter 3 to scientific findings published prior to 2015. In other words, I did not expect to find information written for the general public that had not yet been published in the scientific literature.

To examine news reporting about paternal effects, I used two different search strategies. First, I wanted to create a systematic sample of news coverage at the national level over time, so I worked with Celene to search a leading American newspaper, the *New York Times*, for articles that included "sperm" and its cognates from 1880 to 2018.[13] For the purposes of the *New York Times* content analysis in chapter 4, I analyzed articles published between 1968 and 2018 (N = 138). To ensure I also captured a wider array of news publications, the second search was centered on coverage of two books about paternal effects written for the general public: *The Male Biological Clock*, published in 2004 by urologist and media personality Harry Fisch, and *Do Fathers Matter? What Science Is Telling Us about the Parent We've Overlooked*, published in 2014 by science journalist Paul

Raeburn. Using a technique developed in research with Abigail Saguy on how the media covers science,[14] I used Nexis Uni to search major newspapers, magazines, and television news for mentions of these books in the two years following the publication of each (N = 21 articles for Fisch and 19 for Raeburn, not including duplicate articles that were reprinted in multiple papers).

It was in coding the sample of *New York Times* articles that I read about the March of Dimes public health campaign Men Have Babies Too. I contacted its archivist David Rose about my interest in paternal effects, and he provided expert guidance to the collection, pulling files not only about that campaign but other potentially useful materials.[15] To learn more about the origins of this campaign, in November 2019, I interviewed Jennifer Howse, president of the March of Dimes between 1990 and 2016.

To code all of these materials, I first categorized them as mentioning effects on sperm and/or children, by which I mean the distinction between the effects of men's age, behaviors, and exposures on sperm count, motility, or morphology versus specifically noting that these same factors can damage sperm in such a way that it can affect children's health. I also coded the materials for references to masculinity (including jokes and mentions of embarrassment), race, and class; whether the materials were addressed to women or men or both; mentions of the "newness" of this information; and direct comparisons to the large volume of information about women's reproductive health. Finally, I analyzed these materials based on the advice offered to men, especially whether it involved individual-level solutions or structural solutions or both. PDFs of all materials used in chapter 4 are on file with the author.

It is important to note what this multipronged search strategy does not capture: social media posts (e.g., Twitter, Facebook, blogs) and conversations between clinicians and patients. Social media is now an important medium through which scientific and biomedical information circulates, but the resources I had available for this project did not allow for a systematic search of these platforms. Future research on this topic could certainly explore the similarities and differences in how this information is presented more formally by organizations versus how it is discussed by individuals online. I chose not to observe clinician-patient interactions because the available research suggested that doctors rarely discuss these issues with their male patients,[16] making it unlikely that this form of time-intensive data collection would yield much data. Instead, I asked men in interviews whether their health care providers had ever raised these issues with them.

THE RECEPTION OF BIOMEDICAL KNOWLEDGE

The third part of the study involved qualitative, open-ended interviews with individuals about their views of men's reproduction and their reactions to new biomedical information about paternal effects. With IRB approval from Yale University, I recruited respondents from the general community in a single Northeastern city between 2014 and 2016. The town is both racially and economically diverse; of the 130,000 residents, about 35 percent identify as African American or Black, 32 percent as White, 27 percent as Hispanic or Latinx, and 5 percent as Asian.[17] While the city is home to a research university and academic medical center, which attract a highly educated workforce, more than a quarter of the city's residents live below the poverty line: $24,250 for a family of four in 2015.[18]

In relying on respondents from a single city, I follow the methodological lead of scholars like Emily Martin, whose classic *The Woman in the Body* was based on interviews with women in Baltimore, and Kathryn Edin and Timothy Nelson, whose study of low-income fathers was based on interviews with men in the Philadelphia metropolitan area.[19] As in those studies, my interviews do not constitute data that is representative of the national population. Instead, my goal was to find men from as many different backgrounds as possible in order to capture whatever variety might exist in terms of how people talk about men and reproduction. As a result, I sought men who were diverse in terms of age, parental status, socioeconomic status, and race, all of which I thought might affect their views about reproduction, sperm, and fatherhood. I did not search out men who had experienced infertility because there are already several interview studies with that population.[20] I also avoided recruiting men who were currently trying to have a baby or had a pregnant partner, because I was concerned about the ethics of presenting men with information that might provoke anxiety, especially because there is still uncertainty about the precise risks from paternal effects and how best to address them (see chapter 3 and the Conclusion).

Starting in November 2014, research assistant Todd Madigan posted paper flyers at locations around town: grocery stores, local universities and colleges, libraries, cafes, and bus stops. To avoid men who were particularly interested in reproduction or fatherhood, the flyers were purposely vague in identifying the study as about men's "life experiences." The full text of the ad read:

> YALE STUDY. Male volunteers aged 18–49 needed for a one-hour interview about life experiences. Participants will receive $20 for their time. To learn more and find out if you qualify, please call [phone number] or email us at [address]. This research project is led by faculty in the sociology department of Yale University. Human Subjects [approval number].

I also posted digital ads with the same text on Craigslist in the Gigs section and the Volunteer section. I purposely did not look for men in any sort of medical office. Social scientists have documented men's general unwillingness to go to the doctor,[21] so I thought that men recruited from clinics may be more knowledgeable about and receptive to biomedical information.

As men responded to the ad, Todd screened them by asking their age; race or ethnicity; the highest grade they had completed; whether they were a father or planned to be; if they were employed and what kind of work they did; and how they heard about the study.[22] I set eighteen as the minimum age to avoid IRB restrictions on interviewing minors and also because there are existing interview studies of teen fathers.[23] I set forty-nine as the maximum to mirror the ages used in the category "women of reproductive age" and also because there are relatively few births in the United States to fathers over the age of fifty. I did not ask about gender identity, and nobody raised it in the interviews. My flyer did request "male volunteers," and it is likely that all of my interviewees are cis men.

Recruitment proceeded quickly, and I conducted twenty-five interviews between November 2014 and February 2015. I kept a running tally to ensure the sample remained diverse in terms of the various demographic factors of interest, slightly modifying the flyer as needed to appeal to particular categories of men, such as "college-educated men aged 18–49" or "currently employed men aged 18–49." I became interested in whether men would provide different answers to a male interviewer, so I trained Todd, and he conducted the next nine interviews by the end of February. (At the time, I was also pregnant and beginning to show, and I did not want to have to take into account the added complexity of how men might respond to a pregnant woman interviewing them about reproduction.) In the end, both Todd and I heard similar kinds of responses to the interview questions, including a few fairly misogynistic statements, and our interviews were roughly the same length (on average, mine ran about ten minutes longer). This experience is consistent with previous research on gender-of-interviewer effects, which typically finds that it does not radically change the content of an interview.[24]

Originally, I planned to interview fifty men, but I stopped at thirty-four because I had reached "saturation," a loose qualitative-methods term for hearing the same thing over and over. Half the men were younger (eighteen- to twenty-nine-year-olds), and half were older (thirty- to forty-nine-year-olds). An equal proportion did and did not have children. About half the men had lower SES, a combination measure incorporating information on education, income, and occupation, while half had higher SES. In each of the SES categories, I sought a mix of White, African American, Latino, and Asian respondents.

As I began analyzing the interviews, though, I decided to expand my sample in two ways. First, I noticed that the two gay men in the sample provided surprisingly heteronormative answers to the reproduction question (discussed in chapter 5). These two men also happened to be married to one another, and both were HIV+. (There was no indication they were a couple until I was in the middle of the second interview and figured it out. Luckily, their interviews were one right after the other on a Saturday morning, so the first man did not have any time to debrief the second.) I was intrigued by their responses but certainly could not make any claims about "gay men" on the basis of their two interviews. I decided to talk with additional gay men with the hopes of comparing their answers to those of straight men. I posted paper flyers outside of gay bars and digital flyers on Craigslist and local LGBTQ-oriented Facebook pages; one ad called for "gay men" and the other requested "men who have sex with men" because not all MSMs identify as gay. I conducted six additional interviews with men from these groups in June 2016, bringing to forty the full number of interviews with men.

The second way I expanded the sample was to interview women about their views of men's reproduction. As I analyzed the interviews with men, I kept wondering (and audiences kept asking) whether women would answer questions about their role in reproduction differently. Leaving aside for the moment the point that it would be highly unlikely for audiences to wonder what men would say if it were women being interviewed about reproduction, I did think it was important to conduct a small number of interviews with women to do a truly *gendered* analysis, as I discuss in the Introduction, rather than assuming that men would give different answers than women would. I used the same flyers, the same recruiting techniques, the same sampling strategy, and the same interview guide with women, save for one question I added after the men's-role-in-reproduction question about how they would define a woman's role in reproduction. I interviewed ten women in July 2016, and research assistant Dana Hayward interviewed an additional five women in August 2016 for a total of fifteen.[25] See Table A in chapter 5 and appendix B for more information about the interviewees.

Depending on the day and time, the interviews were conducted either in a small conference room in a university library or at a quiet table in the back of a downtown cafe. They typically lasted around an hour (minimum = 24 minutes, maximum = 110 minutes). I began by presenting each respondent with an IRB consent form, which explained the procedures for maintaining anonymity and confidentiality and requested permission to record. To establish rapport and also to align the interview with the flyer's reference to "life experiences," I began with background questions about the respondent's everyday life, childhood, and experiences at school and work. I then asked several questions about family and children to transition to the topic of men's reproduction. The broad, open-ended questions about reproduction—How would you describe a man's role in reproduction? How would you describe the relationship between a sperm and an egg?— gave respondents the opportunity to express their views in their own words. As is the custom in qualitative interviewing, I returned to significant elements of their answers so that this part of the interview was driven as much as possible by the respondents and not by the researcher.[26]

However, in the latter part of the interview, I used a more researcher-directed approach by asking specific questions about their knowledge of paternal effects and how they had learned it, prompting them to discuss their interactions with clinicians, media sources, family, and friends. Then I presented each respondent with the leaflet reprinted in chapter 6 (figure 15), which I wrote at a tenth-grade reading level based on information and language in three sources: a peer-reviewed journal article by Frey et al. (2008) on the clinical content of preconception care for men, an article on the CDC's website titled "Preconception Health Information for Men" (2015), and a 2012 article titled "Healthy Sperm" on the Mayo Clinic's website. Although I was prepared to read it to anyone whose literacy seemed in doubt, men's subsequent comments and questions assured me they had been able to read and understand it. Only one man needed me to read it, and that was because he forgot his glasses.

I was not sure how much men would have to say about reproduction and sperm, but I was heartened by my own previous interviews with sperm donors, who were quite voluble on these subjects, as well as Edin and Nelson's report that they found it "surprisingly easy to convince fathers to talk with us."[27] Indeed, while there was a lot of laughter in the interviews, and some men certainly expressed surprise that an interview about "life experiences" took an unexpected turn into the topic of healthy sperm, everyone answered the questions. Each interview included a debrief about the current evidence base for the leaflet. At the end, I also offered to answer any questions the respondent had and briefly described the basic goals of the study. Here is the full interview guide.

Interview Guide

Informed consent—Before handing over the form, mention 1) anonymity (changing names and any identifying details they mention) and 2) the goal of the study is to write scholarly articles and a book.

-Thinking about your everyday life right now, please tell me about your life. (Prompts: daily routine, work, family)

  -Can you tell me about your childhood and growing up?

  -Experiences in high school, college?

  -(If dating/married) How did you meet your girlfriend/partner/spouse?

-Do you have any children?

  If yes: How old are they? How old were you when you had your first child? Can you tell me about your life at the time of your first child's birth? Were you trying to have a child? Did you do anything differently while you were trying to conceive a child?

  If no: Would you like to have children one day?

    If yes: How would you like your life to be when you have a child? Would you do anything differently if you were trying to conceive a child?

Now I'm going to ask you some more general questions . . .

-Thinking about the process of having children, if someone asked you to describe a man's role in reproduction, how would you describe a man's role in reproduction?

-If someone asked you to describe the relationship between an egg and a sperm, how would you describe the relationship between an egg and a sperm?

-If a man and a woman are planning to have a child, but they haven't conceived yet, do you know of anything a man can do to increase the chances the child will be healthy?

If yes: Do you remember where you learned this information?

-There are studies that show that older women are more likely to give birth to children with Down syndrome. Do you think a man's age has any effect on the health of the child?

If yes: Do you remember where you learned this information?

-Have you ever spoken with a doctor about conceiving a child?

If yes: Can you walk me through that conversation? What kinds of advice did you get?

-Have you ever spoken to family or friends about conceiving a child?

If yes: Walk me through those conversations.

Now I'd like you to read something and respond in any way you like. There are no right or wrong answers. (Give them the "Healthy Sperm" leaflet to read.)

-Walk me through your responses.

-If you were planning to have a child now, and your doctor gave you this information, how would you respond?

-Would you want your doctor to discuss this information with you?

-How do you think your partner/spouse would react to this information?

-So that is how you would respond. Now I want you to think about the average man you know. How do you think the average man you know would respond to this information?

-[Debrief] I should mention there are different levels of evidence for some of these risks. For example, doctors know that smoking more than two packs of cigarettes a day raises the risk of damaged sperm, but they don't know exactly how unhealthy the diet needs to be or the effects of one drink per day. In other words, doctors are more sure about some of this information than others. Does that affect how you would respond to this information?

-Part of why doctors don't know much about these issues is that they have not been studying men's sperm health for very long. Most of the research on reproduction is about women and pregnancy. Do you have thoughts about why it took doctors so long to begin asking questions about men's sperm health?

Now I have a few summary questions.

-If you had to pick three words to describe the topic of men's role in reproduction, what would those three words be? (Ask them to elaborate on any word that hasn't already been discussed extensively in the interview.)

-Many men are surprised to hear this information because it is new, and it is not being publicized. Imagine that you are put in charge of designing a public health campaign to inform men about this information. How would you go about doing that?

[Clarify any of the following that have not been answered in the course of the interview: age, race, marital status, children, education, occupation, homeowner/renter, religion, sexuality]

-Those are all my questions. Thinking back over the interview, is there anything else you'd like to add? (pause) Is there anything I'm not asking that you think is important to mention?

-We have a small compensation to thank you for your time (hand them envelope with $20 bill). And of course, I'm happy to answer any questions you have about the study.

Qualitative Data Analysis

All fifty-five interviews were recorded and professionally transcribed by Verbal Ink. I double-checked the transcripts by listening to each recording in full and made small edits as necessary. Then I imported the transcripts into Nvivo, a software program that allows for iterative coding. I coded the men's interviews first. Initially, I coded the data by organizing it according to interview questions (e.g., reading all the men's responses to the reproduction question, then all their answers to the egg/sperm question). At the same time, I also read through a random subset of the transcripts to identify emergent themes, e.g., men talking women's bodies, animal analogies, references to race/class/sexuality. I then applied the thematic codes to all the men's interviews. I also conducted text searches for particular words and phrases that appeared over and over (e.g., *fertilize, seed*), but I tried to keep this more mechanical version of coding to a minimum. The same coding structure was applied to the women's transcripts, which are analyzed more fully in a separate article.

By systematically coding men's and women's words, I was able to analyze patterns in their views about men's reproduction and sperm. Specifically, I drew on previous research and theory, as well as emergent themes from the interview data, to generate an analysis that attempted to balance the nuance of individual narratives with patterns across those narratives. One way I work to ensure the rigor of my qualitative analyses is by first identifying a pattern in the interview data and then using counts to verify its prevalence in my sample. For example, when I began noticing the two different sperm stories discussed in chapter 5, I conducted a text search of the word *sperm* (and its cognates, such as *seed, semen,* and *cells*) to identify all instances in which men described sperm. Then, using an Excel spreadsheet, I created counts for the number of men who told the active-sperm-passive-egg story and/or the egg-and-sperm-as-two-halves-of-a-whole story, as well as subsidiary parts of those narratives (e.g., "says sperm enters egg," "references large number of sperm," "references one sperm fertilizing/winning"). Any statistics reported in chapters 5 and 6, as well as my use of quantifying terms (such as "vast majority," "some," or "about half the respondents") are based on counts like this. However, they are not meant to be taken as generalizable to any broader population. Instead, these statistics reflect the propensity (or the lack thereof) of people in my sample to describe reproduction in particular ways. If everyone said something, or if no one said something, then I take this as a rough indicator of the relative prominence or importance of a particular idea. If some proportion of the sample said it, then I looked for patterns by age, race, education, fatherhood status, or other demographics that may have been associated with a particular view.

Interviewees

Table C Interviewees

Pseudonym	Age	Race/Ethnicity	Sexuality	Education	Occupation	SES	Relationship, Children (age)
MEN							
Aaron	43	White	Gay	GED, some college	Student	Higher	Married (to Tom), none
Angelo	39	White	Hetero	Law degree	Lawyer	Higher	Married, son (4)
Antoine	36	African American	MSM	High school diploma	Roofer	Lower	Single, 2 (4, 8?)
Avi	23	White	?	Graduate student	Student	Higher	Single, none
Bobby	35	White	Hetero	4-year college degree	Nonprofit organization	Higher	Married, 3 (2, 6, 8)
Bruce	38	African American	Hetero	High school diploma	Janitor	Lower	Divorced, son (17)
Chad	26	White	Hetero	Master's degree	Unemployed	Higher	Serious girlfriend, none
Craig	46	White	Bisexual	1 year of college	Manufacturer	Lower	Single, none
Daniel	23	Puerto Rican	Hetero	4-year college degree	Researcher	Higher	Dating girlfriend, none
David	48	White	Hetero	One semester of college	Part-time work (on disability)	Lower	Single, none
Deshawn	32	African American	Hetero	High school diploma	Security guard (occasional)	Lower	Serious girlfriend, son (7)
Dustin	27	Puerto Rican	Hetero	High school diploma	Unemployed	Lower	Single, son (removed by state)
Elijah	21	African American	Hetero	Community college student	Student	Lower	Serious girlfriend, none
Gabe	24	African American	Hetero	Some college	Unemployed	Lower	Single, none

Name	Age	Race/Ethnicity	Sexual orientation	Education	Occupation	Income	Relationship status, children (ages)
Gary	41	African American	Hetero	Some college	Forklift driver	Lower	Significant other, 7 (2–18)
George	49	African American	Hetero	11th grade	Handyman	Lower	Significant other, daughter (27)
Henri	28	White	Gay	PhD	Researcher	Higher	Married, none
Hong	29	Chinese	Hetero	Postdoctoral scholar	Researcher	Higher	Married, son (1)
James	19	White	Hetero	University student	Student	Higher	Serious girlfriend, none
John	46	Puerto Rican/White	Hetero	8th grade	Unemployed	Lower	Single, daughter (14)
Josh	33	Indonesian	Hetero	MBA	Student	Higher	Married, 2 (4, 8)
Kenneth	49	White	Hetero	4-year college degree	Office manager	Higher	Divorced, girlfriend, son (25)
Luke	28	White	Hetero	4-year college degree	Non-profit organization	Higher	Single, none
Malik	28	African American	Hetero	High school diploma	Unemployed	Lower	Divorced, girlfriend, 3 (3–7)
Mark	38	White	Hetero	4-year college degree	Nurse	Higher	Single, none
Matt	40	Puerto Rican/White	Het/MSM	8th grade & GED	Clerk	Lower	Single, 2 (removed by state)
Michael	49	White	Hetero	4-year college degree	Sales	Higher	Dating girlfriend, none
Nathan	31	White	Hetero	High school diploma	Unemployed	Lower	Single, none
Neeraj	45	Indian	Hetero	Some college	Nonprofit organization	Higher	Single, none
Nick	33	White	Gay	4-year college degree	Unemployed	Higher	Single, none
Patrick	25	African American	Hetero	Some college	Part-time clerk	Lower	Single, none

(continued)

Pseudonym	Age	Race/Ethnicity	Sexuality	Education	Occupation	SES	Relationship, Children (age)
Paul	29	White	Hetero	High school diploma	Unempl., filing for disability	Lower	Single, 1 (3)
Rob	49	White	Hetero	High school diploma	Part-time work (on disability)	Lower	Single, son (23)
Seth	23	Vietnamese	Gay	4-year college degree	Part-time club host	Higher	Single, none
Tom	33	White	Gay	MPA	City employee	Higher	Married (to Aaron), none
Tony	45	AfAm/Hispanic	Hetero	4-year college degree	Sound tech	Higher	Divorced, son (2?)
Travis	33	White	Hetero	4-year college degree	Unemployed	Higher	Married, none
Victor	43	White	Gay	Master's degree	Unemployed	Lower	Single, none
Wei	24	Chinese	Hetero	Graduate student	Graduate student	Higher	Married, none
Will	18	AfAm/White	Hetero	University student	University student	Higher	Single, none
WOMEN							
Bianca	35	Latina	Hetero	4-year college degree	Housecleaner	Lower	Single, 1
Caitlin	39	White	Hetero	High school diploma	Unemployed	Lower	Married, 4
Carmen	35	White	Hetero	One year of college	Non-profit organization	Higher	Divorced, 2
Heather	27	African American	Hetero	Some college	Unemployed	Lower	Single, 1
Jada	22	African American	Hetero	4-year college degree	Student, bartender	Higher	Single, none
Jennifer	38	White	Hetero	Some college	Unemployed	Higher	Single, none
Joy	29	Chinese	Hetero	Master's degree	Graduate student	Higher	Single, none
Lisa	37	White	Gay	Associate's degree	Musician	Higher	Single, none

Mary	35	White	Hetero	Master's degree	EMT	Higher	Divorced, none
Meg	27	White	Hetero	4-year college degree	Teacher	Higher	Dating boyfriend, none
Monique	30	African American	Hetero	10th grade	Unemployed	Lower	Serious boyfriend, 2 (6, 11)
Sarah	29	White	Hetero	4-year college degree	Stay-at-home mom, nanny	Higher	Married, 1
Sonia	21	Latina	Hetero	Some college	Unemployed	Lower	Single, none
Teresa	37	White	Hetero	GED, some college	Daycare provider	Lower	Married, 4 (6–17)
Tracey	30	African American	Hetero	GED	Cashier	Lower	Sep, living w/ boyfriend, 5 (5–11)

Notes

INTRODUCTION

1. Day et al. 2016; Paul and Robaire 2013.
2. Carey 2012; Kong et al. 2012; Lambert et al. 2006.
3. CDC 2015; Mayo Clinic 2012.
4. Richardson forthcoming.
5. Moscucci 1990.
6. ACOG 2018; ASRM 2013.
7. Markens et al. 1997; Waggoner 2017.
8. Epstein 2007.
9. Ginsburg and Rapp 1991: 330; see also Murphy 2012.
10. Almeling 2015.
11. Ginsburg and Rapp 1991: 330; emphasis added.
12. See, e.g., Hays 1996; Hochschild 1983; Laslett and Brenner 1989; Thorne 1993.
13. See, e.g., Collins 2000; Rubin 1993.
14. Yanagisako and Collier 1990; see also Haraway 1991; Barad 2006.
15. Martin 1991.
16. Oudshoorn 1994; Richardson 2013.
17. Almeling 2011.
18. Fausto-Sterling 2000: 254; Almeling 2015.
19. Jasanoff 2004.

20. Tuana 2004: 195.

21. Proctor and Schiebinger 2008; Frickel et al. 2010; Gross and McGoey 2015.

22. Mills 2007; Oreskes and Conway 2011; Kempner et al. 2011.

23. Condensed excerpt of Croissant's 2014 discussion: 6–9.

24. Fausto-Sterling 2000.

25. See, e.g., Anderson 2006; Braun 2014; De Block and Adriaens 2013; Riessman 1983; Roberts 2011; Shah 2001; Wailoo 2001.

26. Luna and Luker 2013; Roberts 1997; Stern 2005; Davis 2019.

27. Epstein 2007: 52.

28. Epstein 2007; Welch et al. 2012.

29. On gynecology, see Moscucci 1990. On interventions, see Bell 2014; Davis-Floyd 1992; Katz Rothman 1986. On contraception, see Oudshoorn 1994; Watkins 2001. On political clout, see Luker 1984; Joffe et al. 2004.

30. Urology differs from gynecology in that its focus is on the urinary system in both men and women. There are a small number of urologists who subspecialize in male infertility, but the specialty as a whole does not have the same all-encompassing focus on the general topic of men's reproductive health as does gynecology. This was a conscious choice by urologists as they created a formal specialty in the early twentieth century, an episode I discuss in more detail in chapter 1.

31. National Institute of Child Health and Human Development 2013a; see also CDC 2010. This same language was still posted on the NIH website as of November 2019.

32. Oudshoorn 2003.

33. On contraception and abortion, see Gordon 1976; Kligman 1998; Luker 1984; Roberts 1997. On pregnancy, see Bridges 2011; Katz Rothman 1986; Martin 1992; Waggoner 2017. On prenatal testing, see Browner and Press 1995; Rapp 1999. On birth, see Davis-Floyd 1992; Jordan 1983.

34. Daniels 2006; Greene and Biddlecom 2000; Inhorn et al. 2009.

35. On contraception, see Gutmann 2007; Oudshoorn 2003. On infertility, see Barnes 2014; Becker 2000; Inhorn 2012. On birth, see Leavitt 2010; Reed 2005. On sperm donation, see Almeling 2011; Mohr 2018; Wahlberg 2018. Some might add Marsiglio's *Procreative Man* (1998) to this list, but I view it as too biologically deterministic to be consistent with a sociological approach to reproduction.

36. Inhorn et al. 2009; Loe 2004; Mamo and Fishman 2001.

37. Adams and Savran 2002; Pascoe and Bridges 2015.

38. Epstein 2007.

39. See, e.g., Corea 1985; Morgen 2002; Ruzek 1978.

40. To give a concrete example, scholars studying the rollout of genetic testing argued that cultural presumptions around women's deeper connections to family life resulted in heightened feelings of genetic responsibility relative to men (e.g.,

Hallowell 1999). Yet, several of those studies sampled only women, so the authors used assumptions about gender difference to make claims about men. In fact, in follow-up studies, when researchers did collect empirical data from men, they were surprised to find that men too had strong feelings of genetic responsibility to their families in the face of genetic risk (e.g., Hallowell et al. 2006).

41. Wood 2015.

42. Carrigan et al. 1985; Connell 2000.

43. Daniels 2006: 6–7. See also Courtenay 2000; Rosenfeld and Faircloth 2006, for more general discussions of masculinity and health, including the association of men with vigor, invulnerability, and efficiently functioning bodies.

44. Almeling and Waggoner 2013.

45. This point also applies to the fascinating collection of articles in *Scientific Masculinities*, Milam and Nye 2015.

46. Connell 1987: 140.

47. Oudshoorn 1994.

48. Epstein 2007.

49. Richardson 2013.

50. Richardson 2013: 16, 17, 2.

51. I thank Jeff Ostergren for making the images to illustrate this point.

52. See calls from historians for more attention to temporality (Kowal et al. 2013) and *longue durée* perspectives (e.g., Bock von Wülfingen et al. 2015).

53. Benford and Snow 2000; Berger et al. 1973; Mulvey 1999.

54. Tsai et al. 2008; Collins 2012.

55. Hacking 1995: 370; see also Navon 2019. Science studies scholars have developed a rich vocabulary for examining how people, ideas, technologies, and organizations come together in the making of knowledge. For example, Oudshoorn describes "socio-technical networks" as "networks of techniques, knowledge, institutions, experts, and social groups" (2003: 12). Epstein develops the concept of "bio-political paradigms," by which he means "frameworks of ideas, standards, formal procedures, and unarticulated understandings that specify how concerns about health, medicine, and the body are made the simultaneous focus of biomedicine and state policy" (2008: 17). While neither of these scholars discuss feedback loops per se, I think of their concepts as key elements that *constitute* feedback loops. In addition, in keeping with more recent gender scholarship that looks directly at the body, at hormones and chromosomes and gametes, it is important to consider biological processes alongside the cultural and organizational processes catalogued by Oudshoorn and Epstein.

56. Griswold 1987; Petersen and Anand 2004.

57. Duden 1991.

58. Weisz 2006.

59. Daniels 2006; Frey et al. 2008.

CHAPTER 1. WHITHER GUYNECOLOGY?

1. Eyre 2013.

2. Fulsås and Rem 2017: 173; Soloski 2013.

3. Brandt 1985: 12.

4. Ibsen's play centers on a philandering father who transmits syphilis to his son, but Soloski (2013) argues that the exact mode of transmission (e.g., biological, moral, social) was left intentionally vague.

5. The Wassermann test was first described in 1906 (Brandt 1985: 40).

6. Van Buren and Keyes 1874: 541.

7. Fischer 2009.

8. Gamble 1997; Reverby 2009.

9. "Obituary: Thomas Blizard Curling" 1888; Moscucci 1990: 28.

10. Darby 2005.

11. Curling 1843: 437.

12. Porter 2004; Rogers 1998; Starr 1982; Warner 1997.

13. Abbott 1988; Warner 2003; Weisz 2006.

14. Rosen 1944; Stevens 1966; Weisz 2006.

15. On critical junctures, see, for example, Mahoney 2000; Thelen 2000. Sociologists and political scientists working in the tradition of historical institutionalism have developed the concept of "critical junctures" within a broader discussion about path dependence. Whereas they are primarily concerned with political and economic processes, I examine the constitutive role of culture (in the form of gendered cultural norms) in organizational processes within the institution of medicine. I thank Julia Adams for a helpful conversation on this point.

16. Moscucci 1990.

17. Moscucci 1990: 7.

18. Moscucci 1990: 31, quoting Dr. Robert Barnes in *Quain's Dictionary of Medicine* (1882).

19. Moscucci 1990: 34.

20. Moscucci 1990: 157–58.

21. Moscucci 1990: 101–2.

22. Clarke 1998: 38.

23. Today, around 10–15 percent of heterosexual couples experience infertility. Clinicians estimate that "male factors" are the cause in about one third of the cases and "female factors" in another third, while the cause of the remaining third are "unknown" (Chandra et al. 2013; National Institute of Child Health and Human Development 2016).

24. Marsh and Ronner 1999; Pfeffer 1993.

25. Oudshoorn 1994: 17.

26. Oudshoorn 1994: 50, 76–80.

27. Oudshoorn 1994: 26, 53.

28. Oudshoorn 2003; Watkins 2001.

29. Oudshoorn 1994: 80, emphasis added.

30. Gordon 1976.

31. Boston Women's Health Book Collective 1973; Kline 2010; Murphy 2012.

32. Luna and Luker 2013; Ross and Solinger 2017: 9.

33. Darby introduces his 2005 article on spermatorrhea by labeling it "an episode in the history of sexual disease" (284), but given that it was linked to impotence and sterility (287), it could just as easily be labeled a "reproductive" disease. Similarly, Brandt (1985: 6) lists the major themes of his classic study as "sex, disease, and medicine," and none of the following terms appear in the index: *reproduction, fatherhood, children*, or *offspring*.

34. Moscucci (1990: 32), Clarke (1998: 40), and Daniels (2006: 33) mention the editorial but do not provide additional context. Benninghaus's (2012) analysis of how male sterility became a "medical object" includes a subheading "Gynecologists as *Andrologists*" (emphasis added), but she does not discuss any professional societies and writes: "Apparently, turning the male body and its reproductive capacities into an object of modern medicine did not require constituting a new specialization. Gynecologists were quite happy to examine both partners, and experts in dermatology, venereology, psychology and sexology could be called upon if further examinations were deemed necessary" (663).

35. In 1866, Van Buren's professorship was changed from "general and descriptive anatomy" to the "diseases of the genito-urinary system." "University of New York Faculty of Medicine" 1855; "Bellevue Hospital Medical College—City of New York, Sessions for 1866–67" 1866.

36. In an analysis of genito-urinary injuries during the Civil War, Herr (2004) argues that the sheer number of men marred on the battlefield provided physicians of that generation with experience honing their surgical techniques.

37. Keyes 1980: 14–15; Keyes Jr. 1928. For more on Ricord, see Oriel 1989. Some of Keyes's memoirs were republished in abbreviated form in *Urology* in 1977.

38. "Obituary: Edward Lawrence Keyes, MD" 1924; Keyes Jr. 1928; Wishard 1925.

39. Carlisle 1893: 110; Keyes Jr. 1928: 729.

40. Watson (1896: 616) describes Mastin as "Founder of Congress."

41. Weisz 2006: 82.

42. Zorgniotti 1977: 95.

43. The original letter from Mastin to Keyes seems not to have survived (Zorgniotti 1977: 95), but Keyes's responses do. This was not the first time Keyes and Mastin had corresponded. Mastin published an article in the *Boston Medical and Surgical Journal* in 1879, which spurred Keyes to write him a letter that begins nicely enough: "I read your case of prostatic stricture with great interest," but it concludes by noting that if Mastin "could not tell whether or not there was an organic obstruction between the tip of your finger and the bladder—!!!—Well,

if that was the case, all I have to say is, pray give up surgery and take to some other calling. Yours truly, EL Keyes" (Keyes 1882). It is unclear whether this was their first-ever exchange and whether this is a joke or an insult. In any case, it was Keyes to whom Mastin turned four years later when he was looking for someone to organize a genito-urinary society.

44. Keyes 1980: 26.

45. Letters reprinted in Zorgniotti 1977.

46. Bowen 2013.

47. Letters reprinted in Zorgniotti 1977. That same physician, Edward Wigglesworth of Boston, made an identical point during his presidential address that year to the American Dermatological Association when he stated that genito-urinary surgery is a "distinct specialty from that of dermatology, which, of course, includes syphilis" ("American Dermatological Association: The Tenth Annual Meeting" 1886: 301).

48. In addition to Keyes, the attendees included A. T. Cabot and F. B. Greenough (Boston); P. A. Morrow, F. N. Otis, F. R. Sturgis, and R. W. Taylor (New York); F. W. Rockwell (Brooklyn); R. Park (Buffalo); and J. W. White (Philadelphia). Letters and telegrams expressing regret for being absent were received from J. H. Brinton, J. P. Bryson, A. S. Garnett, G. C. Greenway, S. W. Gross, W. H. Hingston, J. N. Hyde, C. H. Mastin, and others.

49. Zorgniotti 1977: 92.

50. Morrow 1886: 380, emphasis added.

51. Transactions of the meeting were published in the *Journal of Cutaneous and Genito-Urinary Diseases*, "Society Transactions: American Association of Genito-Urinary Surgeons"1887: 266–67.

52. Here, I am heeding Frickel's (2014; see also Hilgartner 2014) warning about avoiding teleology in the study of "undone science" by noting when actors (and not just the analyst) identify gaps in knowledge.

53. Black 1875: vi.

54. "Book Review: A Clinical Hand-book on the Diseases of Women" 1882: 513.

55. Wells, "Epidemic of Laparotomy," 1891 in Moscucci 1990: 1.

56. AAGUS 1911: 30.

57. AAGUS 1911: 32. The association's new name was already in use by the July 14, 1890, edition of *Medical News*, which published a paper on urethritis by J. William White, noting it had been read at the American Association of Andrology and Syphilology at Altoona in June 1890.

58. *Gyneco-* (or *gynaeco-*) is a word-forming element meaning "woman, female" from the Latinized form of the Greek *gynaiko-*. The word-forming element *andro-* means "man, male, masculine" from the Greek *andro-* (*Online Etymology Dictionary*, n.d., s.v. "andro-," https://www.etymonline.com/word

/andro-, and s.v. "gyneco-," https://www.etymonline.com/word/gyneco-, accessed February 12, 2020).

59. In 1837, German doctor and professor Moritz Ernst Adolph Naumann wrote in the preface to his *Handbook of the Medical Clinic* of his hopes that a focus on andrology will "exercise a similar fruitful retroactive effect on pathology as a whole, as it has already generally been granted to 'gynecology'" (iv). Naumann's book was favorably reviewed for its "complete andrology, a connected overview of the male genitalia's pathological circumstances" in the *Yearbook of Achievements in the Medical Sciences* the following year (Sachs 1838: 174). In 1878, Ernst Fürstenheim proposed the "newly formed word andrology" at a session of the Berlin medical society as "equitable to the word gynecology." Moreover, he argued that "doctors should be motivated to grant the diseases of the male sex apparatus more attention than had been given thus far" (Waldenburg 1979: 502–3). Fürstenheim's student, Carl Posner, who was named an honorary member of the American Urological Association when it was founded in 1902, also advocated for the use of the term *andrology* in a review of a book about the urinary and reproductive systems (Posner 1884: 1839).

60. I worked with a German-speaking research assistant, Vanessa Bittner, to look for direct connections between the physicians mentioned in the previous footnote and the founding members of AAGUS but could not find any. See Warner (2003) and Bonner (1963) on American physicians traveling to France and Germany.

61. "Memoranda" 1887: 25, emphasis added.

62. Mauss 1973; Oudshoorn 1994; Scheper-Hughes and Lock 1987.

63. Debates about similarities and differences by sex did not begin in the nineteenth century. See Schiebinger 1993 and Laqueur 1990 for analyses of the preceding centuries, which would have informed biomedical discussions of the day.

64. Hopwood 2018; Jordanova 1995. Barbara Duden has argued that prior to the emergence of this new word *reproduction*, "there was simply no term in which insemination, conception, pregnancy, and birth could have been subsumed" (1991: 28).

65. William Acton included a footnote on p. 1 of his *Functions and Disorders of the Reproductive Organs* (1875) stating, "In the following pages the words 'generative,' 'sexual,' 'reproductive,' will be used synonymously; there are some instances in which distinctions may be made between them, but these are so slight I need not further allude to them." See also Niblett 1863, who uses interchangeably the phrases "sexual system" (2), "disorders of the reproductive organs" (3), and "generative organs" (6). Beaney 1883 also uses the terms "organs of reproduction," "sexual systems of women and men," "sexual organs," and "generative organs" interchangeably.

66. Van Buren and Keyes 1874; Acton 1875; Morrow 1893.

67. Examples of texts focused just on men include *A Practical Treatise on Impotence, Sterility, and Allied Disorders of the Male Sexual Organs* (Gross 1887) and *Diseases of the Male Organs of Generation* (Jacobson 1893). Jackson's (1852) *Hints on the Reproductive Organs: Diseases, Causes, and Cure* has separate chapters titled "Men and Their Diseases," which is entirely focused on nocturnal emissions, and "Women and Their Diseases," which covers more territory.

68. Butlin 1892. In some cases, particular parts or diseases became the subject of entire books, as with Curling's *A Practical Treatise on the Diseases of the Testis and of the Spermatic Cord and Scrotum* (1843) and Lallemand's *Practical Treatise on the Causes, Symptoms, and Treatment of Spermatorrhea* (1853). There are a few historical studies of particular aspects of the male body, including the penis (Friedman 2001), circumcision (Darby 2005), and testosterone (Hoberman 2005; Oudshoorn 1994; Sengoopta 2006).

69. Benninghaus (2012) and Vienne (2018) challenge Laqueur's claim that nineteenth-century scientists were primarily focused on sex *difference* by arguing there was also quite a lot of scientific attention to sex similarity. Numerous passages from these medical treatises on men provide additional evidence in support of their argument.

70. Curling 1843.

71. Delaney 1991.

72. Beaney 1883: 33–34. See also Jackson 1852: 29, emphasizing the dissimilarity of women and men.

73. Lee 1890: 289–90.

74. Gasking 1967; Vienne 2018. Nineteenth-century scientists interested in comparative anatomy, zoology, and botany occasionally used the term *spermatology*, which Joseph Thomas defined in his *Comprehensive Medical Dictionary* as "that branch of Physiology that treats of the secretion and nature of semen" (1875: 515).

75. Vienne 2018: 1, emphasis added.

76. Marsh and Ronner 1999; Benninghaus 2012: 647.

77. Moscucci 1990: 2, 32, emphasis in original.

78. Weisz 2006.

79. "Annotations" 1888: 336.

80. "Lancet: London: Saturday, August 25, 1888" 1888: 379.

81. "Lancet: London: Saturday, October 27, 1888" 1888: 826. The *Lancet* returned *again* to the same theme almost fifteen years later, bashing the specialism of "urology or genito-urinary surgeons" and ridiculing Hugh Cabot's presidential address at the tenth annual meeting of the American Urological Association, which "answer[ed] in the affirmative the question, 'Is urology entitled to be regarded as a specialty?'" ("Specialism in General and Genito-Urinary Surgery in Particular" 1912: 398).

82. "Editorial: The American Association of Genito-Urinary Surgeons" 1889: 38–39.

83. "Medical News" 1890a: 1520.

84. "Andrology as a Specialty" 1891: 691.

85. In the opening comments at the first triennial meeting of the Congress, the organizers discussed the need for their umbrella organization precisely because there were too many specialized association meetings to attend, and physicians often had professional interests in more than one area (*Transactions of the Congress of American Physicians and Surgeons: First Triennial Session* 1889: xxiii–xxvii). They promised to be on the lookout for unnecessary specialization by requiring that new societies only be admitted to the Congress if there was a unanimous vote by the Executive Committee ("Minutes" 1888: xxxii).

86. *Transactions of the Congress of American Physicians and Surgeons: Second Triennial Session* 1892: 37–38, emphasis added.

87. *Transactions of the Congress of American Physicians and Surgeons: Second Triennial Session* 1892: 37–38.

88. "Andrology as a Specialty" 1891: 691.

89. Brandt 1985; Hoganson 1998; Kampf 2015; Pfeffer 1993.

90. Rotundo 1993: ch. 8; Kline 2001: 9.

91. See, for example, Sicherman 1977.

92. MacFadden 1900: 5–6; see also Marsh 1988: 177–78.

93. Putney 2001.

94. I thank Carolyn Roberts for a helpful conversation on this point.

95. Foucault 1980; Hall 1983; Largent 2008; Somerville 2000; Stein 2015: 17–18, 23, 147, 245.

96. Stein 2015: 171.

97. Stanton et al. 1973 [1881]; Wollstonecraft 1967 [1792].

98. Brandt 1985: 11–13. Brandt notes that others criticized these numbers as far too high, but the point here is that these diseases were widespread enough to engender concern among the medical profession and public alike.

99. Worboys 2004: 43.

100. Brandt 1985: 9, 16; Pfeffer 1993.

101. Kline 2001: 9.

102. Moscucci 1990: 32; Rosen 1942: 349.

103. Fischer 2009; Porter 2004; Whooley 2013.

104. Ettinger 2006: 6; Leavitt 1986: 62; Whorton 2002: 17; Fischer 2009.

105. Fischer 2009: 191–92.

106. "Editorial: The American Association of Genito-Urinary Surgeons" 1889: 38, emphasis added.

107. Fischer 2009: 2.

108. Fischer 2009: 5.

109. Fischer 2009: 5, 28, 33.

110. This ad was reprinted in the American Medical Association's *Nostrums and Quackery* (Cramp 1921: 387). It is one of many, many examples of ads that appeared in newspapers in the late nineteenth century. See the American Medical Association's Historical Health Fraud and Alternative Medicine Collection, which contains six boxes of advertisements, correspondence, and other materials on the "diseases of men" from 1885–1973.

111. Beaney 1883: v–vi.

112. Lallemand 1853: xii.

113. Evans 1915; Fischer 2009.

114. Fischer 2009.

115. Cooper 1845: 70.

116. Curling 1843: 107.

117. Cooper 1845: 47; Curling 1843: 437, 489.

118. "Andrology as a Specialty" 1891: 691.

119. Andrew Abbott has written about the failure or disappearance of particular medical specialties, such as "railway surgeons," due to technological or organizational changes (1988: 92). Because andrology does not ever become established, I locate the moment of failure at its (attempted) launch rather than after a period of thriving.

120. Mark 1911. "Clap" is slang for venereal disease, usually gonorrhea.

121. Guiteras 1905: 338.

122. Guiteras 1905; Zorgniotti 1976: 283, 287; see also Hay 1910: 1459–60.

123. See lists of founding members for AAGUS in Zorgniotti 1977 and for AUA in Guiteras 1905.

124. Keyes and Keyes Jr. 1906: v–vi.

125. The Keyes Award, AAGUS.org, emphasis added.

126. This is the originating point of Daniels 2006, and is suggested by Clarke 1998: 10, who writes that there were few studies of men's reproduction until the latter part of the twentieth century.

127. Benninghaus 2012: 662; see also Kampf 2015. An early version of this argument appears in Parsons 1977.

CHAPTER 2. ANDROLOGY AGAIN

1. Schirren 1969. Working with a German-speaking research assistant, Vanessa Bittner, we translated the title and first lines of the article from German into English.

2. Krause and Schreiber 2018. See also the "History" (Geschichte) page of the German Society for Andrology (Deutsche Gesellschaft fur Andrologie; https://www.dg-andrologie.de/gesellschaft.html).

3. Likewise, in "Development and Current Status of Andrology in Germany," their article for the new journal, Jordan and Niermann (1969) twice remark on the need for "tight cooperation" between gynecology and andrology. Reflecting on his efforts fifteen years later, Schirren reprises the parallelism between andrology and gynecology: "Nothing is more *natural* then the andrologist and gynecologist cooperating more closely and taking over the care for a childless couple," if possible "under one roof" (1985: 122, emphasis added).

4. Kevles 1995; Kluchin 2009.

5. Oudshoorn 1994.

6. Cutler and Miller 2005; Tomes 1998.

7. The few historical studies that discuss men's reproductive bodies during this period tend to jump from the 1891 *JAMA* editorial to the late 1960s, when the new andrology associations had their initial meetings and published their first journals (e.g., Clarke 1998: 40; Oudshoorn 1994: 79–80). Moscucci (1990) also refers to "andrology clinics" in England during the 1920s and 1930s that were oriented to fertility (33) and mentions a 1923 text by Walker (32–33) that I discuss in note 17. Daniels (2006: 33) refers to an article by Harald Siebke that I examine in this chapter. In all of these studies, though, the history of andrology is dealt with in just a few sentences.

8. Brandt 1985.

9. Oudshoorn 2003: 6.

10. Almeling 2011; Marsh and Ronner 1999.

11. Kline 2001; Richardson forthcoming.

12. Fischer 2009.

13. Dorland 1900: 43. A similar definition appears in the first edition of Gould's *Illustrated Dictionary of Medicine, Biology and the Allied Sciences* (1894): "1. The science of man, especially of the male sex. 2. The science of the diseases of the male genito-urinary organs" (77). Web searches also turn up references to "andrology" in philosophy and anthropology as the "study of man," posed in contrast to, say, the study of geology or theology, but this use of the term was not meant to refer to a medical specialty (e.g., "Cheap Lecturing" 1841; "andrology" in Smith 1909: 48–49; Long 1885).

14. Corner 1910: v. This 1910 edition appears to be a slightly revised version of a book by Corner published by the same publisher just three years earlier, but the earlier version does not contain the same passionate plea in the preface for a specialty oriented to "male diseases." It does, however, contain the same distinction between the "generative tract" and the "urinary tract" and notes that the text focuses on the former (Corner 1907: v).

15. Corner 1910: vi–vii.

16. "Male Diseases" 1913: 670.

17. "Book Notice: Male Diseases in General Practice" 1910: 880. Thirteen years later, Kenneth Walker's *Diseases of the Male Organs of Generation* was

published in the same series as Corner's, Oxford Medical Publications, and began with a similar lament: in contrast to gynecology, andrology "has not yet received the recognition that will one day be accorded to it." Noting his indebtedness to Corner's previous work, Walker (1923: v) offers a similar argument that male diseases should be considered separately from urinary diseases rather than being grouped under the common heading "genito-urinary surgery." Not surprisingly, Walker's call for differentiation provoked a comment about unnecessary specialization in the *British Medical Journal,* which was otherwise complimentary about the content ("Reviews" 1924: 386).

18. Forsbach n.d.

19. Vienne 2006; see also Schultheiss and Moll 2017.

20. Siebke 1951: 635. I am grateful to Vanessa Bittner for her assistance in translating the German to English.

21. Clarke 1998: 10.

22. Jones 2013; May 2013; Patterson 2001.

23. Gordon 2002; Reagan 1998.

24. D'Emilio 1983; Faderman 2015; Reumann 2005.

25. Kline 2010; Morgen 2002.

26. Penny Light 2012: 105; Leavitt 2010.

27. Messner 1997.

28. Kline 2001; Roberts 1997; Schoen 2005; Stern 2005.

29. Feimster 2009; Oswald 2013; Richeson 2009.

30. Murphy 2017.

31. Connelly 2008: 157; Population Council 1978; Sinding 2000; Teitelbaum 1992: 66.

32. Balasubramanian 2018: 43; Oudshoorn 2003: 22.

33. Keettel et al. 1956; Swanson 2012; Swanson 2014.

34. Almeling 2011.

35. Oudshoorn 2003: 250n8.

36. "W. O. Nelson, Expert on Birth Control" 1964; Nelson 1964: 252; Oudshoorn 2003: 71–72.

37. The club's founding is discussed in several sources, each of which identifies a different date: 1965 (Steinberger 1978: 56), 1968 (Rosemberg 1986: 101), or more generally "in the 1960s" (Sherins 2014: 47). Several sources claim that Nelson was involved in its founding, which suggests it must have existed prior to his death in 1964. Steinberger (2010: 115) writes in his memoir about renaming the club in honor of Nelson.

38. Biographical details about Mancini (1914–1977) are from an interview I conducted on August 6, 2018, with his son, Roberto C. Mancini, a physics professor at the University of Nevada. The younger Mancini also kindly provided copies of various documents, such as "Breve Historia del Centro de Investigaciones en Reproducción (1966–2011)," written by Alberto J. Solari, and a tribute to

Mancini published in the *Boletin Informativo*, "Homenaje al Prof. Dr. Roberto E. Mancini (1914–1977)." The goal of the center was to conduct basic and applied research in the study of human reproduction. Copies of these materials are available from the author.

39. Eliasson 1976; Rosemberg 1986.

40. In a 2014 interview, a physician-scientist from France, who had been one of the few researchers working on male infertility in the 1970s and later helped to establish the andrology diploma for that country in the early 1990s, described a series of contacts with international researchers in the 1970s via letters, lab visits, workshops, and meetings. He specifically names many of the people mentioned in this chapter, including Carl Schirren, J. K. Sherman, and Rune Eliasson.

41. Rosemberg and Paulsen 1970: vii.

42. In their introductory pieces to *Andrologie* in 1969, neither Jordan and Niermann or Schirren mention Siebke, the German gynecologist who just the decade before had called for a Männerarzt to parallel a Frauenarzt (Siebke 1951). Rune Eliasson's inaugural presidential address at CIDA in 1976 does refer to Siebke as the person who introduced the term *andrology* (1978: 7–8). By the time Schirren writes a history of his efforts in 1985, he is attributing the term *andrology* to Siebke, noting that "it took many years before those who were then responsible for the examination of the male with respect to reproduction were able to accept this term" (118).

43. Niemi 1987: 201.

44. Eliasson 1978: 7.

45. "Information about ISA, (Formerly CIDA)" 1982: 349.

46. Steinberger 2007: 101–2, 166.

47. Lamb 2009.

48. Lamb 2009; Lukaszyk 2009.

49. Rosemberg 1986: 73.

50. Sherins 2014: 28.

51. Rosemberg 1975.

52. Belker et al. 2006; Bettendorf 1995. In my interview with Mancini's son, he recalled family dinners as a child in Buenos Aires in which Dr. Rosemberg would join as a guest.

53. Mancini et al. 1965.

54. Cooney 2004.

55. Cooney 2004; Rosemberg et al. 1974; Schaffenburg et al. 1981.

56. Rosemberg 1975.

57. Steinberger 1975.

58. ASA Archives & History Committee 2016: 168.

59. Belker et al. 2006.

60. ASA 1975.

61. Steinberger 1978: 57.

62. Steinberger 1978: 57. I had hoped that Steinberger's memoir would offer more details about the founding of the American Society of Andrology, but his recounting of professional events ends with the year 1971.

63. Steinberger 1982: 211, emphasis added.

64. Steinberger 1982: 211.

65. Interview with sperm bank founder, 2006. In a 2014 interview with a physician-scientist from France, he describes similar experiences in that country: "At the end of the 1960s when I wanted to be involved in male infertility, I could not find any place in the medical structure. Then in the '70s, there was a structure developing, and in medical conferences, there were talks about what people are doing in this new field." Later in the interview, he specifies that their focus at the time was on "the mechanics of sperm function and production."

66. Interview with urologist, 2015.

67. ASA Archives & History Committee 2016: 99.

68. Both the *International Journal of Andrology* and the *Archives of Andrology* launched in 1978. The *Archives* remained in print until 2007, and the *International Journal* and *Journal of Andrology* merged both because of financial issues and to improve their "impact factor," a scholarly measure of the visibility and prestige of a journal (Carrell and Rajpert-Meyts 2013; Meistrich and Huhtaniemi 2012).

69. Bartke 2004: 844.

70. ASA Archives & History Committee 2016, "ASA—Our History: 30th Annual Meeting, Seattle, Washington." When reviewing this passage, research assistant Megann Licskai emailed encouraging me to Google "condom hat." I pass this suggestion on to readers.

71. Rosemberg 1986: 74.

72. ASA 2018.

73. ASA Archives & History Committee 2016, "ASA—Our History: 30th Annual Meeting, Seattle, Washington."

74. Clarke 1998; Marks 2001; May 2010; Oudshoorn 1994.

75. The German physicians Jordan and Niermann inaugurated the journal *Andrologie* by pointing to the zeitgeist as one cause of the increasing attention to men's infertility (1969: 3).

76. Ayanian et al. 2002; Brennan et al. 2004; Sahni et al. 2016.

77. Leinster 2014; Detsky et al. 2012; Rosenthal et al. 2005; Thompson et al. 2005.

CHAPTER 3. MAKING KNOWLEDGE
ABOUT PATERNAL EFFECTS

1. As noted in Pechenick et al. 2015, Ngrams based on the Google Books corpus cannot be taken as a direct measure of the popularity of a word or phrase,

particularly because it oversamples scientific literature. I use Ngrams simply to illustrate some general trends.

2. The exact search run in December 2018 using Google's Ngram Viewer was "andrology + andrologist + andrologists + Andrology + Andrologist + Andrologists." The latest year for which data were available at the time of the search was 2008.

3. The exact search run in December 2018 using Google's Ngram Viewer was "male reproductive health + men's reproductive health + male reproduction + men's reproduction, female reproductive health + women's reproductive health + female reproduction + women's reproduction." I would have added capitalized versions of each phrase but the character count is limited by the Ngram tool. The latest year for which data were available at the time of the search was 2008.

4. Marincola 2009.

5. Fawcett 1976: 249.

6. Steinberger 1982: 213.

7. The exact search run in December 2018 using Google's Ngram Viewer was "andrology + andrologist + andrologists, obstetrics + obstetrician + obstetricians, urology + urologist + urologists, gynaecology + gynaecologist + gynaecologists + gynecology + gynecologist + gynecologists." I would have added capitalized versions of each phrase but the character count is limited by the Ngram tool. The latest year for which data were available at the time of the search was 2008.

8. Guzick et al. 2001; WHO 1980. Until the 1930s, sperm motility was the primary criterion for establishing male fertility (Moench 1930). The three basic measures of motility, morphology, and count have been unchanged since the 1940s. In an article about how the electron microscope was being used to assess sperm, Seymour and Benmosche write: "The ordinary refractive microscope revealed nothing more concerning the morphology of sperm than the contour of the head and number and approximate length of tails. All the finer details were hopelessly concealed. Fundamentally, we know little about spermatozoa, and that little can be summed up as 1) motility or nonmotility, 2) general appearance of spermatozoa as seen with magnifications under 2,000, and 3) the numbers of spermatozoa per cubic centimeter of semen" (1941: 2489).

9. Daniels 2006; de Jong et al. 2014; Frey et al. 2008.

10. See, e.g., Brandt 1985 on sexually transmitted diseases; McLaren 2008 and Loe 2004 on erectile dysfunction; Pfeffer 1993 and Marsh and Ronner 1999 on infertility; Oudshoorn 2003 on the male pill.

11. Waggoner 2017; Frey et al. 2008; Almeling and Waggoner 2013.

12. Paltrow and Flavin 2013.

13. Daniels 2006: 112.

14. Brandt 1985; Daniels and Golden 2000; Kampf 2015.

15. Richardson and Stevens 2015.

16. Crean and Bonduriansky 2014; see also Curley et al. 2011: 306, where it is noted that "within the literature, 'paternal effects' on development can have a variety of meanings."

17. Curley et al. 2011.

18. Ramlau-Hansen et al. 2007; Rubes et al. 1998.

19. Scholars and activists working on issues related to disabilities have objected to the term *birth defects* since it suggests that a child is "defective." Unfortunately, this term remains in wide use, and possible substitutions such as *disabilities at birth* or *birth disorders* may obscure the point I am trying to make. As a result, I have retained the term *birth defects* when referring to its use in the medical literature or by organizations (e.g., March of Dimes in the next chapter).

20. On miscarriage, see De La Rochebrochard and Thonneau 2002; Kleinhaus et al. 2006; Lambert et al. 2006. On birth weight, see Shah 2010. On remaining conditions, see Paul and Robaire 2013 for a review. Additional citations on these topics are in notes 29–30, 34–43, 51, 54–58, 60, 63, 56–67, 72, 77, and 80–82.

21. Most often these are retrospective case-control studies, though some investigations of transgenerational effects are historical cohort studies.

22. Friese and Clarke 2012; Pound and Bracken 2014.

23. To survey the scientific and medical literature on paternal effects, research assistant Jenna Healey and I searched PubMed, ScienceDirect, and Google Scholar using terms such as "paternal effect*," "male-mediated developmental toxicology," and "advanced paternal age." Once we identified a high-quality review, we used its bibliography to identify additional studies. We excluded studies focused solely on male infertility and included studies about how men's age, health, behaviors, and exposures can affect reproductive outcomes and children's health.

24. It would be interesting to systematically compare the quality of evidence available for various paternal effects with the evidence supporting claims about maternal effects, such as prohibitions on maternal drinking or concerns about maternal fish consumption during pregnancy.

25. Frey et al. 2012.

26. Porter 2018: 282, 300.

27. Penrose 1955: 313.

28. I thank Rayna Rapp for suggesting this possibility. Since I have not conducted an extensive analysis of this claim, I encourage future researchers to examine more systematically the possibility that when scientists' initial search for paternal effects in chromosomal anomalies came up empty (e.g., Martin and Rademaker 1987), it precluded further research on the question of how men's age and bodily health might affect reproductive outcomes.

29. Friedman 1981; Jones et al. 1975; Murdoch et al. 1972.

30. Goriely and Wilkie 2012.

31. Bordson and Leonardo 1991: 397.

32. American Fertility Society 1991. A survey of sperm banks conducted by the US Office of Technology Assessment in 1987 reported that most sperm banks did require sperm donors be younger than forty (Office of Technology Assessment 1988).

33. For a review, see Paul and Robaire 2013.

34. Choi et al. 2005; Murray et al. 2002.

35. Malaspina 2001; Reichenberg et al. 2006.

36. Carey 2012; Kong et al. 2012.

37. Hultman et al. 2011.

38. Brown et al. 2002.

39. Sipos et al. 2004.

40. Frans et al. 2008.

41. Buizer-Voskamp et al. 2011.

42. Yang et al. 2007.

43. Urhoj et al. 2014.

44. Zhang et al. 2017.

45. Friedman 1981: 748, 745.

46. Toriello and Meck 2008: 457–59; see also Ramasamy et al. 2015.

47. Thacker 2004: 1683.

48. Bray et al. 2006: 852; see also Sartorius and Nieschlag 2010 for a review.

49. van der Zee et al. 2013, emphasis added.

50. Frickel 2004; Sale 1993. The Occupational Safety and Health Act of 1970 led to the establishment of the Occupational Safety and Health Administration (OSHA), as well as a research agency within the CDC called the National Institute for Occupational Safety and Health (NIOSH) (https://www.osha.gov/about.html).

51. Curley et al. 2011; Day et al. 2016.

52. Bonde 2010: 155; Davis 1991: A27.

53. Alexander 2010; Ortiz and Briggs 2003.

54. Aitken 2013; Anderson et al. 2014.

55. DeMarini 2004; Soares and Melo 2008.

56. Laubenthal et al. 2012; Linschooten et al. 2013.

57. Secretan et al. 2009; see also Lee et al. 2009.

58. Milne et al 2012: 52; see also Aitken 2013.

59. La Vignera et al. 2013.

60. Vassoler et al. 2014.

61. Knopik et al. 2009.

62. de Jong et al. 2014; Jensen et al. 2014.

63. Vassoler et al. 2014.

64. Gilardi et al. 2018.

65. Curley et al. 2011; Rando 2012; Schagdarsurengin and Steger 2016.

66. Kaati et al. 2002.

67. Chen et al. 2006.

68. Jimenez-Chillaron et al. 2009.

69. Anderson et al. 2006.

70. Ng et al. 2010.

71. Hepler 2000.

72. Cordier 2008; Daniels 1997; Friedler 1996; Moline et al. 2000.

73. Bingham and Monforton 2001.

74. Friedler 1996.

75. See, e.g., Stevens 1977: 1.

76. Bingham and Monforton 2001.

77. Fabia and Thuy 1974.

78. Daniels 1993: ch. 3.

79. "Sins of the Fathers" 1991; Friedler 1996; Marcus 1990.

80. Savitz et al. 1994.

81. Magnusson et al. 2004.

82. Cohen et al. 1980; Schrader and Marlow 2014. Friedler (1985) found similar effects among mice exposed to nitrous oxide.

83. Dubrova et al. 2002; Dubrova et al. 1996; Gardner et al. 1990; Parker et al. 1999.

84. Anderson et al. 2014; Little et al. 2013; Tawn et al. 2015. It is interesting to note that the initial studies claiming a link are published in high-profile journals—the British Medical Journal, The Lancet, and in the case of Chernobyl radiation, Nature. These findings are then repeatedly refuted by researchers publishing in lower-impact, field-specific journals. As a result, claims about the risk posed by paternal exposures garner significant publicity while null results are less publicized.

85. Miles 1997; Reagan 2016.

86. World Health Organization and United Nations Environment Programme 2013; Levine et al. 2017; Pacey 2013.

87. Anderson et al. 2014: 86; see also Cordier 2008.

88. Clawson and Clawson 1999; Lipton and Ivory 2017.

89. Daniels 2006: 109–115; quotes from 115, 202n14. See also quotes from Dolores Malaspina on how gendered "biases hold us back from scientific advances" in Thacker 2004: 1685.

90. Daniels 2006: 151.

91. Pembrey et al. 2014; see also Braun et al. 2017 and Sharp et al. 2018.

92. Goldin and Katz 2011.

93. Bowles 2018.

94. On this latter point, see Curley et al. 2011: 307.

95. See Link and Phelan 1995 and Phelan et al. 2010 for discussions of how social conditions, and in particular socioeconomic inequalities, are fundamental causes of health and disease. See Almeling and Waggoner 2013 for a discussion of variation in how women's and men's reproductive contributions are considered in medicine.

CHAPTER 4. REPRODUCTIVE HEALTH FOR
HALF THE PUBLIC

1. Fissell and Cooter 2003.

2. Social media, such as Twitter and Facebook, is another important site of contemporary discussions about health and reproduction but is not included in this analysis.

3. Daniels 1997: 602.

4. Campo-Engelstein et al. 2016.

5. LaRossa 1997; Townsend 2002.

6. Although I did not find their article until after I was done with this analysis, I was heartened to see that Campo-Engelstein et al. 2016 uses a similarly narrowing search strategy in their content analysis of newspaper articles about reproductive aging.

7. My sample is larger than Daniels's, who identified just four *New York Times* articles on paternal effects published between 1985 and 1996 (1997: 601). The discrepancy may be due to different search terms or more items having now been digitized and thus easier to search.

8. The count of articles about paternal effects on children is also included in the count of articles about paternal effects on sperm.

9. Associated Press 1976: 23.

10. Nagourney 1999.

11. See, e.g., Kolata 1996b: C1.

12. Brody 1981; Shulevitz 2012: SR1. Brody joined the *New York Times* in 1965 as a medicine and biology reporter; as of November 2018, according to a brief bio on the *New York Times* website, she is still writing the "Personal Health" column, which she has penned on a regular basis since 1976. Several "Personal Health" columns that focus on sperm are included in this sample.

13. WebMD 2014.

14. Mayo Clinic Staff 2012.

15. Bouchez 2006.

16. Campo-Engelstein 2016; Daniels 1997.

17. Angier 2001: F4.

18. Stellman and Bertin 1990: A23.

19. Lewin 1988: A24.

20. Lewin 2001: WK4.

21. Angier 1994: C12.

22. Rabin 2009: A12.

23. Bowles 2018.

24. American Society of News Editors Newsroom Census, www.asne.org.

25. There are forty-nine articles in this category; ten listed no author.

26. Mayo Clinic Staff 2014.

27. Fetters 2015.

28. Greenfield 2013.

29. Sgobba 2015.

30. Heid 2014; Sgobba 2015.

31. What to Expect 2015.

32. Parents.com 2015.

33. Murkoff 2015.

34. Kolata 1996a: E4; Shulevitz 2012.

35. The reader should note that my content analysis of these materials included only the text, not the (often stock) photos of men that accompany many of these articles. For example, the CDC's website on men's preconception health features a photo of a Black man (see figure 12). Future researchers may want to revisit the question of intersections between gender, race, and class with attention to the kinds of images that are chosen to illustrate these issues.

36. Daniels 1997.

37. Associated Press 1991: B8.

38. Kolata 1999: A16.

39. Davis 1991: A27.

40. Crane 2014: ST1.

41. Showalter 1997.

42. Bowles 2018.

43. Goode 2001: A20.

44. Fisch 2004; Healey in preparation. By 2015, health and parenting websites had adopted the metaphor of the male biological clock to discuss the potential consequences of advanced paternal age (e.g., Mayo Clinic's pages "Healthy Sperm" and "Paternal Age"; WebMD's "Men May Have Biological Clocks Too"; and Men's Health "Best Age to Have Kids," which quotes Harry Fisch).

45. Rabin 2005: A5.

46. Jayson 2005.

47. Campo-Engelstein et al. 2016.

48. See, e.g., Lewin 2001.

49. Kong et al. 2012.

50. Carey 2012: A1.

51. Ellin 2016.

52. Belkin 2009: SM12.

53. McGrath 2002: E11.

54. Raeburn 2014a.

55. Editors of *Men's Health* 2015; Fetters 2015.

56. MacKendrick 2018.

57. Epstein 2007.

58. Prins and Bremner 2004.

59. Bowles 2018.

60. National Institute of Child Health and Human Development 2013a.

61. National Institute of Child Health and Human Development 2013b.

62. NIH 2015.

63. CDC 2013.

64. CDC 2014. Federal agencies such as the NIH and CDC link to each other's pages on men's reproductive health, as well as websites of professional organizations, such as the American Society for Reproductive Medicine, and consumer health websites, such as the Mayo Clinic and Planned Parenthood.

65. CDC 2015; Waggoner 2017.

66. CDC 2010: 4.

67. CDC 2010: 21.

68. NIOSH 1996.

69. This same fact sheet is reproduced on the CDC website.

70. NIOSH 1996, emphasis added.

71. See, e.g., Miles 1997; U.S. Department of Defense 1994.

72. ASRM 2012; ACOG 2012.

73. ACOG 2013.

74. ASRM 2015.

75. Messing and Östlin 2006; WHO and United Nations Environment Programme 2013.

76. Barker et al. 2007.

77. Interview with Jennifer Howse, former president of the March of Dimes, November 21, 2019.

78. Male Role Press Conference Suggested Remarks, December 5, 1991, "Male Role in Reproductive Health 1991" folder, Media Relations: 1980–2005, Series 1: Internal Affairs, box 6 of 33, March of Dimes Archives.

79. In a form letter accompanying the new "Men Have Babies Too" brochure sent to media contacts, the public relations manager writes that there have been "hundreds of calls" and gives this as the reason why the Greater New York chapter created the brochure (e.g., Jonathan Moskowitz to Max Gomez, May 18, 1992, "Men Have Babies Too Campaign—Greater New York Chapter 1992" folder, Media Relations: 1980–2005, Series 1: Internal Affairs, box 6 of 33, March of Dimes Archives).

80. The March of Dimes archives include copies of a single-panel brochure produced by the national office called "Dad, It's Your Baby Too," dated February

1982. A brochure with the same title but expanded to three panels is dated October 1991. A memo sent the day before the male role press conference in 1991 includes a typewritten note arguing this brochure should not be included in the press packet because it describes "the father's role [as] simply supportive." A handwritten reply suggests it should be included because it would offer reporters another potential angle on the story. The records do not reveal whether it was included in the press kit or not. (Memo from Martha to Mark, December 4, 1991, "Editorial Luncheon on Environmental Health and Reproductive Risks" folder, Media Relations: 1980–2005, Series 6: National Communications Advisory Committee, box 22 of 33, March of Dimes Archives.)

81. The earliest copy of the brochure in the March of Dimes Archives is dated January 1993 and authorship credit is listed as the Greater New York chapter. There are no copies of the original June 1992 brochure, but two documents suggest that the national office may have made slight changes to the design and text of the brochure before rolling it out as part of a national campaign. First, there is a picture of a newscaster holding up the 1992 brochure in the Greater New York chapter's Fall 1992 newsletter, and the front image of a man holding a child is the same but larger, taking up the entire first page ("New York Chapter's 'Male Role' Campaign Takes Public by Storm," Greater New York March of Dimes Birth Defects Foundation, *Ultra Sound Bites Newsletter*, Fall 1992, pages 1–2). Both that newsletter article and a Greater New York chapter press release ("The Greater New York March of Dimes Releases Information Guide for Fathers-to-Be, June 4, 1992") reprint text from the brochure, and much of the content appears the same in both the June 1992 and January 1993 versions, but I could not compare them word for word. The newsletter and the press release are both in the "Men Have Babies Too Campaign—Greater New York Chapter 1992" folder, Media Relations 1980–2005, Series 1: Internal Affairs, box 6 of 33, March of Dimes Archives.

82. See press releases and correspondence in the folders "Men Have Babies Too Campaign—Media Coverage 1993" and "Men Have Babies Too Campaign—Memos 1993," Media Relations 1980–2005, Series 1: Internal Affairs, box 6 of 33, March of Dimes Archives.

83. See, for example, memos dated February 2, 1993, and April 19, 1993 in the "Men Have Babies Too Campaign—Press Releases and Print PSAs 1993" folder, Media Relations 1980–2005, Series 1: Internal Affairs, box 6 of 33, March of Dimes Archives.

84. Interview with Jennifer Howse, former president of the March of Dimes, November 21, 2019.

85. Personal communication with David Rose, March of Dimes archivist, November 30, 2018. In addition, staffers' notes from marketing meetings and internal lists of "major milestones" from the first half of the 1990s do not list the Men Have Babies Too campaign, suggesting it was not a major focus.

In addition to the Men Have Babies Too campaign, there are only two other times the March of Dimes appears to have focused on men's reproductive health in recent history. The organization had some involvement with the question of whether soldiers' exposure to Agent Orange resulted in their children's disabilities, but that did not involve a large-scale public education campaign (e.g., Toxics, Herbicides, Pesticides, Agent Orange 1979–1984 in the "Office of Government Affairs" folder and Agent Orange 1984 and Agent Orange 1985–1988 in the "Public Relations II" folder, March of Dimes Archives). The March of Dimes has also collaborated with the Alpha Phi Alpha fraternity to encourage "responsibility" among teen fathers of color, but the "leadership binder" does not contain any mention of paternal effects.

86. March of Dimes National Office, "Think Ahead: Is There a Baby in Your Future?" in the "Think Ahead Prepregnancy Campaign 1995–1996" folder, Senior Vice President for Education and Health Promotion Records: 1988–2002, Series 1: Education and Health Program, box 6 of 23, March of Dimes Archives.

CHAPTER 5. SEX, SPERM, AND FATHERHOOD

1. See, e.g., Furstenberg 1988; Marsiglio et al. 2001.

2. LaRossa 1997; Townsend 2002.

3. One potential exception to this claim is the series of studies conducted by William Marsiglio and colleagues on men's "procreative identity" and "procreative consciousness" (e.g., Marsiglio 1998; Marsiglio and Hutchinson 2002). However, these studies are undergirded by an almost essentialist view of biological masculinity, assumptions about heterosexuality, and presumptions of paternal agency that preclude truly open-ended questions. Moreover, although some of their interviewees occasionally discuss sperm and conception, their focus is more on men's views of fatherhood.

4. I conducted thirty-one of the interviews with men, and I hired a male research assistant, Todd Madigan, to do nine of the interviews to test for gender-of-interviewer effects; I describe dismissing this possibility in Appendix A: Methods.

5. Gender scholars may raise an eyebrow at my choice of the word *role*, given that the sex roles approach has been thoroughly debunked due in large part to its portrayal of traits as static and unchanging (e.g., Connell 1987; Lopata and Thorne 1978). However, I wanted to choose a word that could be easily understood by men with all levels of education, and I also wanted to elicit stylized narratives to see if any clear norms emerged in men's answers. Hence, the question was not about their own particular experiences of reproduction. Instead, I asked generally about "a man's" role in reproduction.

6. See Fullwiley 2007 for another example of pauses as data.

7. Abdill 2018; Anderson 1999; Edin and Nelson 2013; Haney 2018.

8. Townsend 2002.

9. Pampers is a brand name for diapers, and Enfamil is a brand name for baby formula.

10. Goldberg et al. 2014; Pew Research Center 2015.

11. Almeling 2015.

12. See, e.g., Schneider 1968.

13. See, e.g., Franklin 2013; Strathern 1992; Thompson 2005. Analogously, social scientists following the latest developments in genetics also find that the meaning of biology is quite malleable. Individuals, far from thinking of DNA as deterministic, incorporate genetic information into their already developed identities, familial relationships, and political commitments (e.g., Gibbon and Novas 2008; Lock et al. 2007).

14. Almeling 2011.

15. Ragoné 1994.

16. For an exception, see Almeling 2011: ch. 5 on sperm donors' views of bio-genetic relatedness.

17. Almeling 2015.

18. To maintain similarity between men's and women's interviews, I asked women about men's role in reproduction before asking them about women's role in reproduction.

19. Almeling 2011; Bangerter 2000; Moore 2007; Wagner et al. 1995.

20. Martin 1991.

21. The technical term for this process is chemotaxis; see Eisenbach and Giojalas 2006 for a review.

22. Nettleton 2015.

23. Unfortunately, I did not think of this question until several interviews had been completed, hence the N of 33 for counts in this section. In asking the question, we alternated word order, asking half the men about "an egg and a sperm" and the other half "a sperm and an egg." As I coded responses to the egg/sperm question, I noticed that some of the men's descriptions of sperm differed from their responses to the reproduction question. To ensure I captured variation *within* interviews of how people talk about sperm, I did a text search of the full transcripts for all fifty-five interviews for "sperm* or semen or cell* or seed." This section also incorporates coding from the results of that text search.

24. Martin 1991. Lest readers think this view among clinicians is a matter of history, I was in the audience of a fertility conference in 2018 when the chair of an ob-gyn department described the process of IVF as "take one egg and about 50,000 sperm, put it in a drop of oil, and let the best man win." When explaining how to do ICSI, he referred to a cartoon character from the 1980s: "take a He-man-looking sperm and inject it directly into an egg."

25. Gasking 1967.

26. See, e.g., McElheny 2012.

27. Delaney 1986.

28. Chavkin 1992; see also the documentary film *Vessel* about Dr. Rebecca Gomperts's organization Women on Waves.

29. See Matthew Gutmann's *Fixing Men* (2007) for a related discussion about how conceptualizations of men as driven by "biological urges" appears to have foreclosed sociological analysis of male sexuality. See also Florence Vienne's (2018: 13) historical analysis of how the animal-like characteristics of sperm have been referred to since the 1850s in describing its agency in fertilization.

30. Almeling and Waggoner 2013.

31. Here the interviewer is the male research assistant introduced in note 4.

32. To define *egalitarianism*, we reviewed questions used in the General Social Survey and the Gender-Equitable-Men Scale (GEMS) developed by the Population Council and Promundo.

33. Research assistant Dana Hayward and I had high intercoder reliability, meaning we agreed on most of the categorizations. We discussed the respondents we were uncertain about and assigned all but seven of them to a category based on our joint determination of which description best fit.

34. Figure includes data for men who were categorizable as more or less egalitarian and who were asked the egg-and-sperm question.

35. See, e.g., Fischer and Hout 2006; Pampel 2011. I did not find differences in egalitarianism by the men's race or the interviewer's gender.

36. Analogously, see Milam 2010 for a historical analysis of the concept of "female choice" in biological studies of sexual selection, in which she argues that the same set of biological "facts" can be interpreted through the lens of gender and result in varying claims about human mating.

37. Schelling 1978: 22.

38. Jaggar 1983.

39. Conrad and Markens 2001.

40. See, e.g., Oudshoorn 1994; Richardson 2013; Roberts 2011.

CHAPTER 6. HEALTHY SPERM?

1. See, e.g., Conrad 1992; Link and Phelan 1995.

2. MacKendrick 2018; Markens et al. 1997; Waggoner 2017.

3. For more on the history of reproduction being located in women's bodies, see the Introduction and chapter 1. For a recent indictment of mother-blame in biomedical research, see Richardson et al. 2014.

4. Paul does have a son, but there is a tendency even among men who are not fathers to envision their potential children as male.

5. Of the thirty-nine men asked this question, five answered there was nothing men could do. Hence, the percentages in this table are based on an N of 34. I do not include actions mentioned by fewer than 15 percent of the men.

6. Healey in preparation.

7. Fisch 2004.

8. Cutler and Lleras-Muney 2010.

9. Given this discourse of "similarity," I thought it was possible that men who were familiar with research on paternal effects might be more likely to tell the second sperm story discussed in chapter 5. However, just two of the nine men did.

10. Bird and Rieker 2008; Courtenay 2000.

11. Daniels 2006.

12. LaRossa 1997; Townsend 2002.

13. Bianchi 2000; Craig et al. 2014.

14. Doucet 2017; Hays 1996; Shirani et al. 2012.

15. Leavitt 2010.

16. A fifth of the men asked whether the information was true.

17. Ajzen 1991; Rosenstock et al. 1988.

18. Clarke et al. 2010; Lupton 1995. Thanks to Liz Roberts for a helpful conversation on this point.

19. Such skepticism has become more pronounced in the few years since I conducted these interviews, as anti-vaccine activism (Reich 2016) and climate change denial (Oreskes and Conway 2011) have gained traction.

20. See, e.g., Benjamin 2016; Reverby 2009.

21. Luna and Luker 2013; Roberts 1997.

22. This was a lengthy quote I edited heavily to remove racist references to African Americans. I have focused on his comments about poverty.

23. See, e.g., Krieger 2001; Link and Phelan 1995; Shim 2014.

24. Reed 2009; see also Inhorn and Wentzell 2011.

25. Conrad and Schneider 1980.

26. Krieger 2001.

27. Lamoreaux in progress; Wahlberg 2018.

28. MacKendrick 2018. See also Valdez 2018 for an analysis of how scientists studying the "environment" and its epigenetic effects still "individualize responsibility" onto pregnant women. The Chemical Youth project led by anthropologist Anita Hardon offers creative new ways of thinking about chemicals and bodies around the world (www.chemicalyouth.org; Hardon et al. 2017).

29. Bayer 2008; Link and Phelan 2001.

30. Landsman 2008; Markens et al. 1997.

CONCLUSION

1. Bettcher 2014; Lampe et al. 2019; Schilt and Lagos 2017.

2. See, e.g., smith 2019.

3. Croissant 2014 (described in "The Making of Non-Knowledge" in the Introduction).

4. Griswold 1987; Petersen and Anand 2004.

5. See, e.g., Lawrence and Weisz 1998.

6. Blair-Loy 2003; Correll et al. 2007; Daniels 2006.

7. Paltrow and Flavin 2013.

8. Kligman 1998.

9. Finer and Zolna 2016; Stevens forthcoming.

10. Ibis Reproductive Health 2017.

11. I ran the search on June 12, 2018. I found a similar ratio of results in a general Google search.

12. I first saw this statement on the NIH webpage "Men's Reproductive Health," www.nichd.nih.gov/health/topics/menshealth, in 2013, and it was still there as of September 2019.

13. Bond et al. 2010; CDC 2010; Frey et al. 2008; Kotelchuck and Lu 2017.

14. Sharp et al. 2018.

15. Garfield 2018: 2, emphasis added.

16. Krieger 2003; Springer et al. 2012.

17. Annandale and Hammarstrom 2011.

18. I did not do a formal count of each category, but they are listed roughly in terms of the frequency with which they were mentioned.

19. Mitchell et al. 2012; Shawe et al. 2019.

20. Bird and Rieker 2008; Courtenay 2000.

21. The US Preventive Services Task Force issues evidence-based recommendations for various preventive services, including cancer screening (www.uspreventiveservicestaskforce.org). At present, it recommends that men be screened for colon cancer starting at age fifty. It recommends *against* screening for testicular cancer in adolescent or adult men. Recommendations for adult women include cervical cancer screening every three to five years, depending on their age.

22. Courtenay 2000.

23. AAFP 2015, emphasis added; see also O'Brien et al. 2018; Warner and Frey 2013.

24. Allen et al. 2017.

25. Epstein and Mamo 2017.

26. MacKendrick 2018.

27. Gavin et al. 2014; Shawe et al. 2019.

28. Healthy People 2020, Topics and Objectives, www.healthypeople .gov/2020/topics-objectives, accessed November 23, 2019.

29. See, e.g., Ross and Solinger 2017.

30. Greene et al. 2006.

31. Legacy, www.givelegacy.com, accessed October 18, 2019.

32. Tuana 2004: 200–209.

APPENDIX A

1. Clarke 1998; Daniels 2006; Moscucci 1990; Pfeffer 1993.

2. Oudshoorn 1994; Sengoopta 2006.

3. Gutmann 2007; Oudshoorn 2003.

4. Vienne 2018.

5. Brandt 1985; Worboys 2004.

6. Carpenter 2010; Darby 2005.

7. Leavitt 2010; Reed 2005.

8. McLaren 2008; Tiefer 1994; Wentzell 2013.

9. Barnes 2014; Becker 2000.

10. Brandt 1985; Messner 1992.

11. Three of these interviews were conducted for my previous book, *Sex Cells* (2011).

12. We did a keyword search for the terms "sperm*" (so as to include results for *spermatozoa, sperms, spermatology*, etc.), which yielded 576 articles; "semen," 205 articles; "seminal fluid," 34 articles; and "insemination," 113 articles. Reading through the titles and abstracts, Jenna culled the sample to 68 potentially relevant articles that we read more closely.

13. To search for articles in the *New York Times,* we searched "Historical Newspapers" from 1860–2011, ProQuest from 2012 to 2013, and Nexis Uni from 2014 to 2018 because each offered the most comprehensive search for those time periods. After experimenting with different search strategies, we eventually settled on separate searches for "sperm*," "seminal," and "semen" during the period 1860–1960; this produced around 3,000 results, and Celene reviewed headlines to narrow it to potentially relevant articles (N = 96). For the period 1960–2018, we searched "sperm* OR semen," which yielded around 5,100 articles (including some duplicates). Celene whittled this sample down to 610 by including only articles focused on how men matter for reproductive outcomes (not articles that were generally about male fertility, sperm donation, in vitro fertilization, etc.). Articles published from the 1880s through the 1960s provided background context and occasionally pointed me to important moments in the history of biomedical attention to men.

14. Saguy and Almeling 2008.

15. Materials I reviewed at the March of Dimes headquarters in White Plains, New York, on November 30, 2018:

Media Relations, 1980–2005, Series 1: Internal Affairs (Box 6 of 33)

Media Relations, 1980–2005, Series 2: Public Affairs (Box 17 of 33)

Media Relations, 1980–2005, Series 6: NCAC (Box 22 of 33)

Senior Vice President for Education and Health Promotion Records: 1988–2002, Series 1: Education and Health Programs (Box 6 of 23)

"Think Ahead" Public Health Campaign kit

Project Alpha binder

Office of Government Affairs (loose folders)

16. Mitchell et al. 2012.

17. U.S. Census Bureau, QuickFacts, www.quickfacts.census.gov.

18. Office of the Assistant Secretary for Planning and Evaluation, U.S. Department of Health and Human Services, 2015 Poverty Guidelines, September 3, 2015, www.aspe.hhs.gov/2015-poverty-guidelines.

19. Martin 1992; Edin and Nelson 2013.

20. See, e.g., Barnes 2014; Becker 2000.

21. Bird and Rieker 2008; Courtenay 2000.

22. The last question was added after I completed the first few interviews because I realized some interview subjects were referring their friends. I did not want to include individuals who may have been briefed regarding the nature of the interview.

23. See, e.g., Kiselica 2008; Weber 2012.

24. See, e.g., Flores-Macias and Lawson 2008; Padfield and Procter 1996.

25. Since the additional interviews with gay men, MSM, and women were conducted after the Zika virus began garnering headlines and journalists began reporting the possibility that it could be transmitted via sperm, I was worried these new respondents would have different things to say about men's reproductive health. In fact, nobody mentioned Zika at any point in the interviews, and their responses were largely similar to those I heard in the first round of interviews.

26. Weiss 1994.

27. Edin and Nelson 2013:15.

Bibliography

AAFP. 2015. "Preconception Care (Position Paper)." American Association of
Family Physicians. www.aafp.org/about/policies/all/preconception-care.html.

AAGUS. 1911. *A Brief History of the Organization and Transactions of the
American Association of Genito-urinary Surgeons, October 16th, 1886 to
October 16th, 1911.* New York: Pub. for the Association.

Abbott, Andrew. 1988. *The System of Professions: An Essay on the Division of
Expert Labor.* Chicago: University of Chicago Press.

Abdill, Aasha M. 2018. *Fathering from the Margins: An Intimate Examination
of Black Fatherhood.* New York: Columbia University Press.

ACOG. 2012. "Evaluating Infertility." American College of Obstetricians and
Gynecologists FAQ 136. Accessed March 29, 2015. www.acog.org.

———. 2013. "A Father's Guide to Pregnancy." American College of Obstetricians and Gynecologists FAQ 032. Accessed March 29, 2015. www.acog.org.

———. 2018. "Well-Woman Visit." American College of Obstetricians and
Gynecologists Committee Opinion no. 755. www.acog.org/Clinical-Guid-
ance-and-Publications/Committee-Opinions/Committee-on-Gynecologic-
Practice/Well-Woman-Visit.

Acton, William. 1875. *The Functions and Disorders of the Reproductive Organs
in Childhood, Youth, Adult Age, and Advanced Life considered in Their
Physiological, Social, and Moral Relations.* London: J. & A. Churchill.

Adams, Rachel, and David Savran, eds. 2002. *The Masculinity Studies Reader.*
Hoboken, NJ: Wiley-Blackwell.

Aitken, R.J. 2013. "Human Spermatozoa: Revelations on the Road to Conception." *F1000 Prime Reports* 5:39.

Ajzen, Icek. 1991. "The Theory of Planned Behavior." *Organizational Behavior and Human Decision Processes* 50(2):179–211.

Alexander, Michelle. 2010. *The New Jim Crow: Mass Incarceration in the Age of Colorblindness.* New York: New Press.

Allen, Deborah, Michele Stranger Hunter, Susan Wood, and Tishra Beeson. 2017. "One Key Question®: First Things First in Reproductive Health." *Maternal and Child Health Journal* 21(3):387–92.

Almeling, Rene. 2011. *Sex Cells: The Medical Market for Eggs and Sperm.* Berkeley: University of California Press.

———. 2015. "Reproduction." *Annual Review of Sociology* 41(1):423–42.

Almeling, Rene, and Miranda R. Waggoner. 2013. "More and Less Than Equal: How Men Factor in the Reproductive Equation." *Gender & Society* 27(6):821–42.

"American Dermatological Association: The Tenth Annual Meeting Held at Greenwich, Conn." 1886. *Journal of Cutaneous Diseases Including Syphilis* 4:10.

American Fertility Society. 1991. "Revised Guidelines for the Use of Semen Donor Insemination: 1991." *Fertility and Sterility* 56(3):396–96.

American Society of Andrology Records, 1975–ongoing, MS 410, Iowa State University Library Special Collections and University Archives, Ames, IA.

Anderson, D., T.E. Schmid, and A. Baumgartner. 2014. "Male-Mediated Developmental Toxicity." *Asian Journal of Andrology* 16(1):81–88.

Anderson, Elijah. 1999. *Code of the Street: Decency, Violence, and the Moral Life of the Inner City.* New York: W.W. Norton.

Anderson, Lucy M., Lisa Riffle, Ralph Wilson, Gregory S. Travlos, Mariusz S. Lubomirski, and W. Gregory Alvord. 2006. "Preconceptional Fasting of Fathers Alters Serum Glucose in Offspring of Mice." *Nutrition* 22(3):327–31.

Anderson, Warwick. 2006. *Colonial Pathologies: American Tropical Medicine, Race, and Hygiene in the Philippines.* Durham, NC: Duke University Press.

"Andrology as a Specialty." 1891. *JAMA* 17(18):691.

ASA. 1975. Sign-up sheet for the inaugural meeting of American Society of Andrology in Detroit 1975. American Society of Andrology Records, 1975– ongoing, MS 410. Iowa State University Library Special Collections and University Archives.

———. 2018. "About the ASA." www.andrologysociety.org.

ASA Archives & History Committee, ed. 2016. *40 and Forward: American Society of Andrology Celebrating 40 Years.* Schaumburg, IL: American Society of Andrology. www.andrologyamerica.org/uploads/2/4/1/9/24198611 /asa40yearsdigitalcompleteb.pdf.

Angier, Natalie. 1994. "Genetic Mutations Tied to Father in Most Cases." *New York Times,* May 17, 1994. www.nytimes.com/1994/05/17/science/genetic-mutations-tied-to-father-in-most-cases.html.

———. 2001. "New Rules in Sperm and Egg's Cat-and-Mouse Game." *New York Times,* February 27, 2001. https://www.nytimes.com/2001/02/27/science/new-rules-in-sperm-and-egg-s-cat-and-mouse-game.html

Annandale, Ellen, and Anne Hammarstrom. 2011. "Constructing the 'Gender-Specific Body': A Critical Discourse Analysis of Publications in the Field of Gender-Specific Medicine." *Health* 15(6):571–87.

"Annotations." 1888. *Lancet* 132(3390):331–40.

ASRM. 2012. "Optimizing Male Fertility." Accessed March 28, 2015. www.asrm.org.

———. 2013. "American Society for Reproductive Medicine's 'Waiting to Have a Baby?' Campaign." Accessed March 28, 2015. www.asrm.org.

———. 2015. "Alcohol and Drug Use." Accessed March 28, 2015. www.asrm.org.

Associated Press. 1976. "Injury to Fetuses Is Traced in Study to Vinyl Chloride." *New York Times,* February 4, 1976: 23. www.nytimes.com/1976/02/04/archives/injury-to-fetuses-is-traced-in-study-to-vinyl-chloride.html.

———. 1991. "Study Links Cancer in Young to Fathers' Smoking." *New York Times,* January 24, 1991. www.nytimes.com/1991/01/24/us/study-links-cancer-in-young-to-fathers-smoking.html.

Atwood, Margaret. 1985. *The Handmaid's Tale.* New York: Fawcett Crest.

Ayanian, John Z., Mary Beth Landrum, Edward Guadagnoli, and Peter Gaccione. 2002. "Specialty of Ambulatory Care Physicians and Mortality among Elderly Patients after Myocardial Infarction." *New England Journal of Medicine* 347(21):1678–86.

Balasubramanian, Savina. 2018. "Motivating Men: Social Science and the Regulation of Men's Reproduction in Postwar India." *Gender & Society* 32(1):34–58.

Bangerter, Adrian. 2000. "Transformation between Scientific and Social Representations of Conception: The Method of Serial Reproduction." *British Journal of Social Psychology* 39(4):521–35.

Barad, Karen. 2006. *Meeting the Universe Halfway: Quantum Physics and the Entanglement of Matter and Meaning.* Durham, NC: Duke University Press.

Barker, Gary, Christine Ricardo, and Marcos Nascimento. 2007. *Engaging Men and Boys in Changing Gender-Based Inequity in Health: Evidence from Programme Interventions.* Geneva: WHO Press.

Barnes, Liberty. 2014. *Conceiving Masculinity: Male Infertility, Medicine, and Identity.* Philadelphia: Temple University Press.

Bartke, Andrzej. 2004. "Early Years of the *Journal of Andrology.*" *Journal of Andrology* 25(6):1.

Bayer, Ronald. 2008. "Stigma and the Ethics of Public Health: Not Can We but Should We." *Social Science & Medicine* 67(3):463–72.

Beaney, James George. 1883. *The Generative System and Its Functions in Health and Disease.* Melbourne: F. F. Baillière.

Becker, Gay. 2000. *The Elusive Embryo: How Women and Men Approach New Reproductive Technologies.* Berkeley: University of California Press.

Belker, Arnold, Jean Fourcroy, Rex Hess, Steve Schrader, Richard Sherins, Carol Sloan, and Anna Steinberger. 2006. "Announcement of the Eugenia Rosemberg Endowment Fund." *Journal of Andrology* 27(3):2.

Belkin, Lisa. 2009. "Your Old Man." *New York Times Magazine,* April 1, 2009. www.nytimes.com/2009/04/05/magazine/05wwln-lede-t.html.

Bell, Ann V. 2014. *Misconception: Social Class and Infertility in America.* New Brunswick, NJ: Rutgers University Press.

"Bellevue Hospital Medical College—City of New York, Sessions for 1866–67." 1866. *American Journal of the Medical Sciences* 52:299.

Benford, Robert D., and David A. Snow. 2000. "Framing Processes and Social Movements: An Overview and Assessment." *Annual Review of Sociology* 26(1):611–39.

Benjamin, Ruha. 2016. "Informed Refusal: Toward a Justice-Based Bioethics." *Science, Technology, & Human Values* 41(6):967–90.

Benninghaus, Christina. 2012. "Beyond Constructivism?: Gender, Medicine and the Early History of Sperm Analysis, Germany 1870–1900." *Gender & History* 24(3):647–76.

Berger, John, Sven Blomberg, Chris Fox, Michael Dibb, and Richard Hollis. 1973. *Ways of Seeing.* New York: Viking Press.

Bettcher, Talia. 2014. "Feminist Perspectives on Trans Issues." In *Stanford Encyclopedia of Philosophy,* spring 2014 ed., edited by Edward N. Zalta. https://plato.stanford.edu/archives/spr2014/entries/feminism-trans/.

Bettendorf, Gerhard. 1995. "Rosemberg, Eugenia." In *Zur Geschichte der Endokrinologie und Reproduktionsmedizin: 256 Biographien und Berichte,* edited by Gerhard Bettendorf, 460–61. Berlin, Heidelberg: Springer Berlin Heidelberg.

Bianchi, Suzanne M. 2000. "Maternal Employment and Time with Children: Dramatic Change or Surprising Continuity?" *Demography* 37(4):401–14.

Bingham, Eula, and Celeste Monforton. 2001. "The Pesticide DBCP and Male Infertility." In *Late Lessons from Early Warnings: The Precautionary Principle 1896–2000,* edited by Poul Harremoës, 203–13. Luxembourg: Office for Official Publications of the European Communities.

Bird, Chloe, and Patricia Rieker. 2008. *Gender and Health: The Effects of Constrained Choices and Social Policies.* New York: Cambridge University Press.

Black, Donald Campbell. 1875. *On the Functional Diseases of the Urinary and Reproductive Organs*. London: J. & A. Churchill.

Blair-Loy, Mary. 2003. *Competing Devotions: Career and Family among Women Executives*. Cambridge, MA: Harvard University Press.

Bock von Wülfingen, Bettina, Christina Brandt, Susanne Lettow, and Florence Vienne. 2015. "Temporalities of Reproduction: Practices and Concepts from the Eighteenth to the Early Twenty-First Century." *History and Philosophy of the Life Sciences* 37(1):1–16.

Bond, M. Jermane, Joel J. Heidelbaugh, Audra Robertson, P. A. Alio, and Willie J. Parker. 2010. "Improving Research, Policy and Practice to Promote Paternal Involvement in Pregnancy Outcomes: The Roles of Obstetricians–Gynecologists." *Current Opinion in Obstetrics and Gynecology* 22(6):525–29.

Bonde, J. P. 2010. "Male Reproductive Organs Are at Risk from Environmental Hazards." *Asian Journal of Andrology* 12(2):152–56.

Bonner, Thomas N. 1963. *American Doctors and German Universities*. Lincoln: University of Nebraska Press.

"Book Notice: Male Diseases in General Practice." 1910. *New York Medical Journal* 91:880–81.

"Book Review: A Clinical Hand-book on the Diseases of Women." 1882. *Ohio Medical Journal* 1(11):513.

Bordson, B. L., and V. S. Leonardo. 1991. "The Appropriate Upper Age Limit for Semen Donors: A Review of the Genetic Effects of Paternal Age." *Fertility and Sterility* 56(3):397–401.

Boston Women's Health Book Collective. 1973. *Our Bodies, Ourselves*. New York: Simon and Schuster.

Bouchez, Colette. 2006. "Men May Have Biological Clocks, Too." WebMD. www.webmd.com/men/features/guys-biological-clock#1.

Bowen, Elliot G. 2013. "Mecca of the American Syphilitic: Doctors, Patients, and Disease Identity in Hot Springs, Arkansas, 1890–1940." PhD diss., State University of New York at Binghamton.

Bowles, Nellie. 2018. "Manosphere in a Panic: Are Your Swimmers in Peril?" *New York Times*, July 26, 2018: D1. www.nytimes.com/2018/07/25/style/sperm-count.html.

Brandt, Allan M. 1985. *No Magic Bullet: A Social History of Venereal Disease in the United States since 1880*. New York: Oxford University Press.

Braun, J. M., C. Messerlian, and R. Hauser. 2017. "Fathers Matter: Why It's Time to Consider the Impact of Paternal Environmental Exposures on Children's Health." *Current Epidemiology Reports* 4(1):46–55.

Braun, Lundy. 2014. *Breathing Race into the Machine: The Surprising Career of the Spirometer from Plantation to Genetics*. Minneapolis: University of Minnesota Press.

Bray, Isabelle, David Gunnell, and George Davey Smith. 2006. "Advanced Paternal Age: How Old Is Too Old?" *Journal of Epidemiology and Community Health* 60(10):851–53.

Brennan, T. A., R. I. Horwitz, F. Duffy, C. K. Cassel, L. D. Goode, and R. S. Lipner. 2004. "The Role of Physician Specialty Board Certification Status in the Quality Movement." *JAMA* 292(9):1038–43.

Bridges, Khiara. 2011. *Reproducing Race: An Ethnography of Pregnancy as a Site of Racialization*. Berkeley: University of California Press.

Brody, Jane E. 1981. "Sperm Found Especially Vulnerable to Environment." *New York Times*, March 10, 1981: C1. www.nytimes.com/1981/03/10/science/sperm-found-especially-vulnerable-to-environment.html.

———. 1991. "Personal Health." *New York Times*, December 25, 1991: 64. www.nytimes.com/1991/12/25/health/personal-health-422091.html.

Brown, A. S., C. A. Schaefer, R. J. Wyatt, M. D. Begg, R. Goetz, M. A. Bresnahan, J. Harkavy-Friedman, J. M. Gorman, D. Malaspina, and E. S. Susser. 2002. "Paternal Age and Risk of Schizophrenia in Adult Offspring." *American Journal of Psychiatry* 159(9):1528–33.

Browner, Carole, and Nancy Press. 1995. "The Normalization of Prenatal Diagnostic Screening." In *Conceiving the New World Order: The Global Politics of Reproduction*, edited by Faye Ginsburg and Rayna Rapp. Berkeley: University of California Press.

Buizer-Voskamp, Jacobine E., Wijnand Laan, Wouter G. Staal, Eric A. M. Hennekam, Maartje F. Aukes, Fabian Termorshuizen, René S. Kahn, Marco P. M. Boks, and Roel A. Ophoff. 2011. "Paternal Age and Psychiatric Disorders: Findings from a Dutch Population Registry." *Schizophrenia Research* 129(2):128–32.

Butlin, Henry T. 1892. "Three Lectures on Cancer of the Scrotum in Chimney-sweeps and Others." *British Medical Journal* 2(1644):1–6.

Campo-Engelstein, Lisa, Laura Beth Santacrose, Zubin Master, and Wendy M. Parker. 2016. "Bad Moms, Blameless Dads: The Portrayal of Maternal and Paternal Age and Preconception Harm in U.S. Newspapers." *AJOB Empirical Bioethics* 7(1):56–63.

Carey, Benedict. 2012. "Father's Age Is Linked to Risk of Autism and Schizophrenia." *New York Times*, August 23, 2012. www.nytimes.com/2012/08/23/health/fathers-age-is-linked-to-risk-of-autism-and-schizophrenia.html.

Carlisle, Robert J, ed. 1893. *An Account of Bellevue Hospital with a Catalog of Medical and Surgical Staff from 1736 to 1894*. New York: Society of the Alumni of Bellevue Hospital. https://archive.org/details/accountofbellevu00carl.

Carpenter, Laura M. 2010. "On Remedicalisation: Male Circumcision in the United States and Great Britain." *Sociology of Health & Illness* 32(4): 613–30.

Carrell, Douglas T., and Ewa Rajpert-Meyts. 2013. "A New Era of 'Andrology.'" *Andrology* 1(1):1–2.

Carrigan, Tim, Bob Connell, and John Lee. 1985. "Toward a New Sociology of Masculinity." *Theory and Society* 14(5):551–604.

CDC. 2010. *Advancing Men's Reproductive Health in the United States: Current Status and Future Directions—Summary of Scientific Sessions and Discussions, September 13, 2010. Atlanta, Georgia.* National Center for Chronic Disease Prevention and Health Promotion, Division of Reproductive Health. www.cdc.gov/reproductivehealth/ProductsPubs/PDFs/Male-Reproductive-Health.pdf.

———. 2013. "Infertility FAQs." Reproductive Health. Accessed March 28, 2015. www.cdc.gov/reproductivehealth/Infertility/index.htm#3.

———. 2014. "Reproductive Health." Accessed March 28, 2015. www.cdc.gov.

———. 2015. "Preconception Health and Health Care: Information for Men." Accessed March 28, 2015. www.cdc.gov/preconception/men.html.

Chandra, Anjani, Casey Copen, and Elizabeth Hervey Stephen. 2013. "Infertility and Impaired Fecundity in the United States, 1982–2010: Data From the National Survey of Family Growth." *National Health Statistics Reports* 67:1–18.

Chavkin, Wendy. 1992. "Women and Fetus: The Social Construction of Conflict." *Women & Criminal Justice* 3(2):71–80.

"Cheap Lecturing." 1841. *New York Herald.* January 4, 1841: 2.

Chen, T. H., Y. H. Chiu, and B. J. Boucher. 2006. "Transgenerational Effects of Betel-Quid Chewing on the Development of the Metabolic Syndrome in the Keelung Community-Based Integrated Screening Program." *American Journal of Clinical Nutrition* 83(3):688–92.

Choi, Ji-Yeob, Kyoung-Mu Lee, Sue Kyung Park, Dong-Young Noh, Sei-Hyun Ahn, Keun-Young Yoo, and Daehee Kang. 2005. "Association of Paternal Age at Birth and the Risk of Breast Cancer in Offspring: A Case Control Study." *BMC Cancer* 5(1):143.

Clarke, Adele. 1998. *Disciplining Reproduction: Modernity, American Life Sciences, and "the Problems of Sex."* Berkeley: University of California Press.

Clarke, Adele, Janet Shim, Laura Mamo, Jennifer Fosket, and Jennifer R. Fishman. 2010. *Biomedicalization: Technoscience, Health, and Illness in the U.S.* Durham, NC: Duke University Press.

Clawson, Dan, and Mary Ann Clawson. 1999. "What Has Happened to the US Labor Movement? Union Decline and Renewal." *Annual Review of Sociology* 25(1):95–119.

Cohen, E. N., H. C. Gift, B. W. Brown, W. Greenfield, M. L. Wu, T. W. Jones, C. E. Whitcher, E. J. Driscoll, and J. B. Brodsky. 1980. "Occupational Disease in Dentistry and Chronic Exposure to Trace Anesthetic Gases." *Journal of the American Dental Association* 101(1):21–31.

Collins, Patricia Hill. 2000. *Black Feminist Thought: Knowledge, Conscious-ness and the Politics of Empowerment*. New York: Routledge.

Collins, Randall. 2012. "C-Escalation and D-Escalation." *American Sociological Review* 77(1):1–20.

Connell, R. W. 1987. *Gender and Power: Society, the Person, and Sexual Politics*. Cambridge, UK: Polity Press.

———. 2000. *The Men and the Boys*. Berkeley: University of California Press.

Connelly, Matthew James. 2008. *Fatal Misconception: The Struggle to Control World Population*. Cambridge, MA: Belknap Press of Harvard University Press.

Conrad, Peter. 1992. "Medicalization and Social Control." *Annual Review of Sociology* 18:209–32.

Conrad, Peter, and Susan Markens. 2001. "Constructing the 'Gay Gene' in the News: Optimism and Skepticism in the US and British Press." *Health* 5(3):373–400.

Conrad, Peter, and Joseph Schneider. 1980. *Deviance and Medicalization: From Badness to Sickness*. Philadelphia: Temple University Press.

Cooney, Elizabeth. 2004. "She Gave Infertile Women Hope, Then Babies." *Worcester (MA) Telegram & Gazette*, June 7, 2004: C1.

Cooper, Astley. 1845. *Observations on the Structure and Diseases of the Testis*. Philadelphia: Lea & Blanchard.

Cordier, S. 2008. "Evidence for a Role of Paternal Exposures in Developmental Toxicity." *Basic & Clinical Pharmacology & Toxicology* 102(2):176–81.

Corea, Gena. 1985. *The Mother Machine: Reproductive Technologies from Artificial Insemination to Artificial Wombs*. New York: Harper and Row.

Corner, Edred M. 1907. *Diseases of the Male Generative Organs*. London: Frowde.

———. 1910. *Male Diseases in General Practice: An Introduction to Andrology*. London: Frowde.

Correll, Shelley, Stephen Benard, and In Paik. 2007. "Getting a Job: Is There a Motherhood Penalty?" *American Journal of Sociology* 112:1297–338.

Courtenay, Will H. 2000. "Constructions of Masculinity and Their Influence On Men's Well-Being: A Theory of Gender and Health." *Social Science & Medicine* 50:1385–401.

Craig, Lyn, Abigail Powell, and Ciara Smyth. 2014. "Towards Intensive Parent-ing? Changes in the Composition and Determinants of Mothers' and Fathers' Time with Children 1992–2006." *British Journal of Sociology* 65(3):555–79.

Cramp, Arthur J. 1921. *Nostrums and Quackery*. Chicago: American Medical Association.

Crane, Dan. 2014. "Banking on My Future as a Father." *New York Times*, April 4, 2014. www.nytimes.com/2014/04/06/fashion/diary-of-a-sperm-banker .html.

Crean, Angela J., and Russell Bonduriansky. 2014. "What Is a Paternal Effect?" *Trends in Ecology & Evolution* 29(10):554–59.

Croissant, Jennifer L. 2014. "Agnotology: Ignorance and Absence or Towards a Sociology of Things That Aren't There." *Social Epistemology* 28(1):4–25.

Curley, J. P., R. Mashoodh, and F. A. Champagne. 2011. "Epigenetics and the Origins of Paternal Effects." *Hormones and Behavior* 59(3):306–14.

Curling, Thomas Blizard. 1843. *A Practical Treatise on the Diseases of the Testis, and of the Spermatic Cord and Scrotum*. Philadelphia: Carey and Hart.

Cutler, David M., and Adriana Lleras-Muney. 2010. "Understanding Differences in Health Behaviors by Education." *Journal of Health Economics* 29(1):1–28.

Cutler, David, and Grant Miller. 2005. "The Role of Public Health Improvements in Health Advances: The Twentieth-Century United States." *Demography* 42(1):1–22.

D'Emilio, John. 1983. "Capitalism and Gay Identity." In *Powers of Desire: The Politics of Sexuality*, edited by Anne Snitow, Christine Stansell, and Sharon Thompson. New York: Monthly Review Press.

Daniels, Cynthia R. 1993. *At Women's Expense: State Power and the Politics of Fetal Rights*. Cambridge, MA: Harvard University Press.

———. 1997. "Between Fathers and Fetuses: The Social Construction of Male Reproduction and the Politics of Fetal Harm." *Signs* 22(3):579–616.

———. 2006. *Exposing Men: The Science and Politics of Male Reproduction*. New York: Oxford University Press.

Daniels, Cynthia R., and Janet Golden. 2000. "The Politics of Paternity: Foetal Risks and Reproductive Harm." In *Law and Medicine: Current Legal Issues 2000*, vol. 3, edited by Michael Freeman and Andrew Lewis. Oxford, UK: Oxford University Press.

Darby, Robert. 2005. *A Surgical Temptation: The Demonization of the Foreskin and the Rise of Circumcision in Britain*. Chicago: University of Chicago Press.

Davis, Dana-Ain. 2019. *Reproductive Injustice: Racism, Pregnancy, and Premature Birth*. New York: New York University Press.

Davis, Devra Lee. 1991. "Fathers and Fetuses." *New York Times*, March 1, 1991: A27.

Davis-Floyd, Robbie. 1992. *Birth as an American Rite of Passage*. Berkeley: University of California Press.

Day, Jonathan, Soham Savani, Benjamin D. Krempley, Matthew Nguyen, and Joanna B. Kitlinska. 2016. "Influence of Paternal Preconception Exposures on Their Offspring: Through Epigenetics to Phenotype." *American Journal of Stem Cells* 5(1):11.

De Block, Andreas, and Pieter R. Adriaens. 2013. "Pathologizing Sexual Deviance: A History." *The Journal of Sex Research* 50(3–4):276–98.

de Jong, A. M., R. Menkveld, J. W. Lens, S. E. Nienhuis, and J. P. Rhemrev. 2014. "Effect of Alcohol Intake and Cigarette Smoking on Sperm Parameters and Pregnancy." *Andrologia* 46(2):112–17.

De La Rochebrochard, Elise, and Patrick Thonneau. 2002. "Paternal Age and Maternal Age Are Risk Factors for Miscarriage: Results of a Multicentre European Study." *Human Reproduction* 17(6):1649–56.

Delaney, Carol. 1986. "The Meaning of Paternity and the Virgin Birth Debate." *Man* 21(3):494–513.

Delaney, Carol Lowery. 1991. *The Seed and the Soil: Gender and Cosmology in Turkish Village Society.* Berkeley: University of California Press.

DeMarini, David M. 2004. "Genotoxicity of Tobacco Smoke and Tobacco Smoke Condensate: A Review." *Mutation Research/Reviews in Mutation Research* 567(2):447–74.

Detsky, A. S., S. R. Gauthier, and V. R. Fuchs. 2012. "Specialization in Medicine: How Much Is Appropriate?" *JAMA* 307(5):463–64.

Dorland, W. A. Newman. 1900. *The American Illustrated Medical Dictionary: A New and Complete Dictionary of the Terms Used in Medicine, Surgery, Dentistry, Pharmacy, Chemistry, and the Kindred Branches, with Their Pronunciation, Derivation, and Definition.* Philadelphia and London: W. B. Saunders.

Doucet, Andrea. 2017. *Do Men Mother?* 2nd ed. Toronto: University of Toronto Press.

Dubrova, Yuri E., G. Grant, A. A. Chumak, V. A. Stezhka, and A. N. Karakasian. 2002. "Elevated Minisatellite Mutation Rate in the Post-Chernobyl Families from Ukraine." *American Journal of Human Genetics* 71(4):801–9.

Dubrova, Yuri E., Valeri N. Nesterov, Nicolay G. Krouchinsky, Vladislav A. Ostapenko, R. Neumann, D. L. Neil, and A. J. Jeffreys. 1996. "Human Minisatellite Mutation Rate after the Chernobyl Accident." *Nature* 380(6576):683–86.

Duden, Barbara. 1991. *The Woman beneath the Skin: A Doctor's Patients in Eighteenth-Century Germany.* Cambridge, MA: Harvard University Press.

Edin, Kathryn, and Timothy J. Nelson. 2013. *Doing the Best I Can: Fatherhood in the Inner City.* Berkeley: University of California Press.

"Editorial: The American Association of Genito-Urinary Surgeons." 1889. *Journal of Cutaneous and Genito-Urinary Diseases* 7:38–40.

Editors of *Men's Health.* 2015. "The Best Foods for Making Babies: Chow Down on This Grub for First-Class Semen." *Men's Health,* March 30, 2014. www.menshealth.com/nutrition/a19532243/the-best-foods-for-your-penis/.

Eisenbach, Michael, and Laura C. Giojalas. 2006. "Sperm Guidance in Mammals—An Unpaved Road to the Egg." *Nature Reviews Molecular Cell Biology* 7(4):276–85.

Eliasson, Rune. 1976. "Presidential Message." *Andrologia* 8(3):i.

———. 1978. "Opening Remarks." *International Journal of Andrology* 1(s1):7–10.

Ellin, Abby. 2016. "Single, 54, and a New Dad." *New York Times,* August 6, 2016.

Epstein, Steven. 2007. *Inclusion: The Politics of Difference in Medical Research.* Chicago: University of Chicago Press.

———. 2008. "Culture and Science/Technology: Rethinking Knowledge, Power, Materiality, and Nature." *American Academy of Political and Social Science* 619:165–82.

Epstein, Steven, and Laura Mamo. 2017. "The Proliferation of Sexual Health: Diverse Social Problems and the Legitimation of Sexuality." *Social Science & Medicine* 188:176–90.

Ettinger, Laura Elizabeth. 2006. *Nurse-Midwifery: The Birth of a New American Profession.* Columbus: Ohio State University Press.

Evans, W. A. 1915. "A Campaign against Quacks." *American Journal of Public Health* 5(1):30–35.

Eyre, Richard. 2013. "In the Spirit of Ibsen." *The Guardian,* September 20, 2013. www.theguardian.com/stage/2013/sep/20/richard-eyre-spirit-ibsen-ghosts.

Fabia, J., and T. D. Thuy. 1974. "Occupation of Father at Time of Birth of Children Dying of Malignant Diseases." *British Journal of Preventive & Social Medicine* 28(2):98–100.

Faderman, Lillian. 2015. *The Gay Revolution: The Story of the Struggle.* New York: Simon & Schuster.

Fausto-Sterling, Anne. 2000. *Sexing the Body: Gender Politics and the Construction of the Body.* New York: Basic Books.

Fawcett, D. W. 1976. "The Male Reproductive System." In *Reproduction and Human Welfare: A Challenge to Research: A Review of the Reproductive Sciences and Contraceptive Development,* edited by Roy Orval Greep, Marjorie A. Koblinsky, and Frederick S. Jaffe, 165–277. Cambridge, MA: MIT Press.

Feimster, Crystal Nicole. 2009. *Southern Horrors: Women and the Politics of Rape and Lynching.* Cambridge, MA: Harvard University Press.

Fetters, K. Aleisha. 2015. "4 Ways to Make Your Sperm Stronger, Faster, and More Fertile." *Men's Health,* March 5, 2015. www.menshealth.com/sex-women/fertility-cheat-sheet.

Finer, Lawrence B., and Mia R. Zolna. 2016. "Declines in Unintended Pregnancy in the United States, 2008–2011." *New England Journal of Medicine* 374(9):843–52.

Fisch, Harry. 2004. *The Male Biological Clock*. New York: Free Press.

Fischer, Claude S., and Michael Hout. 2006. *Century of Difference: How America Changed in the Last One Hundred Years*. New York: Russell Sage Foundation.

Fischer, Suzanne Michelle. 2009. "Diseases of Men: Sexual Health and Medical Expertise in Advertising Medical Institutes, 1900–1930." PhD diss., University of Minnesota. ProQuest.

Fissell, Mary, and Roger Cooter. 2003. "Exploring Natural Knowledge: Science and the Popular." In *The Cambridge History of Science*, vol. 4, *Eighteenth-Century Science*, edited by Roy Porter, 129–58. Cambridge, UK: Cambridge University Press.

Flores-Macias, Francisco, and Chappell Lawson. 2008. "Effects of Interviewer Gender on Survey Responses: Findings from a Household Survey in Mexico." *International Journal of Public Opinion Research* 20(1):100–10.

Forsbach, Ralf. n.d. "'Euthanasie' und Zwangssterilisierungen im Rheinland (1933–1945)." Epochen & Themen, Portal Rheinische Geschichte. www.rheinische-geschichte.lvr.de/.

Foucault, Michel. 1980. *The History of Sexuality*. New York: Vintage Books.

Franklin, Sarah. 2013. *Biological Relatives: IVF, Stem Cells, and the Future of Kinship*. Durham, NC: Duke University Press.

Frans, E. M., S. Sandin, A. Reichenberg, P. Lichtenstein, N. Langstrom, and C. M. Hultman. 2008. "Advancing Paternal Age and Bipolar Disorder." *Archives of General Psychiatry* 65(9):1034–40.

Frey, K. A., Richard Engle, and Brie Noble. 2012. "Preconception Healthcare: What Do Men Know and Believe?" *Journal of Men's Health* 9(1):25–35.

Frey, K. A., S. M. Navarro, M. Kotelchuck, and M. C. Lu. 2008. "The Clinical Content of Preconception Care: Preconception Care for Men." *American Journal of Obstetrics and Gynecology* 199(6 Suppl 2):S389–95.

Frickel, Scott. 2004. *Chemical Consequences: Environmental Mutagens, Scientist Activism, and the Rise of Genetic Toxicology*. New Brunswick, NJ: Rutgers University Press.

———. 2014. "Absences: Methodological Note about Nothing, in Particular." *Social Epistemology* 28(1):86–95.

Frickel, Scott, Sahra Gibbon, Jeff Howard, Joanna Kempner, Gwen Ottinger, and David J. Hess. 2010. "Undone Science: Charting Social Movement and Civil Society Challenges to Research Agenda Setting." *Science, Technology, & Human Values* 35(4):444–73.

Friedler, Gladys. 1985. "Effects of Limited Paternal Exposure to Xenobiotic Agents on the Development of Progeny." *Neurobehavioral Toxicology and Teratology* 7(6):739–43.

————. 1996. "Paternal Exposures: Impact on Reproductive and Developmental Outcome: An Overview." *Pharmacology Biochemistry and Behavior* 55(4):691–700.

Friedman, David M. 2001. *A Mind of Its Own: A Cultural History of the Penis.* New York: Free Press.

Friedman, J. M. 1981. "Genetic Disease in the Offspring of Older Fathers." *Obstetrics & Gynecology* 57(6):745–49.

Friese, Carrie, and Adele E. Clarke. 2012. "Transposing Bodies of Knowledge and Technique: Animal Models at Work in Reproductive Sciences." *Social Studies of Science* 42(1):31–52.

Fullwiley, Duana. 2007. "Race and Genetics: Attempts to Define the Relationship." *BioSocieties* 2(2):221–37.

Fulsås, Narve, and Tore Rem. 2017. *Ibsen, Scandinavia and the Making of a World Drama.* Cambridge, UK: Cambridge University Press.

Furstenberg, Frank. 1988. "Good Dads—Bad Dads: Two Faces of Fatherhood." In *The Changing American Family and Public Policy,* edited by Andrew Cherlin, 193–218. Washington, DC: Urban Institute Press.

Gamble, V. N. 1997. "Under the Shadow of Tuskegee: African Americans and Health Care." *American Journal of Public Health* 87(11):1773–78.

Gardner, M. J., M. P. Snee, A. J. Hall, C. A. Powell, S. Downes, and J. D. Terrell. 1990. "Results of Case-Control Study of Leukaemia and Lymphoma among Young People near Sellafield Nuclear Plant in West Cumbria." *British Medical Journal* 300(6722):423–29.

Garfield, Craig F. 2018. "Toward Better Understanding of How Fathers Contribute to Their Offspring's Health." *Pediatrics* 141(1):e20173461.

Gasking, Elizabeth B. 1967. *Investigations into Generation.* Baltimore: Johns Hopkins University Press.

Gavin, L., S. Moskosky, M. Carter, K. Curtis, E. Glass, E. Godfrey, A. Marcell, N. Mautone-Smith, K. Pazol, N. Tepper, and L. Zapata. 2014. "Providing Quality Family Planning Services: Recommendations of CDC and the U.S. Office of Population Affairs." *MMWR Recommendations and Reports* 63(RR-04):1–54.

Gibbon, Sahra, and Carlos Novas. 2008. *Biosocialities, Genetics and the Social Sciences.* New York: Routledge.

Gilardi, Federica, Marc Augsburger, and Aurelien Thomas. 2018. "Will Widespread Synthetic Opioid Consumption Induce Epigenetic Consequences in Future Generations?" *Frontiers in Pharmacology* 9:702.

Ginsburg, Faye, and Rayna Rapp. 1991. "The Politics of Reproduction." *Annual Review of Anthropology* 20:311–43.

Goldberg, Abbie E., Nanette K. Gartrell, and Gary Gates. 2014. *Research Report on LGB-Parent Families.* Los Angeles: Williams Institute, UCLA Law School.

https://williamsinstitute.law.ucla.edu/wp-content/uploads/lgb-parent-families-july-2014.pdf.

Goldin, Claudia, and Lawrence F. Katz. 2011. "Putting the "Co" in Education: Timing, Reasons, and Consequences of College Coeducation from 1835 to the Present." *Journal of Human Capital* 5(4):377–417.

Goode, Erica. 2001. "Father's Age Linked to Risk of Schizophrenia in Child." *New York Times*, April 12, 2001. www.nytimes.com/2001/04/12/us/father-s-age-linked-to-risk-of-schizophrenia-in-child.html.

Gordon, Linda. 1976. *Woman's Body, Woman's Right: A Social History of Birth Control in America*. New York: Viking Press.

———. 2002. *The Moral Property of Women: A History of Birth Control Politics in America*. Urbana: University of Illinois Press.

Goriely, Anne, and Andrew O. M. Wilkie. 2012. "Paternal Age Effect Mutations and Selfish Spermatogonial Selection: Causes and Consequences for Human Disease." *American Journal of Human Genetics* 90(2):175–200.

Gould, George M. 1894. *An Illustrated Dictionary of Medicine, Biology and Allied Sciences*. Philadelphia: P. Blakiston.

Greene, Margaret E., and Ann E. Biddlecom. 2000. "Absent and Problematic Men: Demographic Accounts of Male Reproductive Roles." *Population and Development Review* 26(1):81–115.

Greene, Margaret, Manisha Mehta, Julie Pulerwitz, Deirdre Wulf, Akinrinola Bankole, and Susheela Singh. 2006. *Involving Men in Reproductive Health: Contributions to Development*. Background paper prepared for United Nations Millennium Project report *Public Choices, Private Decisions: Sexual and Reproductive Health and the Millennium Development Goals*. Washington, DC: Millennium Project. www.unmillenniumproject.org/documents/Greene_et_al-final.pdf.

Greenfield, Paige. 2013. "Strengthen Your Sperm in an Hour." *Men's Health*, October 22, 2013. www.menshealth.com/sex-women/a19536281/strengthen-your-sperm-in-an-hour.

Griswold, Wendy. 1987. "A Methodological Framework for the Sociology of Culture." *Sociological Methodology* 17:1–35.

Gross, Matthias, and Linsey McGoey, eds. 2015. *Routledge International Handbook of Ignorance Studies*. London and New York: Routledge.

Gross, Samuel Weissel. 1887. *A Practical Treatise on Impotence, Sterility and Allied Disorders of the Male Sexual Organs*. Philadelphia: Lea Brothers.

Guiteras, Ramon. 1905. "The American Urological Association." *American Journal of Urology* 1:3.

Gutmann, Matthew. 2007. *Fixing Men: Sex, Birth Control, and AIDS in Mexico*. Berkeley: University of California Press.

Guzick, David S., James W. Overstreet, Pam Factor-Litvak, Charlene K. Brazil, Steven T. Nakajima, Christos Coutifaris, Sandra Ann Carson, Pauline

Cisneros, Michael P. Steinkampf, Joseph A. Hill, Dong Xu, and Donna L. Vogel. 2001. "Sperm Morphology, Motility, and Concentration in Fertile and Infertile Men." *New England Journal of Medicine* 345(19):1388–93.

Hacking, Ian. 1995. "The Looping Effects of Human Kinds." In *Causal Cognition: A Multidisciplinary Debate*, edited by Dan Sperber, David Premack, and Ann James Premack, 351–83. Oxford, UK: Clarendon Press.

Hall, Jacquelyn Dowd. 1983. "'The Mind That Burns in Each Body': Women, Rape and Racial Violence." In *Powers of Desire: The Politics of Sexuality*, edited by Anne Snitow, Christine Stansell, and Sharon Thompson. New York: Monthly Review Press.

Hallowell, Nina. 1999. "Doing the Right Thing: Genetic Risk and Responsibility." *Sociology of Health & Illness* 21:597–621.

Hallowell, Nina, Audrey Arden-Jones, Rosalind Eeles, Claire Foster, Anneke Lucassen, Clare Moynihan, and Maggie Watson. 2006. "Guilt, Blame and Responsibility: Men's Understanding of Their Role in the Transmission of BRCA1/2 Mutations within Their Family." *Sociology of Health & Illness* 28(7):969–88.

Haney, Lynne. 2018. "Incarcerated Fatherhood: The Entanglements of Child Support Debt and Mass Imprisonment." *American Journal of Sociology* 124(1):1–48.

Haraway, Donna. 1991. "A Cyborg Manifesto: Science, Technology and Socialist Feminism in the Late Twentieth Century." In *Simians, Cyborgs and Women: The Reinvention of Nature*, edited by Donna Haraway. New York: Routledge.

Hardon, Anita, and the Chemical Youth Collective. 2017. "Chemical Youth: Chemical Mediations and Relations at Work." Member Voices. *Fieldsights*, November 20, 2017. https://culanth.org/fieldsights/chemical-youth-chemical-mediations-and-relations-at-work.

Hay, Eugene Carson. 1910. "Correspondence: A Proposed Section on Genito-Urinary and Venereal Diseases." *JAMA* 54:2.

Hays, Sharon. 1996. *The Cultural Contradictions of Motherhood*. New Haven, CT: Yale University Press.

Healey, Jenna Caitlin. In preparation. "On Time: Age, Technology, and Reproduction in Modern America." Unpublished manuscript.

Heid, Markham. 2014. "How Your Drinking Habit Could Hurt Your Sperm." *Men's Health*, October 3, 2014. www.menshealth.com/health/a19525769/how-your-drinking-habit-hurts-your-sperm/.

Hepler, Allison L. 2000. *Women in Labor: Mothers, Medicine, and Occupational Health in the United States, 1890–1980*. Columbus: Ohio State University Press.

Herr, Harry W. 2004. "Urological Injuries in the Civil War." *Journal of Urology* 172(5, part 1):1800–1804.

Hilgartner, Stephen. 2014. "Studying Absences of Knowledge: Difficult Subfield or Basic Sensibility?" *Social Epistemology Review and Reply Collective* 3(12):5.

Hoberman, John M. 2005. *Testosterone Dreams: Rejuvenation, Aphrodisia, Doping.* Berkeley: University of California Press.

Hochschild, Arlie. 1983. *The Managed Heart: Commercialization of Human Feeling.* Berkeley: University of California Press.

Hoganson, Kristin L. 1998. *Fighting for American Manhood: How Gender Politics Provoked the Spanish-American and Philippine-American Wars.* New Haven, CT: Yale University Press.

Hopwood, Nick. 2018. "The Keywords 'Generation' and 'Reproduction.'" In *Reproduction: Antiquity to Present Day,* edited by Nick Hopwood, Rebecca Flemming, and Lauren Kassell. Cambridge, UK: Cambridge University Press.

Hultman, C. M., S. Sandin, S. Z. Levine, and P. Lichtenstein. 2011. "Advancing Paternal Age and Risk of Autism: New Evidence from a Population-Based Study and a Meta-analysis of Epidemiological Studies." *Molecular Psychiatry* 16(12):1203.

Ibis Reproductive Health. 2017. "Abortion Coverage Bans on Public and Private Insurance: Access to Abortion Care Limited for Millions of Women." Publications, August 2017. https://ibisreproductivehealth.org/sites/default /files/files/publications/Impact%20of%20insurance%20bans%20formatted %208.17.pdf.

Ibsen, Henrik. 2009 (1881). *Ghosts.* www.gutenberg.org/files/8121/8121-h /8121-h.htm.

"Information about the International Society of Andrology (ISA), (Formerly CIDA)." 1982. *Journal of Andrology* 3(5):349–52.

Inhorn, Marcia. 2012. *The New Arab Man: Emergent Masculinities, Technologies, and Islam in the Middle East.* Princeton, NJ: Princeton University Press.

Inhorn, Marcia, Tine Tjornhoj-Thomsen, and Helene Goldberg, eds. 2009. *Reconceiving the Second Sex: Men, Masculinity, and Reproduction.* New York: Berghahn Books.

Inhorn, Marcia C., and Emily A. Wentzell. 2011. "Embodying Emergent Masculinities: Men Engaging with Reproductive and Sexual Health Technologies in the Middle East and Mexico." *American Ethnologist* 38(4):801–15.

Jackson, James Caleb. 1852. *Hints on the Reproductive Organs: Their Diseases, Causes, and Cure on Hydropathic Principles.* New York: Fowlers and Wells.

Jacobson, W. H. A. 1893. *The Diseases of the Male Organs of Generation.* Philadelphia: Blakiston.

Jaggar, Alison. 1983. *Feminist Politics and Human Nature.* Totowa, NJ: Rowman and Allenheld.

Jasanoff, Sheila, ed. 2004. *States of Knowledge: The Co-Production of Science and Social Order.* London: Routledge.

Jayson, Sharon. 2005. "Is That Ticking Sound a Male Biological Clock?" *USA Today*, March 7, 2005.

Jensen, T. K., S. Swan, N. Jorgensen, J. Toppari, B. Redmon, M. Punab, E. Z. Drobnis, T. B. Haugen, B. Zilaitiene, A. E. Sparks, D. S. Irvine, C. Wang, P. Jouannet, C. Brazil, U. Paasch, A. Salzbrunn, N. E. Skakkebaek, and A. M. Andersson. 2014. "Alcohol and Male Reproductive Health: A Cross-sectional Study of 8344 Healthy Men from Europe and the USA." *Human Reproduction* 29(8):1801–9.

Jimenez-Chillaron, J. C., E. Isganaitis, M. Charalambous, S. Gesta, T. Pentinat-Pelegrin, R. R. Faucette, J. P. Otis, A. Chow, R. Diaz, A. Ferguson-Smith, and M. E. Patti. 2009. "Intergenerational Transmission of Glucose Intolerance and Obesity by In Utero Undernutrition in Mice." *Diabetes* 58(2):460–8.

Joffe, C. E., T. A. Weitz, and C. L. Stacey. 2004. "Uneasy Allies: Pro-Choice Physicians, Feminist Health Activists and the Struggle for Abortion Rights." *Sociology of Health and Illness* 26(6):775–96.

Jones, David. 2013. *Broken Hearts: The Tangled History of Cardiac Care.* Baltimore, MD: Johns Hopkins University Press.

Jones, Kenneth L., David W. Smith, Mary Ann Sedgwick Harvey, Bryan D. Hall, and Linda Quan. 1975. "Older Paternal Age and Fresh Gene Mutation: Data on Additional Disorders." *Journal of Pediatrics* 86(1):84–88.

Jordan, Brigitte. 1983. *Birth in Four Cultures.* Montreal: Eden Press.

Jordan, P., and H. Niermann. 1969. "Entwicklung und gegenwärtiger Stand der Andrologie in Deutschland." *Andrologia* 1(1):2.

Jordanova, Ludmilla J. 1995. "Interrogating the Concept of Reproduction in the Eighteenth Century." In *Conceiving the New World Order: The Global Politics of Reproduction*, edited by Faye D. Ginsburg and Rayna Rapp, 369–86. Berkeley: University of California Press.

Kaati, G., L. O. Bygren, and S. Edvinsson. 2002. "Cardiovascular and Diabetes Mortality Determined by Nutrition during Parents' and Grandparents' Slow Growth Period." *European Journal of Human Genetics* 10(11):682–88.

Kampf, Antje. 2015. "Times of Danger: Embryos, Sperm and Precarious Reproduction ca. 1870s–1910s." *History and Philosophy of the Life Sciences* 37(1):68–86.

Katz Rothman, Barbara. 1986. *The Tentative Pregnancy: Prenatal Diagnosis and the Future of Motherhood.* New York: Viking.

Keettel, W. C., R. G. Bunge, J. T. Bradbury, and W. O. Nelson. 1956. "Report of Pregnancies in Infertile Couples." *JAMA* 160(2):102–5.

Kempner, Joanna, Jon F. Merz, and Charles L. Bosk. 2011. "Forbidden Knowledge: Public Controversy and the Production of Nonknowledge." *Sociological Forum* 26(3):475–500.

Kevles, Daniel J. 1995. *In the Name of Eugenics: Genetics and the Uses of Human Heredity.* Cambridge, MA: Harvard University Press.

Keyes, Edward Lawrence. November 20, 1882. Edward Keyes to Claudius Mastin. Manuscript archives, Doy Leale McCall Rare Book and Manuscript Library, University of South Alabama.

————. 1980. *Memoirs: What I Have Seen and Done in Four and Seventy Years, 1843–1917.* Abridged by E. L. Keyes III. St. Louis: publisher not identified.

Keyes, Edward Lawrence, and Edward Lawrence Keyes Jr. 1906. *The Surgical Diseases of the Genito-urinary Organs.* New York and London: D. Appleton.

Keyes, Edward Lawrence, Jr. 1928. "Master Surgeons of America: Edward Lawrence Keyes." *Surgery, Gynecology, and Obstetrics* 46:3.

Keyes, Edward Lawrence, III. 1977. "Edward Lawrence Keyes (1843–1924)." *Urology* 9(4):484–91.

Kiselica, Mark S. 2008. *When Boys Become Parents: Adolescent Fatherhood in America.* New Brunswick, NJ: Rutgers University Press.

Kleinhaus, K., M. Perrin, Y. Friedlander, and O. Paltiel. 2006. "Paternal Age and Spontaneous Abortion." *Obstetrics and Gynecology* 108(2):369–77.

Kligman, Gail. 1998. *The Politics of Duplicity: Controlling Reproduction in Ceauşescu's Romania.* Berkeley: University of California Press.

Kline, Wendy. 2001. *Building a Better Race: Gender, Sexuality, and Eugenics from the Turn of the Century to the Baby Boom.* Berkeley: University of California Press.

————. 2010. *Bodies of Knowledge: Sexuality, Reproduction, and Women's Health in the Second Wave.* Chicago: University of Chicago Press.

Kluchin, Rebecca M. 2009. *Fit to Be Tied: Sterilization and Reproductive Rights in America, 1950–1980.* New Brunswick, NJ: Rutgers University Press.

Knopik, V. S., T. Jacob, J. R. Haber, L. P. Swenson, and D. N. Howell. 2009. "Paternal Alcoholism and Offspring ADHD Problems: A Children of Twins Design." *Twin Research and Human Genetics* 12(1):53–62.

Kolata, Gina. 1996a. "Measuring Men Up, Sperm by Sperm." *New York Times,* May 5, 1996. www.nytimes.com/1996/05/05/weekinreview/ideas-trends-how-men-measure-up-sperm-for-sperm.html.

————. 1996b. "Sperm Counts: Some Experts See a Fall, Others Poor Data." *New York Times,* March 19, 1996. www.nytimes.com/1996/03/19/science/sperm-counts-some-experts-see-a-fall-others-poor-data.html.

————. 1999. "Experts Unsure of Effects of a Type of Contaminant." *New York Times,* August 4, 1999. www.nytimes.com/1999/08/04/us/experts-unsure-of-effects-of-a-type-of-contaminant.html

Kong, A., M. L. Frigge, G. Masson, S. Besenbacher, P. Sulem, G. Magnusson, S. A. Gudjonsson, A. Sigurdsson, A. Jonasdottir, A. Jonasdottir, W. S. Wong,

G. Sigurdsson, G. B. Walters, S. Steinberg, H. Helgason, G. Thorleifsson, D. F. Gudbjartsson, A. Helgason, O. T. Magnusson, U. Thorsteinsdottir, and K. Stefansson. 2012. "Rate of De Novo Mutations and the Importance of Father's Age to Disease Risk." *Nature* 488(7412):471–75.

Kotelchuck, M., and M. Lu. 2017. "Father's Role in Preconception Health." *Maternal and Child Health Journal* 21(11):2025–39.

Kowal, Emma, Joanna Radin, and Jenny Reardon. 2013. "Indigenous Body Parts, Mutating Temporalities, and the Half-Lives of Postcolonial Technoscience." *Social Studies of Science* 43(4):465–83.

Krause, Walter, and Gerhard Schreiber. 2018. "Warum Andrologie in der Dermatologie." *Der Hautarzt* 69(12):972–76.

Krieger, Nancy. 2001. "Theories for Social Epidemiology in the 21st Century: An Ecosocial Perspective." *International Journal of Epidemiology* 30(4):668–77.

———. 2003. "Genders, Sexes, and Health: What Are The Connections—and Why Does It Matter?" *International Journal of Epidemiology* 32(4):652–57.

La Vignera, S., R. A. Condorelli, G. Balercia, E. Vicari, and A. E. Calogero. 2013. "Does Alcohol Have Any Effect on Male Reproductive Function? A Review of Literature." *Asian Journal of Andrology* 15(2):221–25.

Lallemand, Claude-François. 1853. *A Practical Treatise on the Causes, Symptoms, and Treatment of Spermatorrhoea.* Edited by Henry J. McDougall. Philadelphia: Blanchard and Lea.

Lamb, Dolores. 2009. "Memorial: Emil Steinberger, MD, FACE, 1928–2008." *Journal of Andrology* 30(3):349–50.

Lambert, Sarah M., Puneet Masson, and Harry Fisch. 2006. "The Male Biological Clock." *World Journal of Urology* 24(6):611–17.

Lamoreaux, Janelle. In progress. "Infertile Futures: Epigenetic Environments in a Toxic China." Unpublished manuscript.

Lampe, Nik M., Shannon K. Carter, and J. E. Sumerau. 2019. "Continuity and Change in Gender Frames: The Case of Transgender Reproduction." *Gender & Society* 33(6):865–87.

"Lancet: London: Saturday, August 25, 1888." 1888. *Lancet* 132(3391):378–82.

"Lancet: London: Saturday, October 27, 1888." 1888. *Lancet* 132(3400):825–29.

Landsman, Gail. 2008. *Reconstructing Motherhood and Disability in the Age of "Perfect" Babies.* New York: Routledge.

Laqueur, Thomas. 1990. *Making Sex: Body and Gender from the Greeks to Freud.* Cambridge, MA: Harvard University Press.

Largent, Mark A. 2008. *Breeding Contempt: The History of Coerced Sterilization in the United States.* New Brunswick, NJ: Rutgers University Press.

LaRossa, Ralph. 1997. *The Modernization of Fatherhood: A Social and Political History.* Chicago: University of Chicago Press.

Laslett, Barbara, and Joanna Brenner. 1989. "Gender and Social Reproduction: Historical Perspectives." *Annual Review of Sociology* 15:381–404.

Laubenthal, J., O. Zlobinskaya, K. Poterlowicz, A. Baumgartner, M.R. Gdula, E. Fthenou, M. Keramarou, S.J. Hepworth, J.C. Kleinjans, F.J. van Schooten, G. Brunborg, R.W. Godschalk, T.E. Schmid, and D. Anderson. 2012. "Cigarette Smoke-Induced Transgenerational Alterations in Genome Stability in Cord Blood of Human F1 Offspring." *FASEB Journal* 26(10):3946–56.

Lawrence, Christopher, and George Weisz, eds. 1998. *Greater Than the Parts: Holism in Biomedicine, 1920–1950.* New York: Oxford University Press.

Leavitt, Judith Walzer. 1986. *Brought to Bed: Childbearing in America, 1750 to 1950.* New York: Oxford University Press

———. 2010. *Make Room for Daddy: The Journey from Waiting Room to Birthing Room.* Chapel Hill: University of North Carolina Press.

Lee, Arthur Bolles. 1890. *The Microtomist's Vade-Mecum: A Handbook of the Methods of Microscopic Anatomy.* London: Churchill.

Lee, Kyoung-Mu, Mary H. Ward, Sohee Han, Hyo Seop Ahn, Hyoung Jin Kang, Hyung Soo Choi, Hee Young Shin, Hong-Hoe Koo, Jong-Jin Seo, Ji-Eun Choi, Yoon-Ok Ahn, and Daehee Kang. 2009. "Paternal Smoking, Genetic Polymorphisms in CYP1A1 and Childhood Leukemia Risk." *Leukemia Research* 33(2):250–58.

Leinster, Sam. 2014. "Training Medical Practitioners: Which Comes First, the Generalist or the Specialist?" *Journal of the Royal Society of Medicine* 107(3):99–102.

Levine, H., N. Jorgensen, A. Martino-Andrade, J. Mendiola, D. Weksler-Derri, I. Mindlis, R. Pinotti, and S.H. Swan. 2017. "Temporal Trends in Sperm Count: A Systematic Review and Meta-regression Analysis." *Human Reproduction Update* 23(6):646–59.

Lewin, Tamar. 1988. "Companies Ignore Men's Health Risk." *New York Times,* December 15, 1988. www.nytimes.com/1988/12/15/us/companies-ignore-men-s-health-risk.html.

———. 2001. "Ideas & Trends: Reproductive Gerontology; Ask Not for Whom the Clock Ticks." Week in Review, *New York Times,* April 15, 2001. www.nytimes.com/2001/04/15/weekinreview/ideas-trends-reproductive-geron-tology-ask-not-for-whom-the-clock-ticks.html.

Link, Bruce G., and Jo C. Phelan. 1995. "Social Conditions As Fundamental Causes of Disease." *Journal of Health and Social Behavior* 35:80–94.

———. 2001. "Conceptualizing Stigma." *Annual Review of Sociology* 27:363–85.

Linschooten, J.O., N. Verhofstad, K. Gutzkow, A.K. Olsen, C. Yauk, Y. Oligschlager, G. Brunborg, F.J. van Schooten, and R.W. Godschalk. 2013. "Paternal Lifestyle as a Potential Source of Germline Mutations Transmitted to Offspring." *FASEB Journal* 27(7):2873–79.

Lipton, Eric, and Danielle Ivory. 2017. "Under Trump, E.P.A. Has Slowed Actions Against Polluters, and Put Limits on Enforcement Officers." *New*

York Times, December 10, 2017. www.nytimes.com/2017/12/10/us/politics
/pollution-epa-regulations.html.

Little, M. P., D. T. Goodhead, B. A. Bridges, and S. D. Bouffler. 2013. "Evidence
Relevant to Untargeted and Transgenerational Effects in the Offspring of
Irradiated Parents." *Mutation Research* 753(1):50–67.

Lock, Margaret, Julia Freeman, Gillian Chilibeck, Briony Beveridge, and
Miriam Padolsky. 2007. "Susceptibility Genes and the Question of Embodied
Identity." *Medical Anthropology Quarterly* 21(3):256–76.

Loe, Meika. 2004. *The Rise of Viagra: How the Little Blue Pill Changed Sex in
America.* New York: New York University Press.

Long, J. M. 1885. "Course of Study for the District School." In *New High School
Question Book,* edited by W. H. F. Henry, 390. New York: Hinds, Noble &
Eldredge.

Lopata, Helena Z., and Barrie Thorne. 1978. "On the Term 'Sex Roles.'" *Signs*
3(3):718–21.

Lukaszyk, Andrzej. 2009. "Professor Emil Steinberger (1928–2008)." *Reproductive Biology* 9(1):5.

Luker, Kristen. 1984. *Abortion and the Politics of Motherhood.* Berkeley:
University of California Press.

Luna, Zakiya, and Kristin Luker. 2013. "Reproductive Justice." *Annual Review
of Law and Social Science* 9:327–52.

Lupton, Deborah. 1995. *The Imperative of Health: Public Health and the
Regulated Body.* London: Sage Publications.

Macfadden, Bernarr. 1900. *The Virile Powers of Superb Manhood: How Developed, How Lost, How Regained.* New York: Physical Culture Publishing.

MacKendrick, Norah. 2018. *Better Safe Than Sorry: How Consumers Navigate
Exposure to Everyday Toxics.* Oakland: University of California Press.

Magnusson, L. L., J. P. Bonde, J. Olsen, L. Moller, K. Bingefors, and H. Wennborg. 2004. "Paternal Laboratory Work and Congenital Malformations."
Journal of Occupational and Environmental Medicine 46(8):761–67.

Mahoney, James. 2000. "Path Dependence in Historical Sociology." *Theory and
Society* 29(4):507–48.

Malaspina, Dolores. 2001. "Advancing Paternal Age and the Risk of Schizophrenia." *JAMA* 286(8):904.

"Male Diseases." 1913. *British Medical Journal* 1(2726):670–71.

Mamo, Laura, and Jennifer R. Fishman. 2001. "Potency in All the Right
Places: Viagra as a Technology of the Gendered Body." *Body and Society*
7(4):13–25.

March of Dimes Archives, Administrative Records, March of Dimes headquarters, White Plains, NY.

Mancini, Roberto E., Eugenia Rosemberg, Martin Cullen, Juan C. Lavieri,
Oscar Vilar, Cesar Bergada, and Juan A. Andrada. 1965. "Cryptorchid and

Scrotal Human Testes. I. Cytological, Cytochemical and Quantitative Studies." *Journal of Clinical Endocrinology & Metabolism* 25(7):927–42.

Marcus, Ruth. 1990. "Fetal Protection Policies: Prudence or Bias?" *Washington Post,* October 8, 1990.

Marincola, Elizabeth. 2009. "Don Fawcett (1917–2009): Unlocking Nature's Closely Guarded Secrets." *PLoS Biology* 7(8):e1000183.

Mark, Ernest G. 1911. "Discussion of President's Address." In *Tenth Annual Meeting of the Urological Association,* edited by Charles Greene Cumston. Chicago: Riverdale Press.

Markens, Susan, Carole Browner, and Nancy Press. 1997. "Feeding the Fetus: On Interrogating the Notion of Maternal-Fetal Conflict." *Feminist Studies* 23(2):351–72.

Marks, Lara. 2001. *Sexual Chemistry: A History of the Contraceptive Pill.* New Haven, CT: Yale University Press.

Marsh, Margaret. 1988. "Suburban Men and Masculine Domesticity, 1870–1915." *American Quarterly* 40(2):165–86.

Marsh, Margaret, and Wanda Ronner. 1999. *The Empty Cradle: Infertility in America from Colonial Times to the Present.* Baltimore: Johns Hopkins University Press.

Marsiglio, William. 1998. *Procreative Man.* New York: New York University Press.

Marsiglio, William, and Sally Hutchinson. 2002. *Sex, Men, and Babies: Stories of Awareness and Responsibility.* New York: New York University Press.

Marsiglio, William, Sally Hutchinson, and Mark Cohan. 2001. "Young Men's Procreative Identity: Becoming Aware, Being Aware, and Being Responsible." *Journal of Marriage and Family* 63(1):123–35.

Martin, Emily. 1991. "The Egg and the Sperm: How Science Has Constructed a Romance Based on Stereotypical Male-Female Roles." *Signs* 16(3):485–501.

———. 1992. *The Woman in the Body: A Cultural Analysis of Reproduction.* Boston: Beacon.

Martin, R. H., and A. W. Rademaker. 1987. "The Effect of Age on the Frequency of Sperm Chromosomal Abnormalities in Normal Men." *American Journal of Human Genetics* 41(3):484–92.

Mauss, Marcel. 1973. "Techniques of the Body." *Economy and Society* 2(1):70–88.

May, Elaine Tyler. 2010. *America and the Pill: A History of Promise, Peril and Liberation.* Basic Books.

May, Gary. 2013. *Bending Toward Justice: The Voting Rights Act and the Transformation of American Democracy.* Durham, NC: Duke University Press.

Mayo Clinic Staff. 2012. "Healthy Sperm: Improving your Fertility." Accessed March 29, 2015. www.mayoclinic.org/healthy-living/getting-pregnant/in-depth/fertility/art-20047584?p=1.

———. 2014. "Getting Pregnant." Accessed March 29, 2015. www.mayoclinic.org/healthy-living/getting-pregnant/basics/fertility/hlv-20049462?p=1.

McElheny, Victor K. 2012. *Drawing the Map of Life: Inside the Human Genome Project.* London: Hachette UK.

McGrath, Charles. 2002. "Father Time." The Way We Live Now. *New York Times Magazine,* June 16, 2002. www.nytimes.com/2002/06/16/magazine/the-way-we-live-now-6-16-02-father-time.html.

McLaren, Angus. 2008. *Impotence: A Cultural History.* Chicago: University of Chicago Press.

"Medical News." 1890a. *British Medical Journal* 1(1537):1407–9.

"Medical News." 1890b. *British Medical Journal* 1(1539):1520–22.

Meistrich, M. L., and I. T. Huhtaniemi. 2012. "'ANDROLOGY'—The New Journal of the American Society of Andrology and the European Academy of Andrology." *International Journal of Andrology* 35(2):107–8.

"Memoranda." 1887. *American Lancet* 11:1.

Messing, Karen, and Piroska Östlin. 2006. "Gender Equality, Work and Health: A Review of the Evidence." Geneva: World Health Organization Press.

Messner, Michael. 1992. *Power at Play: Sports and the Problem of Masculinity.* Boston: Beacon Press.

———. 1997. *Politics of Masculinities: Men in Movements.* Thousand Oaks, CA: Sage Publications.

Milam, Erika L. 2010. *Looking for a Few Good Males: Female Choice in Evolutionary Biology.* Baltimore: Johns Hopkins University Press.

Milam, Erika L., and Robert A. Nye, eds. 2015. *Scientific Masculinities.* Chicago: University of Chicago Press.

Miles, Donna. 1997. "VA Center Examines Service Members Reproductive Health." Press release, US Department of Defense. Accessed March 30, 2015. www.defense.gov/news/newsarticle.aspx?id=41049.

Mills, Charles. 2007. "White Ignorance." In *Race and Epistemologies of Ignorance,* edited by Nancy Tuana and Shannon Sullivan, 11–38. Albany: State University of New York Press.

Milne, Elizabeth, Kathryn R. Greenop, Rodney J. Scott, Helen D. Bailey, John Attia, Luciano Dalla-Pozza, Nicholas H. de Klerk, and Bruce K. Armstrong. 2012. "Parental Prenatal Smoking and Risk of Childhood Acute Lymphoblastic Leukemia." *American Journal of Epidemiology* 175(1):43–53.

"Minutes." 1888. *Transactions of the Congress of American Physicians and Surgeons: First Triennial Session, Held at Washington DC.* New Haven, CT: Congress of American Physicians and Surgeons.

Mitchell, E. W., D. M. Levis, and C. E. Prue. 2012. "Preconception Health: Awareness, Planning, and Communication among a Sample of US Men and Women." *Maternal and Child Health Journal* 16(1):31–9.

Moench, Gerard. 1930. "Evaluation of the Motility of the Spermatozoa." *JAMA* 94:478–80.

Mohr, Sebastian. 2018. *Being a Sperm Donor: Masculinity, Sexuality, and Biosociality in Denmark*. New York: Berghahn.

Moline, J. M., A. L. Golden, N. Bar-Chama, E. Smith, M. E. Rauch, R. E. Chapin, S. D. Perreault, S. M. Schrader, W. A. Suk, and P. J. Landrigan. 2000. "Exposure to Hazardous Substances and Male Reproductive Health: A Research Framework." *Environmental Health Perspectives* 108(9):803–13.

Moore, Lisa Jean. 2007. *Sperm Counts: Overcome by Man's Most Precious Fluid*. New York: New York University Press.

Morgen, Sandra. 2002. *Into Our Own Hands: The Women's Health Movement in the United States, 1969–1990*. New Brunswick, NJ: Rutgers University Press.

Morrow, Prince Albert. 1886. "Editorial." *Journal of Cutaneous and Venereal Diseases* 4:1.

——, ed. 1893. *A System of Genito-urinary Diseases, Syphilology, and Dermatology*. New York: Appleton.

Moscucci, Ornella. 1990. *The Science of Woman: Gynecology and Gender in England, 1800–1929*. Cambridge: Cambridge University Press.

Mulvey, Laura. 1999. "Visual Pleasure and Narrative Cinema." In *Film Theory and Criticism: Introductory Readings*, edited by Leo Braudy and Marshall Cohen, 833–44. New York: Oxford University Press.

Murdoch, J. L., B. A. Walker, and V. A. McKusick. 1972. "Parental Age Effects on the Occurrence of New Mutations for the Marfan Syndrome." *Annals of Human Genetics* 35(3):331–36.

Murkoff, Heidi. 2015. "Folic Acid and Male Fertility." *Ask Heidi*. Everyday Health. Accessed March 29, 2015. www.whattoexpect.com/getting-pregnant/ask-heidi/folic-acid-and-male-fertility.aspx.

Murphy, Michelle. 2012. *Seizing the Means of Reproduction: Entanglements of Feminism, Health, and Technoscience*. Durham, NC: Duke University Press.

——. 2017. *The Economization of Life*. Durham, NC: Duke University Press.

Murray, L., P. McCarron, K. Bailie, R. Middleton, G. Davey Smith, S. Dempsey, A. McCarthy, and A. Gavin. 2002. "Association of Early Life Factors and Acute Lymphoblastic Leukaemia in Childhood: Historical Cohort Study." *British Journal of Cancer* 86:356–61.

Nagourney, Eric. 1999. "In Search of a Way to Bolster the Sperm." *New York Times*, June 8, 1999: F7. www.nytimes.com/1999/06/08/health/in-search-of-a-way-to-bolster-the-sperm.html.

National Institute of Child Health and Human Development. 2013a. "Men's Reproductive Health: Overview." Accessed March 28, 2015. www.nichd.nih.gov/health/topics/menshealth/Pages/default.aspx.

——. 2013b. "What Are the Causes of Male Infertility?" Accessed March 28, 2015. www.nichd.nih.gov/health/topics/infertility/conditioninfo/Pages/causes-male.aspx.

————. 2016. "How Common Is Male Infertility, and What Are Its Causes?" Men's Reproductive Health. www.nichd.nih.gov/health/topics/menshealth /conditioninfo/infertility.

Naumann, Moritz Ernst Adolph. 1837. *Handbuch der Medicinischen Klinik.* Berlin: Rücker und Püchler.

Navon, Daniel. 2019. *Mobilizing Mutations: Human Genetics in the Age of Patient Advocacy.* Chicago: University of Chicago Press.

Nelson, Warren O. 1964. "Current Approaches to the Biological Control of Fertility." In *The Population Crisis and the Use of World Resources,* edited by Stuart Mudd. The Hague: W. Junk.

Nettleton, Pamela. 2015. "Brave Sperm and Demure Eggs: Fallopian Gender Politics on YouTube." *Feminist Formations* 27:25–45.

Ng, S. F., R. C. Lin, D. R. Laybutt, R. Barres, J. A. Owens, and M. J. Morris. 2010. "Chronic High-Fat Diet in Fathers Programs Beta-Cell Dysfunction in Female Rat Offspring." *Nature* 467(7318):963–66.

Niblett, Stephen Berry. 1863. *On the Functional Derangements of the Reproductive Organs.* 2nd ed. London: Tallant.

Niemi, Mikko. 1987. "Andrology as a Specialty: Its Origin." *Journal of Andrology* 8(4):201–02.

NIH. 2015. "Aging Changes in the Male Reproductive System." Medline Plus. https://medlineplus.gov/ency/article/004017.htm.

NIOSH. 1996. "The Effects of Workplace Hazards on Male Reproductive Health." Cincinnati, OH: Department of Health and Human Services.

"Obituary: Edward Lawrence Keyes, MD." February 6, 1924. *Medical Journal and Record,* p. 163.

"Obituary: Thomas Blizard Curling." 1888. *British Medical Journal* 1(1419):563–64.

O'Brien, Anthony Paul, John Hurley, Paul Linsley, Karen Anne McNeil, Richard Fletcher, and John Robert Aitken. 2018. "Men's Preconception Health: A Primary Health-Care Viewpoint." *American Journal of Men's Health* 12(5):1575–81.

Office of Technology Assessment, U.S. Congress. 1988. *Artificial Insemination: Practice in the United States: Summary of a 1987 Survey—Background Paper.* Washington, DC: U.S. Government Printing Office. www.princeton .edu/~ota/disk2/1988/8804/8804.PDF.

Oreskes, Naomi, and Erik M. Conway. 2011. *Merchants of Doubt: How a Handful of Scientists Obscured the Truth on Issues from Tobacco Smoke to Global Warming.* London: Bloomsbury.

Oriel, J. D. 1989. "Eminent Venereologists. 3. Philippe Ricord." *Genitourinary Medicine* 65(6):388–93.

Ortiz, Ana Teresa, and Laura Briggs. 2003. "The Culture of Poverty, Crack Babies, and Welfare Cheats: The Making of the 'Healthy White Baby Crisis.'" *Social Text* 21(3):19.

Oswald, Zachary Edmonds. 2013. "'Off with His _____': Analyzing the Sex Disparity in Chemical Castration Sentences." *Michigan Journal of Gender & Law* 19(2):471–503.

Oudshoorn, Nelly. 1994. *Beyond the Natural Body: An Archeology of Sex Hormones.* New York: Routledge.

———. 2003. *The Male Pill: A Biography of a Technology in the Making.* Durham, NC: Duke University Press.

Pacey, Allan A. 2013. "Are Sperm Counts Declining? Or Did We Just Change Our Spectacles?" *Asian Journal of Andrology* 15(2):187–90.

Padfield, Maureen, and Ian Procter. 1996. "The Effect of Interviewer's Gender on the Interviewing Process: A Comparative Enquiry." *Sociology* 30(2):355–66.

Paltrow, L. M., and J. Flavin. 2013. "Arrests of and Forced Interventions on Pregnant Women in the United States, 1973–2005: Implications for Women's Legal Status and Public Health." *Journal of Health Politics, Policy and Law* 38(2):299–343.

Pampel, Fred. 2011. "Cohort Changes in the Socio-demographic Determinants of Gender Egalitarianism." *Social Forces* 89(3):961–82.

Parents.com. 2015. "10 Ways He Can Have Better Baby-Making Sperm." Accessed March 29, 2015. www.parents.com/parents/templates/slideshow/print /member/printableSlideShowAll.jsp?page=1&slideid=/templatedata/parents /slideshow/data/1305560734243.xml.

Parker, L., M. S. Pearce, H. O. Dickinson, M. Aitkin, and A. W. Craft. 1999. "Stillbirths among Offspring of Male Radiation Workers at Sellafield Nuclear Reprocessing Plant." *Lancet* 354(9188):1407–14.

Parsons, Gail. 1977. "Equal Treatment for All: American Medical Remedies for Male Sexual Problems: 1850–1900." *Journal of the History of Medicine and Allied Sciences* 32(1):55–71.

Pascoe, C. J., and Tristan Bridges, eds. 2015. *Exploring Masculinities: Identity, Inequality, Continuity and Change.* New York: Oxford University Press.

Patterson, James T. 2001. *Brown v. Board of Education: A Civil Rights Milestone and Its Troubled Legacy.* New York: Oxford University Press.

Paul, C., and B. Robaire. 2013. "Ageing of the Male Germ Line." *Nature Reviews—Urology* 10(4):227–34.

Pechenick, Eitan Adam, Christopher M. Danforth, and Peter Sheridan Dodds. 2015. "Characterizing the Google Books Corpus: Strong Limits to Inferences of Socio-Cultural and Linguistic Evolution." *PLoS One* 10(10):e0137041.

Pembrey, M., R. Saffery, and L. O. Bygren. 2014. "Human Transgenerational Responses to Early-Life Experience: Potential Impact on Development, Health and Biomedical Research." *Journal of Medical Genetics* 51(9):563–72.

Penny Light, Tracy. 2012. "'Healthy' Men Make Good Fathers: Masculine Health and the Family in 1950s America." In *Inventing the Modern American Family: Family Values and Social Change in 20th Century United States*, edited by Isabel Heinemann. Frankfurt: Campus Verlag.

Penrose, L. S. 1955. "Parental Age and Mutation." *Lancet* 269:312–13.

Petersen, Richard A., and N. Anand. 2004. "The Production of Culture Perspective." *Annual Review of Sociology* 30(1):311–34.

Pew Research Center. 2015. "The American Family Today." Social and Demographic Trends, December 17, 2015. www.pewsocialtrends.org/2015/12/17/1-the-american-family-today/.

Pfeffer, Naomi. 1993. *The Stork and the Syringe: A Political History of Reproductive Medicine*. Cambridge, UK: Polity Press.

Phelan, Jo C., Bruce G. Link, and Parisa Tehranifar. 2010. "Social Conditions as Fundamental Causes of Health Inequalities: Theory, Evidence, and Policy Implications." *Journal of Health and Social Behavior* 51(1, suppl):S28–S40.

Population Council. 1978. "The Population Council: A Chronicle of the First Twenty-Five Years, 1952–1977." New York: Population Council.

Porter, Roy. 2004. *Quacks: Fakers and Charlatans in Medicine*. Stroud: Tempus.

Porter, Theodore. 2018. *Genetics in the Madhouse: The Unknown History of Human Heredity*. Princeton, NJ: Princeton University Press.

Posner, Carl. 1884. "Medicin: Paul Fürbringer, Die Krankheiten der Harn- und Geschlechtsorgane für Aerzte und Studierende dargestellt." *Deutsche Literaturzeitung* 50:1839–40.

Pound, Pandora, and Michael B. Bracken. 2014. "Is Animal Research Sufficiently Evidence Based to Be a Cornerstone of Biomedical Research?" *British Medical Journal* 348:g3387.

Prins, Gail S., and William Bremner. 2004. "The 25th Volume: President's Message: Andrology in the 20th Century: A Commentary on Our Progress during the Past 25 Years." *Journal of Andrology* 25(4):435–40.

Proctor, Robert, and Londa Schiebinger. 2008. *Agnotology: The Making and Unmaking of Ignorance*. Stanford, CA: Stanford University Press.

Putney, Clifford. 2001. *Muscular Christianity: Manhood and Sports in Protestant America, 1880–1920*. Cambridge, MA: Harvard University Press.

Rabin, Roni. 2005. "Is the Clock Ticking for Men, Too?" *New York Newsday*, January 9, 2005.

———. 2009. "Older Fathers Linked to Lower I.Q. Scores." *New York Times*, March 9, 2009. www.nytimes.com/2009/03/10/health/10dads.html.

Raeburn, Paul. 2014a. "Dads' Biological Clocks: The Risks are Huge, or Are They?" *Huffington Post*, August 5, 2014.

———. 2014b. *Do Fathers Matter? What Science Is Telling Us about the Parent We've Overlooked.* New York: Farrar, Straus and Giroux.

Ragoné, Heléna. 1994. *Surrogate Motherhood: Conception in the Heart.* Boulder, CO: Westview Press.

Ramasamy, R., K. Chiba, P. Butler, and D. J. Lamb. 2015. "Male Biological Clock: A Critical Analysis of Advanced Paternal Age." *Fertility and Sterility* 103(6):1402–6.

Ramlau-Hansen, Cecilia Høst, Ane Marie Thulstrup, Lone Storgaard, Gunnar Toft, Jørn Olsen, and Jens Peter Bonde. 2007. "Is Prenatal Exposure to Tobacco Smoking a Cause of Poor Semen Quality? A Follow-up Study." *American Journal of Epidemiology* 165(12):1372–79.

Rando, O. J. 2012. "Daddy Issues: Paternal Effects on Phenotype." *Cell* 151(4):702–8.

Rapp, Rayna. 1999. *Testing Women, Testing the Fetus: The Social Impact of Amniocentesis in America.* New York: Routledge.

Reagan, Leslie J. 1998. *When Abortion Was a Crime: Women, Medicine, and Law in the United States, 1867–1973.* Berkeley: University of California Press.

———. 2016. "'My Daughter Was Genetically Drafted with Me': US-Vietnam War Veterans, Disabilities and Gender." *Gender & History* 28(3):833–53.

Reed, Kate. 2009. "'It's Them Faulty Genes Again': Women, Men and the Gendered Nature of Genetic Responsibility in Prenatal Blood Screening." *Sociology of Health & Illness* 31(3):343–59.

Reed, Richard. 2005. *Birthing Fathers: The Transformation of Men in American Rites of Birth.* New Brunswick, NJ: Rutgers University Press.

Reich, Jennifer. 2016. *Calling the Shots: Why Parents Reject Vaccines.* New York: New York University Press.

Reichenberg, A., R. Gross, M. Weiser, M. Bresnahan, J. Silverman, S. Harlap, J. Rabinowitz, C. Shulman, D. Malaspina, G. Lubin, H. Y. Knobler, M. Davidson, and E. Susser. 2006. "Advancing Paternal Age and Autism." *Archives of General Psychiatry* 63(9):1026–32.

Reumann, Miriam G. 2005. *American Sexual Character: Sex, Gender, and National Identity in the Kinsey Reports.* Berkeley: University of California Press.

Reverby, Susan. 2009. *Examining Tuskegee: The Infamous Syphilis Study and Its Legacy.* Chapel Hill: University of North Carolina Press.

"Reviews." 1924. *British Medical Journal* 1(3296):385–87.

Richardson, Sarah S. 2013. *Sex Itself: The Search for Male and Female in the Human Genome.* Chicago: University of Chicago Press.

———. Forthcoming. *The Maternal Imprint.* Chicago: University of Chicago Press.

Richardson, Sarah S., C. R. Daniels, M. W. Gillman, J. Golden, R. Kukla, C. Kuzawa, and J. Rich-Edwards. 2014. "Society: Don't Blame the Mothers." *Nature* 512(7513):131–32.

Richardson, Sarah S., and Hallam Stevens. 2015. "Beyond the Genome." In *Postgenomics: Perspectives on Biology after the Genome*, edited by Sarah S. Richardson and Hallam Stevens. Durham, NC: Duke University Press.

Richeson, Marques P. 2009. "Sex, Drugs, and . . . Race-to-Castrate: A Black Box Warning of Chemical Castration's Potential Racial Side Effects." *Harvard Blackletter Law Journal* 25:38.

Riessman, Catherine. 1983. "Women and Medicalization: A New Perspective." *Social Policy* 14(1):3–18.

Roberts, Dorothy E. 1997. *Killing the Black Body: Race, Reproduction and the Meaning of Liberty*. New York: Pantheon.

———. 2011. *Fatal Invention: How Science, Politics, and Big Business Re-create Race in the Twenty-First Century*. New York: New Press.

Rogers, Naomi. 1998. *An Alternative Path: The Making and Remaking of Hahnemann Medical College and Hospital of Philadelphia*. New Brunswick, NJ: Rutgers University Press.

Rosemberg, Eugenia. 1975. Eugenia Rosemberg to Emil Steinberger. February 24, 1975. American Society of Andrology Records, 1975–ongoing, MS 410. Iowa State University Library Special Collections and University Archives.

———. 1986. "American Society of Andrology: Its Beginnings." *Journal of Andrology* 7(1):72–75.

Rosemberg, Eugenia, Sandy C. Marks, Jr., Philip Jay Howard, Jr., and Lewis P. James. 1974. "Serum Levels of Follicle Stimulating and Luteinizing Hormones Before and After Vasectomy in Men." *Journal of Urology* 111(5):626–29.

Rosemberg, Eugenia, and C. Alvin Paulsen, eds. 1970. *The Human Testis*. New York: Plenum Press.

Rosen, George. 1942. "Changing Attitudes of the Medical Profession to Specialization." *Bulletin of the History of Medicine* 12:343-54.

———. 1944. *The Specialization of Medicine, with Particular Reference to Ophthalmology*. New York: Froben Press.

Rosenfeld, Dana, and Christopher Faircloth, eds. 2006. *Medicalized Masculinities*. Philadelphia: Temple University Press.

Rosenstock, Irwin M., Victor J. Strecher, and Marshall H. Becker. 1988. "Social-Learning Theory and the Health Belief Model." *Health Education Quarterly* 15(2):175–83.

Rosenthal, Meredith B., Alan Zaslavsky, and Joseph P. Newhouse. 2005. "The Geographic Distribution of Physicians Revisited." *Health Services Research* 40(6, part 1):1931–52.

Ross, Loretta, and Rickie Solinger. 2017. *Reproductive Justice: An Introduction*. Berkeley: University of California Press.

Rotundo, E. Anthony. 1993. *American Manhood: Transformations in Masculinity from the Revolution to the Modern Era*. New York: Basic Books.

Rubes, J., X. Lowe, D. Moore 2nd, S. Perreault, V. Slott, D. Evenson, S. G. Selevan, and A. J. Wyrobek. 1998. "Smoking Cigarettes Is Associated with Increased Sperm Disomy in Teenage Men." *Fertility and Sterility* 70(4):715–23.

Rubin, Gayle. 1975. "The Traffic in Women." In *Toward an Anthropology of Women*, edited by Rayna Reiter. New York: Monthly Review Press.

———. 1993. "Thinking Sex: Notes for a Radical Theory of the Politics of Sexuality." In *The Lesbian and Gay Studies Reader*, edited by Henry Abelove et al. London: Routledge.

Ruzek, Sheryl Burt. 1978. *The Women's Health Movement: Feminist Alternatives to Medical Control*. New York: Praeger.

Sachs, J. J. 1838. *Jahrbuch für die Leistungen der gesammten Heilkunde im Jahre 1837*. Leipzig: W. Engelmann.

Saguy, Abigail C., and Rene Almeling. 2008. "Fat in the Fire? Science, the News Media, and the 'Obesity Epidemic.'" *Sociological Forum* 23(1):53–83.

Sahni, Nikhil R., Maurice Dalton, David M. Cutler, John D. Birkmeyer, and Amitabh Chandra. 2016. "Surgeon Specialization and Operative Mortality in United States: Retrospective Analysis." *British Medical Journal* 354:i3571.

Sale, Kirkpatrick. 1993. *The Green Revolution: The American Environmental Movement, 1962–1992*. New York: Hill and Wang.

Sartorius, G. A., and E. Nieschlag. 2010. "Paternal Age and Reproduction." *Human Reproduction Update* 16(1):65–79.

Savitz, David A., Nancy L. Sonnenfeld, and Andrew F. Olshan. 1994. "Review of Epidemiologic Studies of Paternal Occupational Exposure and Spontaneous Abortion." *American Journal of Industrial Medicine* 25(3):361–83.

Schaffenburg, C. A., A. T. Gregoire, and J. L. Gueriguian. 1981. "Guidelines for the Clinical Testing of Male Contraceptive Drugs." *Journal of Andrology* 2(4):225–28.

Schagdarsurengin, U., and K. Steger. 2016. "Epigenetics in Male Reproduction: Effect of Paternal Diet on Sperm Quality and Offspring Health." *Nature Reviews Urology* 13(10):584–95.

Schelling, Thomas. 1978. *Micromotives and Macrobehavior*. New York: W. W. Norton.

Scheper-Hughes, Nancy, and Margaret Lock. 1987. "The Mindful Body: A Prolegomenon to Future Work in Medical Anthropology." *Medical Anthropology Quarterly* 1(1):6–41.

Schiebinger, Londa. 1993. *Nature's Body: Gender in the Making of Modern Science*. Boston: Beacon Press.

Schilt, Kristen, and Danya Lagos. 2017. "The Development of Transgender Studies in Sociology." *Annual Review of Sociology* 43(1):425–43.

Schirren, Carl. 1969. "Die Andrologie als neues Spezialgebiet der Medizin." *Andrologia* 1(4):2.

———. 1985. "Andrology: Origin and Development of a Special Discipline in Medicine; Reflection and View in the Future." *Andrologia* 17(2):117–25.

Schneider, David. 1968. *American Kinship: A Cultural Account.* Englewood Cliffs, NJ: Prentice-Hall.

Schoen, Joanna. 2005. *Choice and Coercion: Birth Control, Sterilization, and Abortion in Public Health and Welfare.* Chapel Hill: University of North Carolina Press.

Schrader, S.M., and K.L. Marlow. 2014. "Assessing the Reproductive Health of Men with Occupational Exposures." *Asian Journal of Andrology* 16(1):23–30.

Schultheiss, Dirk, and Friedrich H. Moll, eds. 2017. *Urology under the Swastika.* Leuven, Belg.: Davidsfonds Uitgeverij. www.academia.edu/37497997 /UROLOGY_under_the_SWASTIKA.

Secretan, B., K. Straif, R. Baan, Y. Grosse, F. El Ghissassi, V. Bouvard, L. Benbrahim-Tallaa, N. Guha, C. Freeman, L. Galichet, and V. Cogliano. 2009. "A Review of Human Carcinogens—Part E: Tobacco, Areca Nut, Alcohol, Coal Smoke, and Salted Fish." *Lancet Oncology* 10(11): 1033–34.

Sengoopta, Chandak. 2006. *The Most Secret Quintessence of Life: Sex, Glands and Hormones, 1850–1950.* Chicago: University of Chicago Press.

Seymour, Frances, and Moses Benmosche. 1941. "Magnification of the Spermatozoa by Means of the Electron Microscope." *JAMA* 116:2489–90.

Sgobba, Christa. 2015. "7 Signs You've Got Healthy Semen." *Men's Health.* Accessed March 29, 2015. www.menshealth.com/health/a19546830/7-signs-of-healthy-semen/.

Shah, Nayan. 2001. *Contagious Divides: Epidemics and Race in San Francisco's Chinatown.* Berkeley: University of California Press.

Shah, Prakesh S. 2010. "Paternal Factors and Low Birthweight, Preterm, and Small for Gestational Age Births: A Systematic Review." *American Journal of Obstetrics and Gynecology* 202(2):103–23.

Sharp, G.C., D.A. Lawlor, and S.S. Richardson. 2018. "It's the Mother!: How Assumptions about the Causal Primacy of Maternal Effects Influence Research on the Developmental Origins of Health and Disease." *Social Science & Medicine* 213:20–27.

Shawe, Jill, Dilisha Patel, Mark Joy, Beth Howden, Geraldine Barrett, and Judith Stephenson. 2019. "Preparation for Fatherhood: A Survey of Men's Preconception Health Knowledge and Behaviour in England." *PLoS One* 14(3):e0213897.

Sherins, Richard. 2014. "Retrospective on the American Society of Andrology " In *40 and forward: American Society of Andrology Celebrating 40 Years,* edited by ASA Archives & History Committee. Schaumburg, IL: American Society of Andrology.

Shim, Janet K. 2014. *Heart-Sick: The Politics of Risk, Inequality, and Heart Disease*. New York: New York University Press.

Shirani, Fiona, Karen Henwood, and Carrie Coltart. 2012. "Meeting the Challenges of Intensive Parenting Culture: Gender, Risk Management and the Moral Parent." *Sociology* 46(1):25–40.

Showalter, Elaine. 1997. *Hystories: Hysterical Epidemics and Modern Culture*. New York: Columbia University Press.

Shulevitz, Judith. 2012. "Why Fathers Really Matter." Sunday Review. *New York Times*, September 8, 2012. www.nytimes.com/2012/09/09/opinion/sunday /why-fathers-really-matter.html.

Sicherman, Barbara. 1977. "The Uses of a Diagnosis: Doctors, Patients, and Neurasthenia." *Journal of the History of Medicine and Allied Sciences* 32(1):33–54.

Siebke, Harald. 1951. "Gynecological and Andrological Diagnosis of Sterility." *Zentralblatt für Gynäkologie* 73(5a):633-37.

Sinding, S. W. 2000. "The Great Population Debates: How Relevant Are They for the 21st Century?" *American Journal of Public Health* 90(12):1841–45.

"Sins of the Fathers." February 23, 1991. *Economist* 318:109.

Sipos, Attila, Finn Rasmussen, Glynn Harrison, Per Tynelius, Glyn Lewis, David A. Leon, and David Gunnell. 2004. "Paternal Age and Schizophrenia: A Population Based Cohort Study." *British Medical Journal* 329:1070.

Smith, Benjamin E., ed. 1909. *Century Dictionary and Cyclopedia: Supplement*. New York: Century.

smith, s. e. 2019. "Women Are Not the Only Ones Who Get Abortions." *Rewire. News*, March 1, 2019. rewire.news/article/2019/03/01/women-are-not-the-only-ones-who-get-abortions/.

Soares, S. R., and M. A. Melo. 2008. "Cigarette Smoking and Reproductive Function." *Current Opinion in Obstetrics and Gynecology* 20(3):281–91.

"Society Transactions: American Association of Genito-Urinary Surgeons." 1887. *Journal of Cutaneous and Genito-Urinary Diseases* 5:15.

Soloski, Alexis. 2013. "'The Great Imitator': Staging Syphilis in *A Doll House* and *Ghosts*." *Modern Drama* 56(3):287–305.

Somerville, Siobhan B. 2000. *Queering the Color Line: Race and the Invention of Homosexuality in American Culture*. Durham, NC: Duke University Press.

"Specialism in General and Genito-Urinary Surgery in Particular." 1912. *Lancet* 180(4641):1.

Springer, K. W., J. Mager Stellman, and R. M. Jordan-Young. 2012. "Beyond a Catalogue of Differences: A Theoretical Frame and Good Practice Guidelines for Researching Sex/Gender in Human Health." *Social Science & Medicine* 74(11):1817–24.

Stanton, Elizabeth Cady, Susan B. Anthony, and Matilda J. Gage. 1973 [1881]. "Seneca Falls Convention: Selections from History of Woman Suffrage."

In *The Feminist Papers,* edited by Alice S. Rossi. New York: Bantam Books.

Starr, Paul. 1982. *The Social Transformation of American Medicine.* New York: Basic Books.

Stein, Melissa N. 2015. *Measuring Manhood: Race and the Science of Masculinity, 1830–1934.* Minneapolis: University of Minnesota Press.

Steinberger, Emil. 1975. Emil Steinberger to Eugenia Rosemberg. March 12, 1975. American Society of Andrology Records, 1975–ongoing, MS 410. Iowa State University Library Special Collections and University Archives.

———. 1978. "The American Society of Andrology: Its Past, Present and Future." *Andrologia* 10(1):56–58.

———. 1982. "The Past, the Present and the Future of Andrology." *International Journal of Andrology* 5(s5):210–16.

———. 2007. *The Promised Land: Woes of an Immigrant.* Bloomington, IN: AuthorHouse.

———. 2010. *Golden Age and Its Implosion.* Bloomington, IN: AuthorHouse.

Stellman, Jeanne Mager, and Joan E. Bertin. 1990. "Science's Anti-Female Bias." *New York Times,* June 4, 1990. www.nytimes.com/1990/06/04 /opinion/sciences-antifemale-bias.html.

Stern, Alexandra Minna. 2005. *Eugenic Nation: Faults and Frontiers of Better Breeding in Modern America.* Berkeley: University of California Press.

Stevens, Lindsay. Forthcoming. *Planned? Medicine, Inequality, and Pregnancy in the United States.* Oakland: University of California Press.

Stevens, Rosemary. 1966. *Medical Practice in Modern England: The Impact of Specialization and State Medicine.* New Haven, CT: Yale University Press.

Stevens, William K. 1977. "Sterility Linked to Pesticide Spurs Fear on Chemical Use." *New York Times,* September 11, 1977: 1. www.nytimes.com/1977/09/11 /archives/sterility-linked-to-pesticide-spurs-fear-on-chemical-use-sterility .html.

Strathern, Marilyn. 1992. *Reproducing the Future: Anthropology, Kinship and the New Reproductive Technologies.* New York: Routledge.

Swanson, Kara W. 2012. "The Birth of the Sperm Bank." *Annals of Iowa* 71:241–76.

———. 2014. *Banking on the Body: The Market in Blood, Milk, and Sperm in Modern America.* Cambridge, MA: Harvard University Press.

Tawn, E.J., G.B. Curwen, G.S. Rees, and P. Jonas. 2015. "Germline Minisatellite Mutations in Workers Occupationally Exposed to Radiation at the Sellafield Nuclear Facility." *Journal of Radiological Protection* 35(1):21–36.

Teitelbaum, Michael S. 1992. "The Population Threat." *Foreign Affairs* 71(5):63–78.

Thacker, P.D. 2004. "Biological Clock Ticks for Men, Too." *JAMA* 291(14):1683–85.

Thelen, Kathleen. 2000. "Timing and Temporality in the Analysis of Institutional Evolution and Change." *Studies in American Political Development* 14(1):101–8.

Thomas, Joseph. 1875. *A Comprehensive Medical Dictionary: Containing the Pronunciation, Etymology, and Signification of the Terms Made Use of in Medicine and the Kindred Sciences.* Philadelphia: Lippincott.

Thompson, Charis. 2005. *Making Parents: The Ontological Choreography of Reproductive Technologies.* Cambridge, MA: MIT Press.

Thompson, Matthew J., Dana Christian Lynge, Eric H. Larson, Pantipa Tachawachira, and L. Gary Hart. 2005. "Characterizing the General Surgery Workforce in Rural America." *Archives of Surgery* 140(1):74–79.

Thorne, Barrie. 1993. *Gender Play: Girls and Boys in School.* New Brunswick, NJ: Rutgers University Press.

Tiefer, Leonore. 1994. "The Medicalization of Impotence: Normalizing Phallocentrism." *Gender & Society* 8(3):363–77.

Tomes, Nancy. 1998. *The Gospel of Germs: Men, Women, and the Microbe in American Life.* Cambridge, MA: Harvard University Press.

Toriello, H. V., and J. M. Meck. 2008. "Statement on Guidance for Genetic Counseling in Advanced Paternal Age." *Genetics in Medicine* 10(6): 457–60.

Townsend, Nicholas. 2002. *The Package Deal: Marriage, Work, and Fatherhood in Men's Lives.* Philadelphia: Temple University Press.

Transactions of the Congress of American Physicians and Surgeons: First Triennial Session, Held at Washington D.C. 1889. New Haven, CT: Congress of American Physicians and Surgeons.

Transactions of the Congress of American Physicians and Surgeons: Second Triennial Session, Held at Washington D.C. 1892. New Haven, CT: Congress of American Physicians and Surgeons.

Tsai, Tony Yu-Chen, Yoon Sup Choi, Wenzhe Ma, Joseph R. Pomerening, Chao Tang, and James E. Ferrell. 2008. "Robust, Tunable Biological Oscillations from Interlinked Positive and Negative Feedback Loops." *Science* 321(5885):126–29.

Tuana, Nancy. 2004. "Coming to Understand: Orgasm and the Epistemology of Ignorance." *Hypatia* 19(1):194–232.

United Automobile Workers v. Johnson Controls, Inc. 1991. 499 U.S. 187 (1991).

"University of New York Faculty of Medicine." 1855. *American Journal of the Medical Sciences* 30:7.

U.S. Department of Defense. 1994. "Birth Outcome Studies: Studies Completed." Accessed March 30, 2015. www.defense.gov/news/fact_sheets/f941205_brthstds.html.

Urhoj, S. K., L. N. Jespersen, M. Nissen, L. H. Mortensen, and A. M. Nybo Andersen. 2014. "Advanced Paternal Age and Mortality of Offspring under 5 Years of Age: A Register-Based Cohort Study." *Human Reproduction* 29(2):343–50.

Valdez, Natali. 2018. "The Redistribution of Reproductive Responsibility: On the Epigenetics of 'Environment' in Prenatal Interventions." *Medical Anthropology Quarterly* 32(3):425–42.

Van Buren, W. H., and E. L. Keyes. 1874. *A Practical Treatise on the Surgical Diseases of the Genito-urinary Organs including Syphilis: Designed as a Manual for Students and Practitioners.* New York: D. Appleton.

van der Zee, B., G. de Wert, E. A. Steegers, and I. D. de Beaufort. 2013. "Ethical Aspects of Paternal Preconception Lifestyle Modification." *American Journal of Obstetrics and Gynecology* 209(1):11–6.

Vassoler, F. M., E. M. Byrnes, and R. C. Pierce. 2014. "The Impact of Exposure to Addictive Drugs on Future Generations: Physiological and Behavioral Effects." *Neuropharmacology* 76, part B:269–75.

Vienne, Florence. 2006. "Der Mann als medizinisches Wissensobjekt: Ein blinder Fleck in der Wissenschaftsgeschichte." *N.T.M.* 14:222–30.

———. 2018. "Eggs and Sperm as Germ Cells." In *Reproduction: Antiquity to the Present Day,* edited by Nick Hopwood, Rebecca Flemming, and Lauren Kassell. Cambridge, UK: Cambridge University Press.

Waggoner, Miranda. 2017. *The Zero Trimester: Pre-Pregnancy Care and the Politics of Reproductive Risk.* Oakland: University of California Press.

Wagner, Wolfgang, Fran Elejabarrieta, and Ingrid Lahnsteiner. 1995. "How the Sperm Dominates the Ovum—Objectification by Metaphor in the Social Representation of Conception." *European Journal of Social Psychology* 25(6):671–88.

Wahlberg, Ayo. 2018. *Good Quality: The Routinization of Sperm Banking in China.* Oakland: University of California Press.

Wailoo, Keith. 2001. *Dying in the City of the Blues: Sickle Cell Anemia and the Politics of Race and Health.* Chapel Hill: University of North Carolina Press.

Waldenburg, D. L. 1979. "VI. Verhandlungen ärztlicher Gesellschaften: Hufeland'sche Gesellschaft in Berlin." *Berliner Klinische Wochenschrift* 16(33):502–3.

Walker, Kenneth M. 1923. *Diseases of the Male Organs of Generation.* London: H. Frowde and Hodder & Stoughton.

Warner, J. N., and K. A. Frey. 2013. "The Well-Man Visit: Addressing a Man's Health to Optimize Pregnancy Outcomes." *Journal of the American Board of Family Medicine* 26(2):196–202.

Warner, John Harley. 1997. *The Therapeutic Perspective: Medical Practice, Knowledge, and Identity in America, 1820–1885.* Princeton, NJ: Princeton University Press.

———. 2003. *Against the Spirit of the System: The French Impulse in Nineteenth-Century American Medicine.* Baltimore, MD: Johns Hopkins University Press.

Watkins, Elizabeth Siegel. 2001. *On the Pill: A Social History of Oral Contraceptives*. Baltimore, MD: Johns Hopkins University Press.

Watson, Irving Allison. 1896. *Physicians and Surgeons of America (Illustrated): A Collection of Biographical Sketches of the Regular Medical Profession*. Concord, NH: Republican Press Association.

Weber, Jennifer Beggs. 2012. "Becoming Teen Fathers: Stories of Teen Pregnancy, Responsibility, and Masculinity." *Gender & Society* 26(6):900–21.

WebMD. 2014. "Sperm FAQ." Reviewed by Trina Pagano, MD. Accessed March 29, 2015. www.webmd.com/infertility-and-reproduction/guide/sperm-and-semen-faq.

Weinberg, Wilhelm. 1912. "Zur Vererbung des Zwergwuchses." *Archiv für Rassen- und Gesellschafts-Biologie* 9:710–17.

Weiss, Robert. 1994. *Learning from Strangers: The Art and Method of Qualitative Interview Studies*. New York: Free Press.

Weisz, George. 2006. *Divide and Conquer: A Comparative History of Medical Specialization*. New York: Oxford University Press.

Welch, L. C., K. E. Lutfey, E. Gerstenberger, and M. Grace. 2012. "Gendered Uncertainty and Variation in Physicians' Decisions for Coronary Heart Disease: The Double-Edged Sword of 'Atypical Symptoms.'" *Journal of Health and Social Behavior* 53(3):313–28.

Wentzell, Emily A. 2013. *Maturing Masculinities: Aging, Chronic Illness, and Viagra in Mexico*. Durham, NC: Duke University Press.

What To Expect. 2015. "Fertility Foods for Men and Women." Infographic. Accessed March 29, 2015. www.whattoexpect.com/tools/photolist/fertility-foods-for-men-and-women-infographic.

WHO. 1980. *WHO Laboratory Manual for the Examination of Human Semen and Semen-Cervical Mucus Interaction*. Singapore: Press Concern.

WHO and United Nations Environment Programme. 2013. *State of the Science of Endocrine Disrupting Chemicals—2012*. Geneva: WHO Press.

Whooley, Owen. 2013. *Knowledge in the Time of Cholera: The Struggle Over American Medicine in the Nineteenth Century*. Chicago: University of Chicago Press.

Whorton, James C. 2002. *Nature Cures: The History of Alternative Medicine in America*. New York: Oxford University Press.

Wishard, William M. 1925. "Memorial to Edward L Keyes." *Transactions of the American Association of Genitourinary Surgeons* 18:515–17.

Wollstonecraft, Mary. 1967 [1792]. *A Vindication of the Rights of Woman*. New York: W. W. Norton.

"W. O. Nelson, Expert on Birth Control, 58." 1964. *New York Times*, October 20, 1964: 32. www.nytimes.com/1964/10/20/w-o-nelson-expert-on-birth-control-58.html.

Wood, Christine Virginia. 2015. "Knowledge Ecologies, 'Supple' Objects, and Different Priorities across Women's and Gender Studies Programs and Departments in the United States, 1970–2010." *Journal of the History of the Behavioral Sciences* 51(4):387–408.

Worboys, Michael. 2004. "Unsexing Gonorrhoea: Bacteriologists, Gynaecologists, and Suffragists in Britain, 1860–1920." *Social History of Medicine* 17(1):41–59.

Yanagisako, Sylvia, and Jane Collier. 1990. "The Mode of Reproduction in Anthropology." In *Theoretical Perspectives on Sexual Difference,* edited by Deborah Rhode. New Haven, CT: Yale University Press.

Yang, Q., Q. Yang, S. W. Wen, A. Leader, and X. K. Chen. 2007. "Paternal Age and Birth Defects: How Strong Is the Association?" *Human Reproduction* 22(3):696–701.

Zhang, Chiyuan A., Yash S. Khandwala, Michael L. Eisenberg, and Ying Lu. 2017. "The Age of Fathers in the USA Is Rising: An Analysis of 168,867,480 Births from 1972 to 2015." *Human Reproduction* 32(10):2110–16.

Zorgniotti, A. W. 1976. "The Creation of the American Urologist, 1902–1912." *Bulletin of the New York Academy of Medicine* 52(3):283–92.

———. 1977. "Three Important Holograph Letters by Edward Lawrence Keyes concerning the Founding of the American Association of Genito-Urinary Surgeons (1886–1887)." *Transactions of the American Association of Genitourinary Surgeons* 68:91–95.

Index

Note: Page numbers in *italics* denote a figure or table.

Abbott, Andrew, 210n119
abortion: banning of, 172; as feminist issue, 32–33, 133; potential for further erosion of access by emphasizing men's involvement in reproduction, 173
Academy of Nutrition and Dietetics, 186
achondroplasia, 79, 80
Acton, William, 207n65
addiction, law and policy to address, 103
Affordable Care Act (2010), 103
age of interviewees, 188–89
age of parents: overview, 77, 78
—MATERNAL: and Down syndrome risk, 79, 148; men's awareness of risks of, 144, 145; news coverage of, 92, 101; rate of, as equal to paternal effects, 80; warnings about, vs. downplaying of paternal age effects, 82
—PATERNAL: overview, 79–82; and achondroplasia, 79, 80; child mortality rates and, 81; chromosomal aneuploidies not found in, 79, 216n28; consumer website coverage of, 96; disease risk to children, 78, 79–81, 101, 102; early-life, 78; and epigenetic effects, 77; erectile dysfunction and, 105; genetic disorders, 79–80; interviewee conceptions of, 148–49; interviewee knowledge of, 149; interviewee lack of mentions of, 128–29; and new mutations, 77, 80, 81, 102; news coverage of, 92, 94–95, 97–98, 101–2; rate of, as equal to maternal effects, 80; reassurances in published sources about, 82, 101–2, 105; risks of, 80–81; risks of, debate about informing, 81–82; sperm bank age limits imposed due to, 80, 217n32; sperm fertility and, 96, 105; studies about, generally, 78
Agent Orange, 86, 94, 107, 222–23n85
agnotology. *See* non-knowledge
alcohol consumption: alcoholism, medicalization of, 162; and maternal effects, 97, 216n24; nineteenth-century campaigns against, emphasizing effects on children's health, 77; and paternal effects, 83–84, 97, 108; recommendation for warning labels about paternal effects of, 97, 178; and sperm fertility, 83–84, 93, 106, 108
American Academy of Family Physicians, 108, 177, 186
American Andrological Association, 36, 40, 44–45. *See also* American Association of Andrology and Syphilology; American Association of Genito-Urinary Surgeons

American Association for the Advancement of Science, 85

American Association of Andrology and Syphilology, 40, 44, 206n57

American Association of Genito-Urinary Surgeons, 36, 38–39, 40, 43–45, 48, 51

American Association of Tissue Banks, 80

American College of Medical Genetics, 81, 108, 186

American College of Obstetricians and Gynecologists, 108, 186

American Dermatological Association, 206n47

American Fertility Society, 80. *See also* American Society for Reproductive Medicine

American Illustrated Medical Dictionary (Dorland), 56

American Journal of Urology, 51

American Lancet (journal), 41

American Medical Association (AMA): and advertisement of services, 48; Congress of American Physicians and Surgeons as competitor to, 37; and European training of physicians, 29; founding of, 29; lack of information about paternal effects on website of, 107–8; and methodology, 186; and "quacks," 50, 52, 210n110

American Society for Men's Health, 186

American Society for Reproductive Medicine (ASRM, formerly American Fertility Society), 80, 101, 108, 186, 221n64

American Society of Andrology (ASA): affiliations and interests of members, 62, *64*, 66–67; Distinguished Andrologist Award, 62; first meeting of (1975), 62–63, *64*, 66; founding of, 61–62; humor and, 65–66, *66*, 214n70; as largely unknown in the U.S., 66–67; logo of, *64*, 65, *66*; and methodology, 184; number of members, 66; and specialty, discussion about necessity of, 62–63, 65, 214n65. *See also Journal of Andrology*

American Urological Association: as distinct from andrology, 51; excising "genito-" from name of, 51; founding of, 51, 207n59; and methodology, 186; ridicule of, 208n81; Urology Care Foundation, 186; website of, lack of information on paternal effects, 108

Andrologie/Andrologia (journal), 54, 211n3; founding of, 54, 55, 60, 214n75; and Keyes's effort to organize andrology, 60; and methodology, 184; as official publica-

tion of various national associations, 60, 65

andrology: overview, 21–22, 67–69; continued lack of specialty since the 1970s, 88–89; and cooperation with gynecology, 57, 211n3; definitions, etymology, and use of term, 35, 40, 45, 56–57, 61, 67, 206–7nn58–59, 211–12nn13,14,17, 213n42; early-twentieth-century proposals for, 55–57, 211–12nn7,13,14,17; increasing awareness over time of, 73–75, *74–75*; and methodology, 184–85; ridicule of, 43–45, 56, 68, 208n81. *See also* genito-urinary surgeons; medical specialization in men's reproductive health; organizational infrastructure; urology

—LATE 1880S ATTEMPT TO ESTABLISH: overview, 21–22; and advertising, refusal to allow, 48; American Urological Association as distinct from, 51; and anxiety about White male virility, 46–47; and dermatology, 37, 38, 39, 44, 206n47; failure of, 21n119, 50; female patients seen by, 39, 41; genito-urinary diseases as focus of, 35–36; *JAMA* editorial lauding the inception of, 33–36, *34*, 39, 44, 45–46, 60, 205n34, 211n7; the male body as focus of, 35, 38–39; as market failure, 52–53; members/invitees, 37, 38, 206n48; name of the specialty, 38, 40, 43–45, 206n57, 207n59; and "quacks" and charlatans, 47–50, 52, 210n110; and respectability, quest for, 45–46, 50, 68; ridicule of, 43–45, 208n81; scope of the specialty, 37–39; uncertainty about differences and similarities in male and female bodies and, 41–43, 207nn63–65, 208nn67–69,74; and venereal disease, stigma of, 28–29, 47–51, 48–50, 68, 210n120

—LATE 1960S ESTABLISHMENT OF: overview, 22, 54–55; and cooperation with gynecology, 211n3; founding of, 59–61, 212–13nn38,40; humor and, 65–66, *66*, 214n70; Male Reproductive Biology Club, 59, 61, 212n37; national associations, loosely organized international network of, 60; and organizational infrastructure, creation of, 68, 89; scope of specialty, 61; social context for, 58–59, 67–68, 89, 169, 214n75; and specialty, discussion about necessity of, 62–63, 65, 214n65; as unaware of late-nineteenth-century efforts, 60, 68, 213n42. *See also* American Society

of Andrology (ASA); Comité Internacional de Andrología (CIDA); International Society of Andrology
—PARALLELISM WITH GYNECOLOGY, 56, 57, 166, 174, 211–12n17; dualistic/binary conceptions of gender and rhetoric of, 40, 57, 68, 166, 174; late 1880s organizing effort and, 35, 39–40, 41, 42, 68, 206n52; late 1960s organizing effort and, 54, 60–61, 68, 211n3
Andrology. See Journal of Andrology (now *Andrology*)
Angier, Natalie, 97–98
animal studies, 78, 216n23
anti-vaccine activism, 226n19
Archives of Andrology, 214n68
Argentina, and andrology, 1960s establishment of, 55, 60, 212–13nn38,42,52
Aristotle, 133
Arnot, Robert, 112
ASA. *See* American Society of Andrology
assisted reproductive technologies: and biological vs. social relationships, 125; egg donors, 125; intracytoplasmic sperm injection (ICSI), 11, 224n24; surrogacy, 125; in vitro fertilization (IVF), 11, 224n24
attention deficit hyperactivity disorder (ADHD), 83, 102
Atwood, Margaret, *The Handmaid's Tale*, 172
autism and paternal effects: overview, 78; age and, 80, 81, 82, 102; news coverage of, 94, 102

Bailey, Janice L., 87
Beaney, James George, 42, 48–49, 207n65
behavioral abnormalities, and paternal effects, 83, 84, 97
behaviors of parents: overview, 77–78; definition of, 77–78
—MATERNAL: alcohol consumption, 97, 216n24; fish consumption, 216n24; incarceration of women for, 76, 171; individualization of risk, 163, 226n28; men's awareness of risks of, 144, 146
—PATERNAL: overview, 82–83; alcohol consumption, 83–84, 97, 108; body mass index (BMI), 79; diet, 79, 84; drugs, illegal, 84, 108; and epigenetic effects, 77, 82; exercise, 79; and germ-line mutations, 83; interviewee guesses about, 146–48; interviewees' prior knowledge of, 150, 163; and new mutations, 77; news media coverage

of, 93, 94; risks of, informing, 83; smoking, 79, 83, 100, 108; sperm fertility and, 83–84; studies about, generally, 78–79
Belkin, Lisa, 102
Bellevue Hospital Medical College (New York), 36–37, 205n35
Benninghaus, Christina, 53, 205n34, 208n69
betel nuts, 84
binary conceptions of gender. *See* dualistic/binary conceptions of gender
biological clock: female, 3, 149; male, 2, 3, 96, 101, 102, 220n44; male, interviewee awareness of, 148, 149. *See also* age of parents
biological stories/sperm stories: animal analogies in, 135, 140, 225n29; cultural notions of masculinity and, 132, 134, 135, 140; cultural understandings of biology as malleable, 138–39, 140, 225n26; egalitarian gender attitudes and sperm stories, 138–39, *139*, 140–41, 161, 225nn32–35; equalizing reproductive risk as new story told by interviewees, 161, 167; the male as agent in, 135, 162; methodology and, 137, 138, 193–94, 224n23, 225nn32–35; the "natural" and, 139; and non-knowledge about men's reproductive health, 140; political work of, 140; scientific knowledge-making and influence of, 129–30, 224nn21,24; of social scientists, 140; Sperm story #1: active sperm and passive egg, 129–35, 137, *139*, 167, 224n24, 225n29; Sperm story #2: sperm and egg as two halves of a whole, 130, 135–39, *139*, 140–41, 167; women's versions of sperm stories, 137–38. *See also* eggs and sperm
biological ties and social relationships, 125, 224n13
biomedical infrastructure. *See* organizational infrastructure
biomedical knowledge. *See* knowledge-making; non-knowledge
biomedical research: dualism of sex and hierarchy/inequality, 9–10; establishment of rules requiring the inclusion of women and people of color in, 3, 16, 104; gender norms as shaping, 6, 16–17, 129–30, 224n21; the "inclusion and difference paradigm" (Epstein) and, 16; the male body as standard in, 10–11; recommendations to include paternal effects in, 173–76
biopolitics, and mandatory response of acquiescence to health messages, 157

bipolar disorder and paternal effects: age and, 80, 81; news coverage of, 94, 102

birth defects: definition and use of term in this text, 216n19; federal requirement adding folic acid to grain products for prevention of, 103; maternal blame for, 97–98, 146

—PATERNAL EFFECTS AND: overview, 78; age and, 81; alcohol consumption, 83

birthweight, paternal effects and, 78, 83, 84

Black, Donald Campbell, 39

bodies as gendered. *See* dualistic/binary conceptions of gender; gender as relational

bodies as standard or reproductive: all bodies as reproductive, as paradigm shift, 172–73; all bodies as reproductive, cautions regarding, 172, 173; historical context of, 41; uncertainty about similarities and differences between male and female, 41–43, 207nn63–65, 208nn67–69,74. *See also* dualistic/binary conceptions of gender; female body as reproductive; male body as standard

body mass index (BMI), and paternal effects, 79

Boston Medical and Surgical Journal, 205–6n43

Bowles, Nellie, 98, 100–101

Brandt, Allan M., 205n33, 209n98

British Medical Journal, 44, 211–12n17, 218n84

Brody, Jane, "Personal Health" column, 112, 219n12

Bunge, Raymond, 59

Cabot, Hugh, 208n81

Campo-Engelstein, Lisa, 92, 101, 219n6

cancer, chimney sweep's, 42

cancer and paternal effects: age and, 80; early-onset breast cancer, 80; hepatoblastoma, 83; leukemia, 80, 83; retinoblastoma, 80; smoking by father, 83, 100

cardiovascular disease. *See* heart disease

Catholic immigrants, 46

CDC. *See* Centers for Disease Control and Prevention

Ceauçescu, Nicolae, 172

Centers for Disease Control and Prevention (CDC): individual-level actions recommended by, 105; links to other websites, 221n64; meeting about men's reproductive health (2010), and report summarizing, 106; and methodology, 186, 191,

220n35; "Preconception Health Information for Men" (2015), 105, *106,* 142–43, 191, 220n35; women's bodies and health as focus of, 105. *See also* National Institute for Occupational Safety and Health

Centro de Investigación de Reproducción (Buenos Aires), 60, 212–13n38

Chang, Min-Chueh, 62

chemical exposures: overview, 84–85; Agent Orange and unspecified battlefield chemicals, 86, 94, 107, 222–23n85; carcinogens (in science labs), 85; chemical body burden, 163; DBCP (dibromochloropropane) pesticide, 85, 93; DDT, 94; hydrocarbons, 85; and lack of testing of chemicals, 107; lead, 85; March of Dimes brochure on, 113; nitrous oxide (laughing gas), 85, 218n82; recommendation for warning labels about paternal effects of, 178; vinyl chloride, 94. *See also* behaviors; environmental exposures; exposures of parents; occupational exposures; radiation exposures

Chemical Youth project, 226n28

chemotaxis. *See* eggs and sperm

Chernobyl disaster (1986), 86, 218n84

childbirth, father's presence at, 58, 151

child-free by choice, 172

child mortality rates, paternal age and, 81

children, effects on. *See* maternal effects; paternal effects

China, paternal effects publicized in, 163

chromosomes, gender norms and scientific designation of X and Y as "sex chromosomes," 6, 16–17

churches, and public health messaging on men's reproductive health, 180

CIDA. *See* Comité Internacional de Andrología

circulation of biomedical knowledge about men's reproductive health: overview, 22–23, 91–93, 114–16; breadth vs. depth of this study, 21; diffusion model compared to, 91; increasing attention over time to men's reproductive health, 73–75, *74–75*; lack of, and lack of organizational infrastructure, 109, 114, 115, 167, 170; methodology of data collection, 73–74, 93–96, 185–87, 214–15nn1–3,7, 219nn6–8,12, 220n35, 228nn12–13; tripartite framework and, 21, 169–70. *See also* consumer websites for health and parenting; federal health agencies and circulation of

knowledge about paternal effects; Men Have Babies Too (March of Dimes public health campaign on paternal effects); news media and circulation of knowledge about paternal effects; professional medical associations and circulation of knowledge about paternal effects
civil rights movement, 58–59
Civil War, 36, 205n36
"clap," as slang for venereal disease, 210n120
Clarke, Adele, 31, 184, 205n34, 210n126
class: and barriers to behavioral changes to prevent paternal effects, 159; and medical abuses of poor people, 10, 28; medical surveillance and, 171; and "men's specialty clinics," 50; news media recommendations for men's reproductive health as ignoring issues of, 103; and STI treatment, 28. See also intersectional analysis
climate-change: denial of, 226n19; non-knowledge and, 8
clinical trials: establishment of rules requiring the inclusion of women and people of color in, 3, 16; the male body as standard in, 3. See also biomedical research
cocaine, 84, 106
Comité Internacional de Andrología (CIDA): founding of, 60; International Congress of Andrology, 61; and methodology, 185. See also International Society of Andrology; Mancini, Roberto; Puigvert, Antonio
conception: the male as agent in, 135; the male as seed and the female as soil, 133; preformation/homunculus (18th century), 133. See also biological stories/sperm stories; eggs and sperm
condoms, 11, 66
Congress of American Physicians and Surgeons, 37, 44–45, 209n85
Connell, R. W., 15
consumer websites for health and parenting: federal agencies linking to, 221n64; gender in coverage of men's reproductive health, 98–99; on male biological clock, 220n44; and methodology, 95–96, 185, 186, 191, 220n35; paternal age coverage by, 96; recommendation to include information on men's reproductive health, 180; slang used by, 99; sperm fertility as focus of, vs. effects on children's health, 96, 115

continuing education requirements including men's reproductive health, 177
contraception: birth control programs, 59; as feminist issue, 32–33, 58
—FEMALE, the pill, 32, 62
—MALE: condoms and vasectomy as only forms of, 11; pill for, as "technology-in-the-making," 11, 32, 76
Conway, Erik, 8
Cooper, Astley, 50
Cooter, Roger, 91
Corner, Edred Moss, 56, 57, 211–12nn14,17
Croissant, Jennifer, 8, 169
Crouzon syndrome, 80
Curley, James P., 216n16
Curling, Thomas Blizard, 28, 42, 50, 208n68

Daniels, Cynthia, 15, 86–87, 92, 100, 205n34, 210n126, 219n7
Darby, Robert, 205n33
Davis, Devra Lee, 87, 100
DBCP (dibromochloropropane), 85, 93
DDT, 94
Department of Defense (DoD): discounting paternal effects of chemical exposures, 107; and methodology, 186. See also chemical exposures; war
Department of Health and Human Services, and methodology, 186
depressive disorders and paternal effects, age and, 81
dermatology, 37, 38, 39, 44, 57, 206n47
developmental origins of health and disease (DOHaD), and paternal effects, 87, 175
developmental toxicity, 78–79. See also behaviors of parents; exposures of parents
diabetes: and paternal effects, 84; and sperm fertility, 104
diet: law and policy to improve, 103; and paternal effects, 79, 84
diffusion of knowledge, 91. See also circulation of biomedical knowledge
diseases and disorders. See ADHD; autism; behavioral abnormalities; cancer; diabetes; genetic disorders; glucose tolerance, impaired; heart disease; learning disabilities; metabolic syndrome; psychological disorders
Distinguished Andrologist Award, 62
DNA. See paternal effects; entries at "genetics"
DoD. See Department of Defense
Dow Chemical, 85
Down syndrome, 79, 146, 148

drugs, illegal: interviewees on structural problem of, 159; March of Dimes brochure on, 113; paternal effects and, 84, 108; sperm fertility and, 93. *See also* pharmaceuticals

dualistic/binary conceptions of gender: medical knowledge-making and, 6, 16–17, 129–30, 168–69, 224n21; medical nonknowledge and, 15, 17, 168–69; and protective labor laws and policies, 84, 97; and rhetorical move of positioning andrology as a parallel to gynecology, 40, 57, 68, 166, 174; sex as, 9–10, 13, 168; the study of women OR men as, 15; "the male as standard and the female as reproductive" as, 12–13. *See also* bodies as standard or reproductive; gender

Duden, Barbara, 21, 207n64

dwarfism (achondroplasia form), 79, 80

Edin, Kathryn, 188, 191

education: association with health knowledge, 149; high school health or sex education courses, 180. *See also* medical schools and training programs; socioeconomic status

eggs and sperm: active egg (chemotaxis) biology of, 129–30, 224n21; and debates about difference and similarity, 42–43; donors of, gendered norms and valuation of, 6; embryology and view of equal reproductive contributions of, 43; gender norms and scientific conceptions of, 6, 129–30, 224n24; the male as seed and the female as soil, 133; "preformation"/homunculus, 133. *See also* biological stories/sperm stories; conception

Eliasson, Rune, 61, 213nn40,42

employees. *See* occupational exposures

endocrine-disrupting chemicals, 86, 94, 100, 179–80

endocrinology, 32, 61–63, 65–67, 95, 166, 175

environmental exposures: endocrine-disrupting chemicals, 86, 94, 100, 179–80; and individualization of risk and responsibility, 163, 226n28; interviewees on difficulty of avoiding, 159–60; lack of federal health agency warnings on, 107; news coverage of, 94, 95. *See also* chemical exposures; exposures of parents; radiation exposures

environmental factors. *See* structural and environmental barriers standing between

individual men and the goal of healthy sperm; structural and environmental contributors to disease

Environmental Protection Agency (EPA): and methodology, 186; no mention of paternal effects from exposures, 107; population-level risk reductions possible via, 103

environmental regulations, evisceration of, 86

EPA. *See* Environmental Protection Agency

epidemiological studies, 78–79, 216nn21,23

epigenetics, 77, 78, 82, 150, 226n28. *See also* maternal effects; paternal effects; *entries at "genetics"*

Epstein, Steven, 10, 16, 203n55

erectile dysfunction (impotence): age and, 105; as included in late-nineteenth-century attempt to establish andrology, 36

estrogen and testosterone. *See* hormone model

eugenics: and anxiety about White male virility, 47; concern with men's reproductive health, 55, 79, 166; consumer website language influenced by, 96; fall out of favor of, 54; history of, and ongoing discrimination against people with disabilities, 181; and language of "sperm quality," 96, 181; and mass murder in Nazi Germany, 54–55; and mass sterilization, 54; "population control" rhetoric and undertones of, 59; and professionalization of medicine, 30

Europe, training of American physicians in, 29, 36, 40

exercise, and paternal effects, 79

Exploring Masculinities, 12

exposures of parents: overview, 78; definition of, 78; laws and policies protecting women and not men, 84, 97

—MATERNAL, lead, 85

—PATERNAL: epigenetics and, 77; interviewees' prior knowledge of, 150, 158; new mutations and, 77; risk assessment and uncertainty, 79, 86, 218n84; studies about, generally, 78–79. *See also* chemical exposures; environmental exposures; occupational exposures; radiation exposures

fatherhood: changing cultural norms around, 58, 119, 151; excluded in social scientific literature on masculinity, 12; interviewee descriptions of, 121–24; methodology of interviewee recruitment and status of,

121, 188–89, 226n4. *See also* interview study of views on men's reproduction

Fausto-Sterling, Anne, 6, 9

Fawcett, Don W., 74

FDA. *See* Food and Drug Administration

federal health agencies: recommendations for, 178–80; risk-reduction laws and policies, 103

federal health agencies and circulation of knowledge about paternal effects: overview, 92–93, 104; funding as focused on women's health, 104; lack of focus on paternal effects, 104–7, 115, 167; and lack of organizational infrastructure for publicizing knowledge, 115, 167; methodology and, 185–86; OSHA reference to children's health effects, 107; recommendations for expanding research into men's reproductive health, 175; sperm fertility as focus of, vs. paternal effects, 104–7, 115, 167

feedback loops: of association between reproductive knowledge and women's bodies as precluding such association with men's bodies, 18, 20, 30–31, 33, 168–69, 203n55; and biological, cultural, and institutional processes, 18, 203n55; categories of "men" and "reproductive health" now linked by weak feedback loop, 90; and classifications of people, 20; metaphor of the photographer with, 18, 20, 203n55; and organizational infrastructure, lack of, 53, 115, 168; and possibility of change, 169; social movements of the 1960s and '70s and interruption of, 68; temporality and, 18

"female" and "female body," as terms in this text, 10

female body as reproductive: overview, 11; biomedical research and assumption of, 11, 12; as dualism with "male body as standard," 12–13; and feedback loop from early medical specialization, 31–32, 33; feminism and reinforcement of, 32–33; and lack of knowledge about men, 12; social science literature and assumption of, 11, 12; and study of women OR men but calling it gender, 13–15, 202–3n40; the ubiquity of the contraceptive pill and, 32. *See also* male body as standard

femininity: as rooted in the ovaries, 32; as social construction, 6. *See also* gender

feminism: and anxiety about White male virility, 47, 58; on biological sex differ-

ences, 6, 140; and competing cartographies of the clitoris, 181–82; and conception story of male as seed and female as soil, 133; and contraception and abortion, 32–33, 58; early-twentieth-century andrology proposals referencing, 56; in news coverage of inequalities in reproductive risk, 97–98; and reinforcement of the female body as reproductive, 32–33; reproductive justice movement, 32–33, 179; and social change movements of the 1960s and '70s, 58–59, 169; women's studies programs, 14

fertility. *See* infertility; sperm fertility/ infertility

Finland, and andrology, 1960s establishment of, 60

Fischer, Suzanne, 48

Fisch, Harry, 95, 101, 186–87

Fissell, Mary, 91

folic acid, added to grain products, 103

Food and Drug Administration (FDA), inclusion rules for women and people of color in biomedical research, 3

"forbidden knowledge" as non-knowledge, 8

Forsbach, Ralf, 57

Foucault, Michel, 157

France: and andrology, 1960s establishment of, 213n40, 214n65; training of American physicians in, 36, 40

Frans, E. M., 81

Freidman, Jan M., 81

Frey, Keith A., 190–91

Frickel, Scott, 206n52

Friedler, Gladys, 86, 87

Fürstenheim, Ernst, 207n59

gap in knowledge. *See* non-knowledge; non-knowledge about men's reproductive health

gay men/MSM (men who have sex with men) as interviewees: and heteronormative views of men's reproductive role, 124, 158–59; and methodology, 120, *121*, 189–90. *See also* homosexuality

gender: egalitarian attitudes about, and sperm story about equal contributions of sperm and egg, 138–39, *139*, 225nn32–35; medical knowledge-making as shaped by dualism/norms of, 6, 16–17, 129–30, 224n21; medical non-knowledge as shaped by dualism/norms of, 15, 17, 168–69; and methodology, 189, 190; and news

gender *(continued)*
    coverage of paternal effects, 96, 97–99,
        100–101; nonbinary conceptions of, inter-
        sex and trans scholarship and activism
        and, 10, 169; politics of, as reshaped by
        new knowledge about men's reproductive
        health, 24, 171; "sex" as differentiated
        from, 5–6; "sex hormone" model and
        norms of, 6, 16, 32; the study of women
        OR men but calling it gender, 13–15, 202–
        3n40; as term in this text, 10. *See also*
        dualistic/binary conceptions of gender;
        femininity; gender as relational; intersec-
        tional analysis; masculinity; women
gender as relational: blame of women for
        birth defects and genetic disorders,
        97–98, 146; as both content and process,
        16–17, 20; defined as the study of the
        dynamic processes in construction of
        women/men, male/female, masculinity/
        femininity, 15; and morbidity/mortality
        rates, 151; non-knowledge of men's repro-
        ductive health as shaped by, 15, 17–20,
        168–69; research approaches and, 16–17,
        20–21; shift from the study of women OR
        men to the study of gender, 15, 17, 171. *See
        also* dualistic/binary conceptions of gen-
        der; non-knowledge about men's repro-
        ductive health (relationality of gender
        resulting in reproductive knowledge
        about women and non-knowledge about
        men); organizational infrastructure and
        knowledge-making about reproduction
gender studies. *See* women's studies
generation/generative organs, as term, 41,
        207n65
genetic disorders: achondroplasia (form of
        dwarfism), 79, 80; Down syndrome, 79,
        146, 148; maternal blame for, 97–98, 146;
        paternal age effect disorders, 80; sickle
        cell trait, 128
genetic science: and awareness of diseases that
        "run in families," 77; epigenetic modifica-
        tions, 77, 78, 82, 150, 226n28; germ-line
        mutations, 83; new mutations (de novo),
        77, 80, 81, 102; recommendations for, 175
genetics, interview study and mentions of:
        and egalitarian thinking about concep-
        tion, 136–37; scarcity of references to
        paternal effects, 128, 129
genetic studies, 78–79, 89, 169, 216n23
genetic testing: men's feelings of responsibil-
        ity to their families for genetic risk, 161,

        202–3n40; and paternal age effect disor-
        ders, identification of, 79–80; and study
        of women and calling it gender,
        202–3n40
genital conditions: shame and stigma
        attached to, 28–29. *See also* STIs (sexually
        transmitted infections, "venereal disease")
genitals: clitoris, competing cartographies of,
        181–82; female, and pathologization of
        women, 31, 43; male, as not believed to
        define men's nature, 43
genito-urinary surgeons: and early-twentieth-
        century proposals for andrology, 211–
        12n17; and the late-nineteenth-century
        attempt to establish andrology, 37–41,
        43–45, 48–50, 51, 205–6nn36,43,47,
        208n81. *See also* andrology; medical spe-
        cialization in men's reproductive health;
        urology
German Society for the Study of Fertility and
        Sterility, 54
Germany: and andrology, 1960s establish-
        ment of, 54, 60, 211n3, 213n42, 214n75;
        and andrology, twentieth-century propos-
        als for, 56–57; Nazi Germany, 54–55, 57,
        61; training of American physicians in,
        40, 207n60; and use of the term "androl-
        ogy," 40, 207n59
Gifford, Frank, 112
Ginsburg, Faye, 4, 5
glucose tolerance, impaired, 84
gonorrhea, 47, 210n120. *See also* STIs
Gould, George M., 211n13
government agencies. *See* federal health
        agencies
Greece, Classical, 77, 133
Guiteras, Ramon, 51
Gulf War: toxic exposures of soldiers in, 86,
        107. *See also* Department of Defense; war
Gutmann, Matthew, 225n29
gyms, and public health messaging on men's
        reproductive health, 180
gynecology: overview, 30–31; among the first
        medical specialties, 3, 29–30, 31, 52;
        dominance of, and attempts to profes-
        sionalize genito-urinary surgery, 39–40;
        etymology and use of term "gynecology,"
        40, 206–7nn58–59; and feedback loop of
        the female body as reproductive, 31–32,
        33; increasing awareness over time of, 75,
        75; male infertility treated in, 205n34;
        merged into single specialty with obstet-
        rics, 31; pathologization of female biology

and, 31; urology distinguished from, 202n30. *See also* andrology—parallelism with gynecology; obstetrics; organizational infrastructure and knowledge-making about reproduction

Hacking, Ian, 20
Hales, Barbara, 86, 87
Hardon, Anita, 226n28
Healey, Jenna, 77–79, 185, 216n23
health care: preventive services recommendations, 227n21; recommendations to include men's reproductive health in, 173–76; reluctance of men to obtain, 151, 158, 176, 227n21
Healthy People 2020, 179
"Healthy Sperm" leaflet created for interviews (Almeling): men's reactions to the notion of, 151–60; methodology of, 142–43, *143*, 190–91
heart conditions (congenital), and paternal effects, 84
heart disease: and the male body as standard and lack of knowledge about women, 10, 12, 13; and paternal effects, 84
Heidelberg Medical Institute (Reinhardt brothers), 48, *49*, 50
Herr, Harry W., 205n36
heterosexuality: and heteronormativity, 124, 158–59; the late 1960s and questioning inevitability of, 58
high school health or sex education courses, and men's reproductive health, 180
homeopaths, 47–48
homosexuality: and anxiety about White male virility, 46–47, *47*, 58; liberation movement of the 1960s and '70s, 58–59; search for the "gay gene," 140. *See also* gay men/ MSM (men who have sex with men)
Honig, Stanton, 106
hormone model: and delay of discovery of testosterone, 32; estrogen and testosterone present in both male and female bodies, 16, 32; search for testosterone, 55; twentieth-century paradigm shift to, 55
—"SEX HORMONE" MODEL: and development of the female contraceptive pill, 32; gender norms and, 6, 16, 32; organizational infrastructure and, 32
Howse, Jennifer, 110–12, 187
human-rights framework for healthy communities, 179

humor and embarrassment: and American Society of Andrology, 65–66, *66*, 214n70; in interview study of views on men's reproduction, 122, 123, 126; methodology and, 187; in news coverage of paternal effects, 92, 97, 98–99; ridicule of the late 1880s attempt to establish andrology, 43–45, 56, 68, 208n81
hydrocarbons, 85
hysteria, 100

Ibsen, Henrik, *Ghosts*, 27, 28, 47, 204n4
ignorance studies. *See* non-knowledge
immigrants: Catholic, and Protestant anxiety about male virility, 46; and STI treatments, 50
impotence. *See* erectile dysfunction (impotence)
individualization of risks: blame and stigma for failure to achieve health, 163–64, 171; of maternal effects, 144, 146, 163, 226n28; medicalization and, 162; new knowledge about men's reproductive health and reframing of, 171–72; and personal responsibility for wellness, 162–63, 226n28. *See also* paternal effects— individualization of risks
industrialization, and anxiety about White male virility, 46
infertility: contemporary understanding of, as equally occurring among men and women, 31, 204n23; medicalization of, 162; rate of, 204n23. *See also* assisted reproductive technologies; sperm fertility/infertility
—FEMALE, focus on, and the female body as reproductive, 11, 31–32
—MALE: and andrology, need for specialty of, 63, 65, 214nn65,75; and artificial insemination by donor, 55; and cooperation of andrology and gynecology, proposed, 57, 211n3; early-twentieth-century treatment of, 55; gynecologists as treating, 205n34; lack of funding for, 104; late-nineteenth-century treatment of, 53; men's reproductive health and focus on, 11; pharmaceutical companies looking to profit from, 94; treatments for, as limited, 11, 53; urology subspecialization in, 202n30; view of sperm/egg as equally sharing hereditary material, 43. *See also* sperm fertility/infertility
insanity, removal of ovaries as treatment of, 31

institutional review boards (IRBs), and reproductive risks to men, 176
International Agency for Research on Cancer,
83
International Congress of Andrology, 61, 63,
74–75
International Journal of Andrology (journal): merger with the *Journal of Andrology*, 65–66, 214n68; and methodology,
184
International Society of Andrology: and definition of "andrology" as specialty, 61; and
methodology, 184, 185. *See also* Comité
Internacional de Andrología (CIDA)
intersectional analysis: definition of, 6; and
news coverage of men's reproductive
health and lack of, 99, 220n35; and the
pathologization of varying bodies, 9–10;
reproductive justice, 32–33, 179
interview study of views on men's reproduction: overview, 23, 119, 167; lack of previous research, 119–20, 128, 223n3; non-
knowledge about men's reproductive
health and, 140; sources of men's information on men's reproductive health, 176,
227n18
—METHODOLOGY: overview, 120–21; gendered analysis, 190; and gender-of-interviewer effects, 189, 223n4, 225n35;
"Healthy Sperm" leaflet created for interviews, 142–43, *143*, 190–91; interviewee
recruitment and demographics, 120, *121*,
187–90, *196–99*, 223n4, 229nn22,25;
interview guide, 191–93; interviewing
approach and process, 120–21, 190–91,
223n5; mandatory response of acquiescence to health messaging, 157; qualitative data analysis, 121, 193–94; and saturation, 189; and social desirability bias,
158; sperm stories, 137, 138, 193–94,
224n23, 225nn32–35; table of men's
awareness of actions to take for healthy
children, *147*, 226n5; women interviewees, *121*, 128, 190, 193, 224n18, 224n21
—PATERNAL EFFECTS: overview, 142–44, 167;
age of father, conceptions of, 148–49;
awareness of maternal effects, 144–46;
awareness of possible actions to increase
the chances of healthy children, 146–47,
147, 226n5; barriers (social and structural) that stand between individual men
and healthy sperm, 23, 144, 152, 153, 155–
56, 157–60; equalizing risk and responsi-

bility, 160–61; guesswork about, 147–48;
"Healthy Sperm" leaflet created for use in,
142–43, *143*, 190–91; individualized risks
vs. structural/environmental causes, 144,
147, *147*, 151, 162–64, 226n28; morality
and, 156, 157; prior knowledge of, 149–51,
163, 226n9; and provider/enforcer narratives, 145; statements of intention vs.
actual actions, 157; uncertainty about
risks, 150–51, 156–57; willingness to
improve children's health, 23, 144, 151–53,
154–55, 156–57
—ROLE OF MEN IN REPRODUCTION: overview,
119–22, 167; biological/physical aspects,
120–23, 125–27; humor and embarrassment about biological aspects of, 122,
123, 126; paternal effects, lack of references to, 128–29, 167; provider role
as cultural script, 123–24, 127, 145,
167; and "reproduction" as word choice,
120–21; and "role" as word choice,
223n5. *See also* biological stories/sperm
stories
—WOMEN'S RESPONSES: on men's role in
reproduction, 128; methodology and,
121, 128, 190, 193, 224n18, 224n21; on
paternal effects, 128–29; and sperm/egg
biological stories, 137–38; on women's
role in reproduction, 127–28
intracytoplasmic sperm injection (ICSI), 11,
224n24
in vitro fertilization (IVF): ICSI as also
requiring, 11; and sperm story of active
sperm and passive egg, 224n24. *See also*
assisted reproductive technologies
Iowa, University of, 59, 61
IQ scores and paternal effects, 94
Italy, and andrology, 1960s establishment of,
60
IVF. *See* in vitro fertilization

Jackson, James Caleb, 208n67
*JAMA. See Journal of the American Medical
Association*
Jasanoff, Sheila, 7
Jordan, P., 211n3, 213n42, 214n75
Journal of Andrology (now *Andrology*):
founding of, 65; merger with the *Interna-
tional Journal of Andrology*, 65–66,
214n68; and methodology, 184; reprint-
ing 1891 *JAMA* editorial, 60
*Journal of Cutaneous and Genito-Urinary
Diseases*, 38, 39, 44

Journal of the American Medical Association (JAMA): editorial lauding the inception of andrology (1891), 33–36, *34*, 39, 44, 45–46, 52, 60, 205n34, 211n7; and methodology, 185, 228n12; and paternal age, informing of risks, 82

Karolinska Institute (Stockholm), 61
Kempner, Joanna, 8
Keyes, Edward Lawrence: overview, 36–37; and andrology, 19th century attempt to establish, 28–29, 36–39, 43–45, 206n48; and Claudius Mastin, 37, 205–6n43; and parallelism between andrology and gynecology, 40, 41, 43; and syphilis treatment, 27–28, 36–37; and textbook on genitourinary diseases, 27–28, 36, 38, 51
Keyes Medal, 51
Kinsey Report, 58
kinship, 125
knowledge circulation. *See* circulation of biomedical knowledge about men's reproductive health
knowledge gap. *See* non-knowledge; non-knowledge about men's reproductive health
knowledge-making: gender dualism/norms and, 6, 16–17, 129–30, 224n21; new findings and other interpretations of, 181–82; and organizational infrastructure, importance of, 88–89; and science and society as irreducible, 7. *See also* non-knowledge about men's reproductive health (relationality of gender resulting in reproductive knowledge about women and non-knowledge about men); organizational infrastructure and knowledge-making about reproduction
Kong, A., 102

laborers. *See* occupational exposures
labor unions, and occupational exposures, 85, 86
Lallemand, Claude-François, 49–50, 208n68
Lamb, Dolores, 106
Lancet, The (journal), 43–44, 79, 208n81, 218n84
Laqueur, Thomas, 208n69
laughing gas (nitrous oxide), 85, 218n82
law and policy: Affordable Care Act coverage for women's preconception health appointments, 103; folic acid required to be added to grain products, 103; incarceration of women for behavior during pregnancy, 76; occupational protections for women but not men, 84, 97; recommendation for regulation of chemicals and other pollutants, 178; recommendation for warning labels notifying men of risk of paternal effects, 178; regulation of health behaviors of individuals, 103; structural and environmental risk reduction approaches via, 103
lead exposures, 85
learning disabilities, 84
LeBlond, Charles, 59
Lewin, Tamar, 97
LGBTQ. *See* gay men/MSM (men who have sex with men); homosexuality
Lipshultz, Larry, 101

MacFadden, Bernarr, 46
McGrath, Charles, 102
MacKendrick, Norah, 163
Malaspina, Dolores, 82, 87, 97, 98, 101, 218n89
"male" and "male body," as terms in this text, 10
male body as standard: and biomedical research, 10–11; as dualism with "female body as reproductive," 12–13; and establishment of inclusion rules for biomedical research and clinical trials, 3; and lack of heart disease knowledge about women, 10, 12; and the pathologization of varying bodies, 9–10; puzzle of, when compared to non-knowledge about men's reproductive contributions, 12–13; social science research and, 11–12; and study of women OR men but calling it gender, 13–15, 202–3n40; women's health activists and critique of, 3, 10. *See also* female body as reproductive
male-mediated developmental toxicity, 79. *See also* behaviors of parents; exposures of parents
Male Reproductive Biology Club, 59, 61, 212n37
male reproductive body: as ignored, 11; Nazi Germany and, 57. *See also* andrology; interview study of views on men's reproduction; male body as standard; sperm
Mancini, Roberto Eusebio: and founding of andrology in the late 1960s, 60; and methodology, 185, 212–13nn38,52; and Rosemberg, 62, 213n52

March of Dimes: and "birth defects" as term, 216n19; founding of, 109; Male Role Press Conference (1991), 112; "Real Men Do Get Pregnant" editorial luncheon, 112; recommendations for messaging on men's reproductive health, 178; and soldiers' exposure to Agent Orange, 222–23n85; and teen fathers of color, 222–23n85; women's preconception health as primary focus of, 114, 222–23n85. *See also* Howse, Jennifer; Men Have Babies Too (March of Dimes public health campaign on paternal effects)

Marfan syndrome, 80

marijuana, 84, 108

market: and failure to launch medical specialty, 52–53; for sperm-related products, 94, 180

Marsiglio, William, 202n35, 223n3

Martin, Emily, 6, 129, 131, 188

masculinity: biological stories and cultural notions of, 132, 134, 135, 140; humor in public health messaging and risk of reinforcing, 179; humorous allusions to, in news coverage about paternal effects, 92, 97, 98–99; and male invulnerability, 158–59; and mid-twentieth-century changes in the role of men and fathers, 58; and reluctance to seek medical care, 151, 158, 176, 227n21; "reproductive masculinity" (Daniels), 15; as rooted in the testicles, 32; as social construction, 6; social scientific literature on, men's reproductive contributions excluded in, 11–12. *See also* gender; virility/emasculation

Masculinity Studies Reader, 12

Mastin, Claudius, 36, 205–6n43

masturbation, 28

maternal effects: overview, 76; men's awareness of public health messaging about, 144–46; quality of evidence for claims of, 216n24

—RISKS OF: individualization of, vs. structural and environmental causes, 144, 146, 163, 226n28; interaction with paternal factors, 87, 174; portrayed as "certain and known" vs. "uncertainty" of paternal effects, 92, 97–98, 100

Mayo Clinic (website): federal agencies linking to, 221n64; "Healthy Sperm" (2012), 98, 191; on male biological clock, 220n44; male fertility as focus of, 96; and methodology, 96–97, 186, 191

media. *See* consumer websites for health and parenting; news media

medicalization, 162, 171

medical journals: articles suggesting more attention to men's reproductive health, 174–75; dynamics of risk assessment of paternal exposures in, 218n84; impact factor, 214n68; ridicule of andrology in, 43–45, 56, 68, 208n81. *See also Journal of the American Medical Association (JAMA); other specific journals*

medical knowledge. *See* knowledge-making; non-knowledge

Medical News (journal), 206

medical schools and training programs: continuing education requirements including men's reproductive health, 177; recommendations for expansion into men's reproductive health, 174–75. *See also* medical textbooks

medical specialization: overview, 29–30, 68–69; "critical juncture" of the late 19th century in, 29–30, 52, 53, 204n15; failures of specialties, 210n119; lack of, consequences of, 69, 170; multiplying professional meetings due to increasing number of, 37; organizational infrastructure as accompanying, 67, 166; overspecialization, concerns about, 43, 45, 69, 170, 209n85, 211–12n17. *See also* gynecology; organizational infrastructure

medical specialization in men's reproductive health, lack of: overview, 69, 166–68, 174; circulation of knowledge as limited by, 170; continuing since the 1970s, 89; news coverage and, 95; paucity of materials produced by federal agencies and professional organizations and, 109; recommendation against instituting, in favor of incorporating men's reproductive health into preexisting organizational infrastructure, 174. *See also* andrology; genito-urinary surgeons; organizational infrastructure and knowledge-making about reproduction; urology

medical surveillance, 171

medical textbooks: andrology as term in, 56, 211–12nn14,17; gendered norms and conceptions of passive eggs and aggressive sperm, 6; Keyes and, 27–28, 36, 51; reduced focus on venereal disease in, 51; syphilis in, 27–28; and uncertainty about differences and similarities between male and female bodies, 42, 208nn67–69 men, as term in this text, 10

Men Have Babies Too (March of Dimes public health campaign on paternal effects): overview, 109; brochure, *110-11*, 112-14, 221-22nn79-81; development of, 110-12; and difficulty of institutionalizing men's reproductive health information, 114; methodology and, 187; as minor focus, 114, 222-23n85. *See also* Howse, Jennifer; March of Dimes

Men's Health (website): gender in men's reproductive health coverage, 98; magazine form of, 96; on male biological clock, 220n44; and methodology, 96, 186; slang used by, 99

men's reproductive health: overview, 2-4; focus on, and the potential to influence gender politics, 24, 171; increasing awareness over time of, 73-75, *74-75*; language recommendations for use in, 180-81; limited scope of, 11, 22, 104-5. *See also* infertility—male; interview study of views on men's reproduction; paternal effects; sperm fertility/infertility

men's rights activists, 101, 173

men's specialty clinics. *See* "quacks" and charlatans, men's reproductive health and

menstrual pain, removal of ovaries as treatment of, 31

metabolic syndrome, 84

metaphor of the photographer. *See* nonknowledge about men's reproductive health (relationality of gender resulting in reproductive knowledge about women and non-knowledge about men)—metaphor of the photographer

methodology: overview, 183; breadth over depth, emphasis on, 21; circulation of biomedical knowledge, 73-74, 93-96, 185-87, 214-15nn1-3,7, 219nn6-8,12, 220n35, 228nn12-13; Google Ngrams, 73-74, 214-15nn1-3,7; production of biomedical knowledge, 183-85; review of medical and scientific literature on paternal effects, 216n23; social media excluded from analysis, 187, 219n2; tripartite analytical framework, 21, 169-70. *See also* interview study of views on men's reproduction—methodology

midwives, 47-48

Milam, Erika L., 225n36

Mills, Charles, 8

Milne, Elizabeth, 83

miscarriage, paternal effects and, 78, 94

morality: and interview study of views on men's reproduction, 153, 156, 157; and medicalization, 162, 171; venereal disease as moral failing, 28, 45-47, 50, 52-53

morbidity/mortality rates, 151

Morrow, Prince Albert, 38, 47, 50

Moscucci, Ornella, 31, 40, 43, 184, 205n34, 211n7

MSM. *See* gay men/MSM (men who have sex with men) as interviewees

Murkoff, Heidi, 99

National Institute for Occupational Safety and Health (NIOSH), 85, 94, 217n50. *See also* Occupational Safety and Health Administration (OSHA)

National Institutes of Health (NIH): budget of, 104; and contraceptive development, 62; inclusion rules for women and people of color in biomedical research and clinical trials, 3, 104; on lack of attention to men's reproductive health, 173; lack of research funding for men's reproductive health, 104; and methodology, 186; scarcity of information on men's reproductive health, 11, 104-5, 202n31; women's health as focus of, 104

National Research Council, 100

Nature: on diet and paternal effects, 84; on equal proportion of paternal and maternal effects, 80; on nuclear exposures, paternal effects of, 218n84; on paternal age and children's disease risk, 102

Naumann, Moritz Ernst Adolph, 207n59

Nazi Germany, 54-55, 57, 61

Nelson, Timothy, 188, 191

Nelson, Warren O., 59, 61, 212n37

neurasthenia, 46

New Republic, 95

news media: advertising for men's specialist clinics, *49*, 210n110; and exposure of fraudulent medical claims, 50; on maternal effects, 92

news media and circulation of knowledge about paternal effects: overview, 92-93; book reviews/articles, 95, 101; children's health effects, percentage of mentions, 93-94, *94*, 95; gender as frame in, 96, 97-99, 100-101; humorous allusions to masculinity in, 92, 97, 98-99; lack of specialty for men's reproductive health reflected in, 95, 167; male panic, 100-101,

news media and circulation *(continued)*
102; and March of Dimes public health
messaging, 112, 113–14, 221n79; and
methodology, 93–96, 185, 186–87,
219nn6–8,12, 228n13; on occupational
exposures, 85; previous studies of, 92;
reassurance of men in, 101–2; risks as
minimized in, 92, 96, 99–102, 103; and
risks, individualization of, 96, 102–3;
sperm fertility as focus of, vs. effects on
children's health, 92, 93–94, *94*, 96, 146–
47. *See also* consumer websites for health
and parenting
New York Genito-Urinary Society, 51
New York Medical Journal, 56
New York Times, and methodology, 93–95,
186, 187, 219nn6–8,12, 228n13
Ngrams. *See* methodology
Niblett, Stephen Berry, 207n65
Niemi, Mikko, 60
Niermann, H., 211n3, 213n42, 214n75
NIH. *See* National Institutes of Health
nitrous oxide (laughing gas), 85, 218n82
non-knowledge: overview, 7–8; avoiding teleology in the study of, 206n52; case studies in, 8; gender dualism/norms as shaping, 15, 17; and history of controlling and
delegitimizing women's sexuality and
pleasure, 181–82; politics of knowledge-
ignorance, 181–82; temporality and, 169–
70; and the tripartite analytical framework, 169–70; typology of (Croissant), 8,
169. *See also* non-knowledge about men's
reproductive health
non-knowledge about men's reproductive
health: overview, 4, 8–9, 165–68; gender
as relational and, 15, 17–20; and the politics of reproduction, 24, 182; and "reproductive masculinity" (Daniels), 15. *See
also* non-knowledge about men's reproductive health (relationality of gender
resulting in reproductive knowledge
about women and non-knowledge about
men)
non-knowledge about men's reproductive
health (relationality of gender resulting in
reproductive knowledge about women
and non-knowledge about men): overview, 168–69; and biological stories, 140;
and difficulty of talking about men's
reproductive risk, 146; as feedback loop,
18, 20, 30–31, 33, 168–69, 203n55; funding of research and, 104; Google searches

illustrating, 173, 227n11; lack of a medical
specialty in men's reproduction and,
30–31; meddling in men's bodies despite,
52–53
—METAPHOR OF THE PHOTOGRAPHER: overview, 17–18, *19*, 30; demographic characteristics of the observer and, 18; feedback
loop and, 18, 20, 203n55; and relation to
"seeing," "framing," and "male gaze," 20,
169; and "training" to view the body, 18;
weak feedback loop associating men and
reproductive health, 90. *See also* feedback
loops

obstetrics: among the first medical specialties, 29–30; increasing awareness over
time of, 75, *75*; merged into single specialty with gynecology, 31. *See also*
gynecology
occupational exposures: overview, 84–87,
218nn82,84; agricultural workers, 85;
battery manufacturing, 85; chemical
plant workers, 85, 97; dentists, 85; doctors, 85; electronics workers, 97; interviewees on difficulty of avoiding, 154–55,
158; lab scientists, 85; laws and policies
protecting women and not men, 84, 97;
March of Dimes brochure on, 113;
mechanics, 85; miners, 85; National
Occupational Research Agenda Statement on Reproductive Hazards, 107;
news media coverage of, 93, 94, 97;
nuclear plant workers, 85–86; painters,
85; recommendation for warning labels
about paternal effects from, 178; soldiers
on battlefields, 86, 94, 107, 222–23n85.
See also chemical exposures; exposures of
parents; National Institute for Occupational Safety and Health (NIOSH); Occupational Safety and Health Administration (OSHA); radiation exposures
Occupational Safety and Health Administration (OSHA): establishment of, 217n50;
and methodology, 186; population-level
risk reduction possible via, 103; warnings
about reproductive health and paternal
effects of chemical exposures, 107
Ohio Medical Journal, 39–40
opioids, 84
Oreskes, Naomi, 8
organizational infrastructure: as accompanying the process of medical specialization,
67, 166; andrologists of the late 1960s and

creation of, 68, 89; continued weakness of, 88–89; definition of, 89; lack of, and lack of circulation of knowledge about men's reproductive health, 109, 114, 115, 167, 170; recommendation for incorporating men's reproductive health into preexisting, 174–76. *See also* organizational infrastructure and knowledge-making about reproduction

organizational infrastructure and knowledge-making about reproduction: overview, 30, 32; and contraceptive research, 32; and failure to launch andrology, 53, 57, 67; and feedback loop associating women with reproduction, 31–32, 33, 68, 168; and the "sex-hormone" model, 32. *See also* dualistic/binary conceptions of gender

organs, uncertainty about similarities and differences between male and female, 41–43, 207nn63–65, 208nn67–69,74

organs-based model of the body, 41, 55

OSHA. *See* Occupational Safety and Health Administration

Oudshoorn, Nelly, 16, 32, 203n55

Our Bodies, Ourselves, 181–82

ovaries: femininity as rooted in, 32; removal of, to treat physical and emotional problems, 31, 40

ovulation-tracking software, 180

Parents.com: and methodology, 96, 186; print magazine form of, 96

paternal effects: overview, 22–23, 75–79; definition of (as yet unsettled), 77, 216n16; distinguished from sperm fertility, 75–76; epigenetic modifications, 77, 78, 82, 150, 226n28; factors of age, behaviors, and exposures, 77–78; genetic, epidemiological, and animal studies, 78–79, 216nn21–24; language used to describe, 180–81; methodology and, 216n23; spontaneous new mutations (de novo), 77, 80, 81, 102; study of, difficulty of getting support for, 86–88, 166–67; study types, generally, 78–79. *See also* age of parents; behaviors of parents; circulation of biomedical knowledge about men's reproductive health; exposures of parents; interview study of views on men's reproduction—paternal effects; Men Have Babies Too (March of Dimes public health campaign on paternal effects)

—RISKS OF: age, 80–82; behaviors, 83; cumulative risk assessment, 87, *88*, 174; debate about informing men of risks, 81–82, 83; debate about uncertainty of risk, 79, 86, 100–102, 107, 218n84; exposures, 79, 86, 218n84; and institutional review boards (IRBs), 176; interaction with maternal factors, 87, 174; interviewees on the need for equalization of, 160–61; interviewees on the need to act despite the uncertainty of, 150–51, 156–57; news media's focus on uncertainty of risk, 92, 96, 99–102, 103; OSHA and warnings about risk, 107; reduction of, while understanding the elimination of all risk is impossible, 181; as "uncertain" vs. maternal effects as "certain and known," 92, 97–98, 100. *See also* reproductive equation, including men as part of

—INDIVIDUALIZATION OF RISKS: federal health agency websites and, 105; insistence on uncertainty of risk and, 103; and mandatory response of acquiescence to health messaging, 157; methodology and analysis for, 187; news coverage of paternal effects and, 96, 102–3; public health messaging and focus on, 144, 146, 160, 162–64; structural and environmental factors ignored in favor of, 144, 160, 162–64

patients' rights movement, 58

Paulson, C. Alvin, 60, 62

Pechenick, Eitan Adam, 214–15n1

pediatricians, and men's reproductive health, 177

Pediatrics (journal), 175

Penrose, Lionel, 79

people of color: and anxiety about White male virility, 46–47, 58; castration of male prisoners, 59; civil rights movement, 58–59; and forced sterilization, 10, 59; history of medical abuse of, 28, 59, 158; history of social control of reproduction of, 59, 159, 171; inclusion rules for biomedical research and clinical trials, 3, 16, 104; March of Dimes campaign for teen fathers, 222–23n85; and "population control" programs, 59

pesticides: DBCP, 85, 93; DDT, 94

Pfeiffer syndrome, 80

pharmaceuticals: as barrier to behavioral changes to avoid paternal effects, 158; recommendation for warning labels about

pharmaceuticals *(continued)*
  paternal effects of, 178; and sperm fertility, 94, 104, 105
philanthropic organizations, recommendations for expanding research into men's
  reproductive health, 175
photographer metaphor. *See* non-knowledge
  about men's reproductive health (relationality of gender resulting in reproductive
  knowledge about women and non-knowledge about men)—metaphor of the
  photographer
physical culture, and anxieties about virility, 46
Pincus, Gregory, 62
Planned Parenthood, 32, 178, 221n64
politics of reproduction: analyses of, as
  focused on women's reproduction, 5; definition of, 4; knowledge about men's
  reproductive health as vital to, 24, 182;
  nesting-doll metaphor of biological and
  social processes, 6–7, 160; publicizing
  information about paternal effects and
  ramifications for, 161. *See also* gender
population control rhetoric, 59
Population Council, 59, 60, 62
Posner, Carl, 207n59
preconception health: CDC webpage, 105,
  106, 142–43, 191, 220n35; expansion of
  resources to men, 76; men's health care
  appointments, 176–77; most attention
  and resources directed at women, 76, 105.
  See also maternal effects; paternal effects
preformation, 133. *See also* conception
pregnancy apps, men's reproductive health
  messaging via, 180
pregnancy, paternal effects on outcomes. *See*
  birth defects; birthweight; miscarriage;
  stillbirths
Preventive Services Task Force, U.S., 227n21
prisoners, castration, 59
production of biomedical knowledge about
  men's reproductive health: overview,
  21–22; and breadth vs. depth of this study,
  21; methodology of data collection, 183–
  85; tripartite framework and, 21, 169–70.
  See also andrology; non-knowledge about
  men's reproductive health; organizational
  infrastructure and knowledge-making
  about reproduction; paternal effects
professional medical associations: "men as
  partners" positioning of, 109; methodology and, 185, 186. *See also specific
  associations*

professional medical associations and circulation of knowledge about paternal effects:
  overview, 92–93, 104; federal agencies
  linking to websites of, 221n64; lack of
  information about paternal effects, 107–9,
  115, 167; and lack of organizational infrastructure for publicizing knowledge, 115,
  167; recommendations for increasing
  attention to men's reproductive health, 175.
  See also American Society of Andrology
  (ASA); andrology; International Society of
  Andrology; *other specific associations*
Protestants, and calls for "muscular Christianity," 46
psychological disorders. *See* bipolar disorder;
  depressive disorders; schizophrenia
public health: individual risks and responsibilities as focus of, vs. structural and environmental causes, 144, 146, 160, 162–64;
  mandatory response of acquiescence to
  messages of, 157; recommendations for
  improved messaging about men's reproductive health, 178–80; sanitary measures
  and improvements in, 55; structural and
  environmental factors, focus on, 178. *See
  also* Men Have Babies Too (March of
  Dimes public health campaign on paternal effects)
Public Health Service (U.S.), Tuskegee Study,
  28
Puigvert, Antonio, 60

"quacks" and charlatans, men's reproductive
  health and: *JAMA* 1891 editorial citing,
  35–36, 45–46, 52; medical profession distinguished from, 48, 52, 53; men's specialist clinics, 48–50, *49*, 52, 53, 55, 210n110;
  "quacks" as term, and professionalization
  of medicine, 47–48
qualitative research. *See* interview study of
  views on men's reproduction

Rabin, Roni Caryn, 98
race: and anxiety about White male virility
  and racial dominance, 46–47, 58; and definitions of "older" fathers, 148–49; and
  egalitarian attitudes about gender in biological stories, 225n35; and interviewee
  recruitment, 120, *121*, 188–89; the late
  1960s and questioning of biology-based,
  58; and STI treatment, 28. *See also* intersectional analysis; people of color;
  whiteness

radiation exposures: and paternal effects, 85–86, 94, 218n84; and sperm fertility, 104. *See also* chemical exposures; environmental exposures; exposures of parents

Raeburn, Paul, 95, 102, 186–87

Rapp, Rayna, 4, 5, 216n28

reception of biomedical knowledge about men's reproductive health: overview, 23; and breadth vs. depth of this study, 21; tripartite framework and, 21, 169–70. *See also* interview study of views on men's reproduction

Reed, Kate, 161

Reinhardt brothers (Heidelberg Medical Institute), 48, *49*, 50

reproduction, as term, 4–5, 41, 120–21, 207nn64–65

reproductive bodies. *See* bodies as standard or reproductive

reproductive equation, including men as part of, 87, *88*, 174

reproductive health/reproductive medicine, inclusion of men's reproductive health in, 175

reproductive justice. *See* intersectional analysis

reproductive plans: health care appointments and questions about, 177, 178; IRBs and gender-neutral question on, 176

reproductive sciences, emergence of field of, 31–32

Richardson, Sarah, 16–17

Ricord, Philippe, 36

risks. *See* individualization of risks; maternal effects—risks of; paternal effects—risks of

Robaire, Bernard, 86

Romania, and social control of reproduction, 172

Roosevelt, Franklin D., 109

Rose, David, 187

Rosemberg, Eugenia, 60, 62, 213n52

Rubin, Gayle, 6

rural areas: and concerns about overspecialization, 69; and "men's specialty clinics" of the 19th century, 50

Saguy, Abigail, 187

Sanger, Margaret, 32

sanitation, and improvements in public health, 55

Schelling, Thomas, 140

Schirren, Carl, 54, 55, 60, 211n3, 213nn40, 42

schizophrenia and paternal effects: overview, 78; age and, 80, 81, 82, 102; news coverage of, 94, 97, 101, 102

sex: avoidance of biological essentialism in men's reproductive health, 175–76; differentiated from gender, 5–6; dualistic/ binary conceptions of, 9–10, 13, 168; late 1880s and uncertainty about similarities and differences in, 41–43, 207nn63–65, 208nn67–69,74; late 1960s and changing cultural norms about "naturalness" of differences in, 58; as opposites, 9, 13; as term in this text, 10

sex education courses (high school), 180

sexology, 46–47, 58

sex roles approach, 223n5

sexual health, 11, 12, 22, 105, 166, 175

sexuality, men's: historical approaches to, 36, 52; in social scientific literature, 12

sexually transmitted infections. *See* STIs (sexually transmitted infections, "venereal disease")

Seymour, Frances, 215n8

shame and stigma: of andrology, and quest for respectability, 45–46, 50, 68; of genital conditions, 28–29; of individualized conditions and failure to achieve health, 163–64, 171; of venereal disease, 27, 28, 47–51, 52, 53, 210n120

Sherins, Richard, 61–62

Sherman, Jerome K., 59, 213n40

sickle cell trait, 128

Siebke, Harald, 57, 211n7, 213n42

skepticism of science and medical expertise, 153, 158, 159, 226n19

smoking tobacco: March of Dimes brochure on, 113; men's awareness of maternal effects and, 145, 146; non-knowledge about, 8; and paternal effects, 79, 83, 100, 108; recommendation for warning labels about paternal effects from, 178; sperm fertility and, 83, 106, 108

social media, excluded from research, 187, 219n2

social movements of the 1960s and '70s: and rise of andrology, 58–59, 67–68, 89, 169, 214n75. *See also* civil rights movement; feminism

Society for Male Reproduction and Urology, 108

Society for the Study of Male Reproduction, 65, 108, 186

Society of Toxicology, and methodology, 186

socioeconomic status (SES): definition of, 189; and interviewee recruitment, 120, *121*, 188–89, *196–99*

Solari, Alberto J., 212–13n38

Soloski, Alexis, 204n4

Spain, and andrology, 1960s establishment of, 55, 60

specialization. *See* medical specialization

sperm: belief as "forever young" and subsequent denial of paternal effects, 77, 86–87; crucial period for epigenetic damage to, 78; early-life exposures and effects on health of, 78; health of sperm distinguished from fertility of, 76. *See also* biological stories/sperm stories; eggs and sperm; paternal effects; sperm banks; sperm fertility/infertility

spermatology, 208n74

spermatorrhea, 28, 30, 36, 48, 49–50, 205n55

sperm banks: age limits on donors, 80, 217n32; commercializing the male biological clock, 180; rise of, 59

sperm fertility/infertility: age and, 96, 105, 148; alcohol and, 83–84, 93, 106, 108; assessed by motility, morphology, and count, 75–76, 215n8; cocaine and, 106; consumer websites and focus on, vs. paternal effects, 96, 115; diseases causing, 104, 105; endocrine-disrupting chemicals and, 86; federal health agencies as focused on, vs. paternal effects, 104–7, 115, 167; health of sperm distinguished from, 76; illegal drug use and, 93; news media as focused on, vs. paternal effects, 92, 93–94, *94*, 96, 146–47; pesticide DBCP and, 85, 93; pharmaceuticals and, 94, 104, 105; radiation and, 104; smoking and, 83, 106, 108; steroid use and, 94, 106, 108. *See also* infertility—male; paternal effects

sperm stories. *See* biological stories/sperm stories

Steinberger, Emil, 61–63, 74–75, 212n37, 214n62

Stein, Melissa, 47

sterility. *See* infertility

sterilization: and the Population Council, 59. *See also* sterilization, forced and coerced

sterilization, forced and coerced: eugenics and mass sterilization, 54; of male prisoners, 59; in Nazi Germany, 57; and the pathologization of varying bodies, 10; of

poor women, 10, 59; of racial minorities, 10, 59; and reproductive justice, 32–33

steroids, 94, 106, 108

stigma. *See* shame and stigma

stillbirths, paternal effects and, 94

STIs (sexually transmitted infections, "venereal disease"): andrology and focus on, 35–36, 205n33; and anxiety about White male virility, 47; "clap" as slang for, 210n120; and dermatology, 37, 38, 57, 206n47; late-nineteenth-century spread of, 47, 209n98; men's reproductive health and focus on, 11; "men's specialist clinics" and treatment of, 48–50, *49*, 210n110; as moral failing, 47, 50; nineteenth-century campaigns emphasizing health effects on children, 77; shame and stigma attached to, 27, 28, 47–51, 52, 53, 210n120; uncertainty about treatment, 27–28; urology and excision from practice of, 51; World War I recruitment of soldiers and prevalence of, 55. *See also* gonorrhea; syphilis

structural and environmental barriers standing between individual men and the goal of healthy sperm, 23, 144, 152, 157–58, 159–60

structural and environmental contributors to disease: vs. individualization of risk as focus in public health messaging, 144, 160, 162–64; law and policy approaches to, 103; methodology and analysis for, 187; recommendations for biomedical research into, 174; recommendations for emphasizing and benefits of addressing, 171–73; recommendations for public health messaging on, 178

Supreme Court, U.S., *Johnson Controls* decision, 85, 93, 100

Swan, Shanna, 98

Sweden, and andrology, 1960s establishment of, 60

syphilis: dermatology and, 37, 206n47; Edward L. Keyes and treatment of, 27–28, 36–37; lack of testing for, 27–28, 204n5; portrayed in Henrik Ibsen's *Ghosts*, 27, 28, 47, 204n4; rates of, 47. *See also* STIs

Taylor, Robert W., 45

testicles: hesitation of men to get care for problems with, 50; masculinity as rooted in, 32; problems with, as assault on male virility, 50

testosterone. *See* hormone model

Texas–Houston, University of, 61
Thomas, Joseph, 208n74
thyroid problems, and sperm fertility, 104
toxic exposures. *See* exposures
trans scholarship and activism, and nonbinary conceptions of gender, 10, 169
Tuana, Nancy, 7–8, 181
Tuskegee Study, 28

United Autoworkers Union v. Johnson Controls Inc., 85, 93, 100
urology: excision of "genito-" from, 51; gynecology distinguished from, 202n30; increasing attention over time to, 75, *75*. *See also* American Urological Association; andrology; genito-urinary surgeons; medical specialization in men's reproductive health

Valdez, Natali, 226n28
Van Buren, William H., 27–28, 36, 38, 205n35
vasectomy, 11. *See also* contraception—male
venereal disease. *See* STIs (sexually transmitted infections, "venereal disease")
Vienne, Florence, 43, 57, 208n69, 225n29
Vietnam War: chemical exposures of soldiers in, 86, 107, 222–23n85. *See also* Department of Defense; war
Vij, Sarah, 104
vinyl chloride exposures, 94
virility/emasculation: interviewee anxiety about, 134; men's rights activists and worry about, 101; White anxiety about, 46–47, 58

Waggoner, Miranda, 105, 136–37
Walker, Kenneth, 211–12nn7,17
war: chemical exposures of soldiers in, 86, 94, 107, 222–23n85; World War I recruitment and prevalence of venereal disease, 55. *See also* Department of Defense
Washington, University of, 60
WebMD (website): on male biological clock, 220n44; and methodology, 95–96, 186; on paternal age, 96
websites. *See* consumer websites for health and parenting
Weinberg, Wilhelm, 79
Wells, Thomas Spencer, 40
What to Expect When You're Expecting (website): book form of, 96; and methodology, 96, 186; recommendation to include

men's reproductive health information, 180; slang used by, 99
White, J. William, 206n57
whiteness: anxiety about male virility and racial dominance, 46–47, 58; normativity of, 46–47; "white ignorance" as non-knowledge, 8
Wigglesworth, Edward, 206n47
women: as blamed for birth defects and genetic disorders, 97–98, 146; burden on, to pass information to male partners, 99, 163, 178, 180; health care appointments covering information about men's reproductive health, 178; inclusion rules for biomedical research and clinical trials, 3, 16, 104; lack of research on views of women's reproductive contributions, 128; as news reporters covering paternal effects, 98; as paternal effects researchers, 87; as term in this text, 10. *See also* feminism; gender; interview study of views on men's reproduction—women's responses; non-knowledge about men's reproductive health (relationality of gender resulting in reproductive knowledge about women and non-knowledge about men); organizational infrastructure and knowledge-making about reproduction
women's clinics. *See* gynecology
women's health activists: critique of the male body as standard, 3, 10; and the uneven power dynamic between doctor and patient, 58
women's reproductive health, ubiquity of focus on, 3, *74–75, 75*, 175
women's studies programs, 14
Worcester, Medical Research Institute of, 60, 62
workers and workplaces. *See* occupational exposures
World Health Organization (WHO): on chemical exposures, 108–9; and methodology, 186
World War I, venereal disease prevalence and, 55

X and Y chromosomes. *See* chromosomes

Yearbook of Achievements in the Medical Sciences, 207n59

Zika virus, 229n25

Founded in 1893,
UNIVERSITY OF CALIFORNIA PRESS
publishes bold, progressive books and journals
on topics in the arts, humanities, social sciences,
and natural sciences—with a focus on social
justice issues—that inspire thought and action
among readers worldwide.

The UC PRESS FOUNDATION
raises funds to uphold the press's vital role
as an independent, nonprofit publisher, and
receives philanthropic support from a wide
range of individuals and institutions—and from
committed readers like you. To learn more, visit
ucpress.edu/supportus.